Primary health care and continuous quality improvement

An evidence-based guide

Alison Laycock, Lynette O'Donoghue and Ross Bailie

SYDNEY UNIVERSITY PRESS

First published by Sydney University Press
© Alison Laycock, Lynette O'Donoghue and Ross Bailie 2025
© Sydney University Press 2025

Sydney University Press
Fisher Library F03
Gadigal Country
University of Sydney NSW 2006
AUSTRALIA
sup.info@sydney.edu.au
sydneyuniversitypress.com

A catalogue record for this book is available from the National Library of Australia.

NATIONAL
LIBRARY
OF AUSTRALIA

ISBN 9781743329269 paperback
ISBN 9781743329276 epub
ISBN 9781761540103 pdf

Cover design: Nathan Grice
Graphics: Studio Elevenses (studioelevenses.com.au)

We acknowledge the traditional owners of the lands on which Sydney University Press is located, the Gadigal people of the Eora Nation, and we pay our respects to the knowledge embedded forever within the Aboriginal Custodianship of Country.

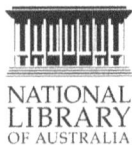

Systems awareness and systems design are important for health professionals, but they are not enough. They are enabling mechanisms only. It is the ethical dimensions of individuals that are essential to a system's success. Ultimately, the secret of quality is love. You have to love your patient, you have to love your profession, you have to love your God. If you have love, you can then work backward to monitor and improve the system.

Avedis Donabedian

Contents

Contents

List of Figures

List of Tables

Foreword

Adjunct Professor Tarun Weeramanthri

New approaches to health care are constantly needed in rural and remote Australia – to build on existing strengths, fill gaps and ensure access and quality. Such approaches need to be applied in situations with high patient needs, constant staff turnover and limited resources. These factors end up being drivers of innovation, and many "new models" can later be more widely applied in a range of settings, urban as well as rural, in Australia and overseas.

However, it is one thing to come up with effective and efficient approaches in research and pilot programs and quite another to scale them up and sustain them over time, and across large jurisdictions and whole health systems. It is the *continuous* in continuous quality improvement that is the hardest bit.

The Northern Territory has long been a place where health research and health policy applicable to Aboriginal and Torres Strait Islander populations have been developed and trialled. This carries a historic legacy, both good and bad. Part of the positive legacy is a modern-day commitment to proper ethical partnerships between communities and researchers, and between government services and Aboriginal community controlled health organisations.

The work described in this volume is notable for its direct relevance to primary health care (PHC), its rigour and (frankly) its longevity over decades and through various institutional arrangements. It started with the Audit and Best Practice in Chronic Disease (ABCD) program in the early 2000s, which linked with the Northern Territory Preventable Chronic Disease Strategy (PCDS) that began a few years earlier in the late 1990s and continues to this day. The basic architecture of the strategy remains intact but has been modified and improved over time, as a result of a commitment to ongoing research and evaluation and an attention to meaningful partnerships. These are the same principles that underpin the continuous quality improvement work in primary health care, which has now been expanded nationally and extended in scope to cover a range of chronic conditions, preventive as well as clinical care, and mental health.

So, if you are looking to enhance your knowledge of continous quality improvement (CQI) or PHC, or build some health architecture to stand the test of time, there will be many useful lessons and practical tools to be found in this volume. The gains may be modest initially, but such hard-won improvements sustained over time and built into a new base of primary care practice will be worthwhile in the long run for a large number of patients.

The public health dimension of PHC is also writ large – we might start with individual risk factors for chronic disease, but we very soon see the absolute need to link such care to a broader risk environment (social and economic) at the family, community and population health level. And anyone reading, writing or thinking about Aboriginal health in Australia will quickly realise that the "culture" word should first be applied to the organisation of health services, and to the broader society, before it is used to "blame and explain" unacceptable gaps in health outcomes.

There are many people, some of whom are longstanding personal friends and colleagues, who have contributed substantively to the success of this program of work. All have been motivated by a passion for equity and a desire to improve health care and health outcomes. They have been willing to work together as a team, to learn together by sharing information, data, perspectives and insights, and to sustain collaborations over the long term. The leadership and co-mentoring provided by people in a range of roles and levels within the collaboration have been essential ingredients in building trusted research-policy-practice partnerships, unique in Australia and relevant everywhere.

Tarun Weeramanthri is a public health physician and President of the Public Health Association of Australia. He lived and worked in the Northern Territory for 17 years, as a researcher with the Menzies School of Health Research in Darwin (1991–95), as Community Physician with the Northern Territory Centre for Disease Control (1996–2003) and as the Northern Territory Chief Health Officer (2004–07). He was Chief Health Officer in Western Australia from 2008 to 2018. His awards include the Sidney Sax Medal by the Public Health Association of Australia for his contribution to public health in Australia.

Professor Ian Anderson

One of the earliest jobs in my career was working at an Aboriginal community controlled health service. These services were created from the 1970s through Aboriginal and Torres Strait Islander activism to address our people's poor access to health care, and the racism they experienced when seeking care. I began to work as an Aboriginal health worker over the summer of 1986 at the Victorian Aboriginal Health Service when I was still a medical student at university. After my graduation, I worked as a general practitioner and as the chief executive officer at the same service. These early work experiences convinced me of the importance of providing quality primary health care to improve Indigenous health outcomes more generally.

Later in my career, as a health services researcher, I became aware of the broader body of research that investigated the relationship between coordinated and integrated primary health care and population health outcomes. In Indigenous health there are important questions that arise from this. For example, does both the routine screening of chronic disease risks and the integration of prevention activity with clinical interventions improve chronic disease outcomes for Aboriginal and Torres Strait Islander peoples? The answers to such questions have important implications for clinical operations, primary care services and policymakers.

From 2003 onwards, the Cooperative Research Centre for Aboriginal Health (and its later iterations) developed both a primary healthcare research program and a connected program in health systems research. Within this context we fostered a research focus on continuous quality improvement in Aboriginal and Torres Strait Islander primary healthcare services. This was a key stimulus for some of the research work outlined in this volume. It also had an influence on Indigenous health policy thinking, such as the health investment program associated with the Council of Australian Governments' Closing the Gap initiatives that has been active since 2008.

It is exciting to see the ongoing evolution of this field of work, described in detail in this book, as it continues to impact and improve health services' practice, thereby contributing to better health outcomes for Aboriginal and Torres Strait Islander peoples.

Professor Ian Anderson, Order of Australia, is a Palawa man and the Deputy Vice-Chancellor at the University of Tasmania. He was previously the Foundation Chair, Indigenous Higher Education; Pro Vice-Chancellor (Engagement), the Foundation Chair of Indigenous Health at the University of Melbourne and Deputy Vice-Chancellor at the Australian National University. His academic, policy and practice roles in Indigenous health include Director of Research for the Lowitja Institute and related Cooperative Research Centre for Aboriginal Health and Chair of the National Indigenous Health Equality Council.

About the authors

Alison Laycock (DipT, BEd, BFA, PhD) is a research fellow at the University Centre for Rural Health, University of Sydney. She has led knowledge translation programs for two quality improvement research networks funded by Australia's National Health and Medical Research Council (NHMRC) – the Centre for Research Excellence: Strengthening Systems for Indigenous Health Care Equity (CRE-STRIDE) and the Centre for Research Excellence in Integrated Quality Improvement (CRE-IQI). The focus of her health services research and evaluation work is improving the translation of evidence into practice, using participatory methods to strengthen care systems and improve health and wellbeing outcomes. Alison has worked collaboratively with health service, community and research partners to develop quality improvement tools and training resources, and guides for health promotion practice and health research in Aboriginal and Torres Strait Islander primary healthcare settings. Prior to joining academia, she worked in policy and program coordination roles in public health, health promotion and primary health care.

Ross Bailie (MD, MBChB, FAFPHM) is Professor of Rural Health with the University of Sydney School of Public Health and the University Centre for Rural Health, based in Lismore, Northern NSW. Ross's research has been centred on increasing availability of information for policy and service planning for Aboriginal and Torres Strait Islander health and for rural and remote communities. He has built practice-based research networks to support quality improvement in Indigenous primary health care over more than two decades. In his role as scientific director for the Centre for Primary Health Care Systems at the Menzies School of Health Research, Ross established the National Centre for Quality Improvement in Indigenous Primary Health Care (One21seventy). He is co-lead for the Rural and Remote Theme of the Healthy Environments and Lives (HEAL) National Research Network and co-lead of the NHMRC-funded Centre for Research Excellence: Strengthening Systems for Indigenous Health Care Equity (CRE-STRIDE). Ross has worked in South Africa, New Zealand and Australia.

Lynette O'Donoghue (GradDipIndigHProm, BSc) is a proud Yankunytjatjara and Warumungu-Warlpiri woman, and a research fellow at the University Centre for Rural Health, University of Sydney. She has contributed significantly to Indigenous leadership of the NHMRC-funded Centre for Research Excellence: Strengthening Systems for Indigenous Health Care Equity, advocating meaningful engagement of Aboriginal and Torres Strait Islander communities and services in the design, implementation and translation of research activities. Lynette has a wealth of experience in quality improvement research and practice, health promotion, primary healthcare program evaluation, participatory research approaches with health service partners, and mentoring non-Indigenous colleagues in culturally safe practice.

She had a key role in pioneering participatory quality improvement approaches in Aboriginal and Torres Strait Islander primary health care and has facilitated many workshops and training opportunities in continuous quality improvement and community-based health promotion.

♥

The authors have long worked together in quality improvement and primary healthcare projects and have been recipients of an Australian Evaluation Society Award for Excellence in Indigenous Evaluation. This work has always been part of a wider team effort.

Positioning ourselves as authors is essential in this space. We write as one Aboriginal and two non-Indigenous authors, drawing respectfully on the work of many Aboriginal and Torres Strait Islander and non-Indigenous colleagues. We acknowledge the dominance of Western research and knowledge traditions in academia and recognise the strength and authority of Indigenous research and knowledge traditions.

Acknowledgements

In the spirit of respect, we acknowledge the people and the Elders of the Aboriginal and Torres Strait Islander Nations who are the traditional custodians of the land and waters of Australia, and the rights of First Nations peoples worldwide.

This book would not have been possible without the clinicians, other health services staff and managers, communities, policymakers, health support agencies and academics who have supported or contributed directly to continuous quality improvement (CQI) research and practice. We thank the health services that provided de-identified data on CQI and appreciate the extensive and varied contribution of so many people to the work that is reflected in this book. We also thank all authors of the peer-reviewed publications, tools and other knowledge translation products we have drawn upon.

We acknowledge the active support, enthusiasm and commitment of founding members of the Audit and Best Practice for Chronic Disease (ABCD) research program on CQI, and all later partners and collaborators in the ABCD National Research Partnership, the Centre for Research Excellence in Integrated Quality Improvement (CRE-IQI) and the Centre for Research Excellence: Strengthening Systems for Indigenous Health Care Equity (CRE-STRIDE). Thanks to the dedicated managers and staff of One21seventy, the National Centre for Quality Improvement in Indigenous Primary Health Care at Menzies School of Health Research, who provided CQI support and training to health services over several years.

Most of the research has been funded by the National Health and Medical Research Council of Australia and the Australian Research Council, with in-kind support from partner institutions. One21seventy was supported with funding from the Lowitja Institute and from government and community controlled primary healthcare services.

We are grateful to the Aboriginal and Torres Strait Islander Reference and Management Committees of the Centre for Research Excellence: Strengthening Systems for Indigenous Health Care Equity and to Kerryn Harkin for project support. Thank you to Adjunct Professor Tarun Weeramanthri and Professor Ian Anderson for contributing the Foreword.

Many people suggested resources and references, contributed to stories, gave permission for their words to be included or shared expertise in other ways. We thank them all.

Chapter reviewers

Almost all chapters have been reviewed by at least two people. Thank you to these reviewers:

Andrew Carson-Stevens, Cardiff University

Barbara Nattabi, University of Western Australia

Christine Connors, Top End Health Services, Northern Territory Health

Dan McAullay, Edith Cowan University

Danielle Cameron, University of Sydney

David Pieris, The George Institute

Elizabeth Ramsay, University of Technology Sydney

Gillian Harvey, Flinders University

Hugh Taylor, University of Melbourne

Jacqueline Boyle, Monash University

Janya McCalman, Central Queensland University

Jodie Bailie, University of Sydney

Judy Katzenellenbogen, University of Western Australia/Telethon Kids

Judy Taylor, James Cook University

Karen Carlisle, James Cook University

Kerry Copley, Aboriginal Medial Services Alliance Northern Territory (NT)

Kerryn Harkin, University of Sydney

Kristy Clancy, James Cook University

Louise Patel, Aboriginal Medial Services Alliance NT

Marea Fittock, Northern Territory Department of Health

Megan Williams, University of Technology Sydney

Melanie Gibson-Helm, Victoria University of Wellington

Paul Burgess, Northern Territory Department of Health

Roxanne Bainbridge, University of Queensland

Sandra Campbell, Central Queensland University

Sandra Thompson, University of Western Australia

Sarah Larkins, James Cook University

Stefanie Puszka, Australian National University

Tessa Benveniste, Central Queensland University

Veronica Matthews, University of Sydney

Vicki Saunders, Central Queensland University

People who shared experiences and stories, provided tips or project information

Aboriginal and Torres Strait Islander Reference Committee, Centre for Research Excellence: Strengthening Systems for Indigenous Health Care Equity

Amanda Robinson, Top End Health Service, Northern Territory Health

Danielle Cameron, University of Sydney

Danielle Jordan, Top End Health Service, Northern Territory Health

David Thomas, Menzies School of Health Research/Aboriginal Medial Services Alliance Northern Territory

Edward Strivens, Queensland Department of Health

Julie Brimblecombe, Monash University

Kathleen Conte, DePaul University/University of Sydney

Kerry Copley, Aboriginal Medial Services Alliance Northern Territory

Leslie Baird, National Centre for Family Wellbeing

Louise Patel, Aboriginal Medial Services Alliance Northern Territory

Mark Ramjan, Top End Health Service, Northern Territory Health

Megan Passey, University of Sydney

Nalita Turner, James Cook University

Shawn Cartwright, Top End Health Service, Northern Territory Health

Theresa Paterson, Aboriginal Medial Services Alliance Northern Territory

Note: Many contributors have dual affiliations (for example, with research institutions and health services). We have listed their main affiliation.

Thank you to peer reviewers

We are grateful to three anonymous reviewers who provided constructive feedback on the draft manuscript.

Use of terms

The term "Aboriginal and Torres Strait Islander" is used respectfully and inclusively throughout this book, acknowledging that there are many cultural differences between and within Aboriginal and Torres Strait Islander communities. The terms "Indigenous" and "First Nations" are generally used to refer to Indigenous peoples globally. For ease of reading, the term "non-Indigenous" is used to refer to people who do not identify as Indigenous.

Throughout this book, we use the term "client" rather than "patient". This is consistent with the conception of PHC as more than clinical care, and the shift from a medical-centric model of care in which patients "receive treatment" to models that empower people in decisions about their health-related needs and care.

How to use this book

While the concepts and principles of continuous quality improvement (CQI) in health care are universal, specific approaches have been developed in response to the principles and characteristics of primary health care (PHC). This book provides an accessible contemporary guide on implementing CQI in PHC settings, with guidance for health services and their staff, policymakers, researchers, funders and support organisations. It draws together two decades of practical experience and established leadership in this field to position our work in Aboriginal and Torres Strait Islander health in Australia in an international context. The applied research described is based on participatory principles and engagement with community-based organisations and different levels of government. True to this approach, many of the people involved in the CQI work have generously reviewed chapters and had input as the book was developed.

We firmly believe that "continuous quality improvement is everybody's business" and have intentionally written for a diverse audience. We recognise that different parts of the book will be of greater or lesser interest according to the context in which you work, your role and experience in the PHC system, or your area of study, research or teaching. There are four interlinked parts.

Part I

Part I identifies core concepts underpinning PHC and CQI. It explains why CQI is necessary in PHC and how CQI approaches in PHC differ from approaches used in other parts of the health system. Three chapters provide a foundation for understanding the PHC system context, CQI tools, processes and contemporary perspectives presented in parts II to IV.

Part II

Part II provides guidance for implementing CQI in PHC, with information of greatest relevance for health service providers and those developing CQI policy and support. The five chapters explain how to generate, present and analyse CQI data and how to adapt CQI tools and techniques to improve care quality in PHC settings. We introduce a CQI cycle that acknowledges the complexity of improving comprehensive PHC and steps readers through its application. Practical examples or stories from the field illustrate each phase: for example, how to present data for analysis; how to understand and address variation in care quality; and how to use systems thinking and local knowledge to interpret data and to plan improvement strategies. Some key CQI resources are recommended. The final chapter in Part II focuses on ways to embed an organisational culture of CQI.

Part III

Part III shares what has been learnt from applying the CQI approach described in parts I and II. Use of this CQI approach over two decades has produced data on clinical performance and change over time in a wide range of Australian Aboriginal and Torres Strait Islander PHC services, thus providing a strong evidence base for its use. Ten chapters demonstrate the successes and challenges experienced in implementing CQI for important clinical conditions, such as diabetes, or life stages, such as child health, with reference to the determinants that affect care and outcomes. Each chapter provides internationally relevant background, information about recommended care, CQI findings, and key messages for improving the quality of PHC. Implications for improving care in Aboriginal and Torres Strait Islander settings are included for Australian readers. The lessons offered in Part III may be particularly relevant for health service providers, policymakers and communities implementing CQI in low- and middle-income countries and in settings where healthcare inequity persists between population groups.

Part IV

Part IV discusses the wide-scale application of CQI and contemporary collaborative approaches to PHC research, with a focus on strengthening systems to improve PHC equity. In these three chapters, we describe some approaches for engaging stakeholders at different levels of the health system and across sectors in CQI. We also outline the principles and methodologies informing culturally safe, strengths-based and transformative CQI research in Indigenous PHC settings and describe strategies for strengthening links between communities and health services. Several innovative evaluations are included. The examples presented in these chapters are complex interventions or strategies implemented within complex systems, offering transferable lessons for quality improvement work in a range of systems, services and communities. Researchers and policymakers who may be commissioning research or developing CQI policies and plans may find these chapters useful.

Throughout chapters, shaded boxes are used to highlight important messages.

Over the past two decades, through the many individuals, PHC teams, services and communities involved in this CQI work, we have learnt a lot about implementing quality improvement in PHC settings. There is much more to learn if we are to transform systems to achieve more equitable people-centred care and meet the healthcare challenges of the future.

List of abbreviations

ABCD	Audit and Best Practice for Chronic Disease
ACCHO	Aboriginal community controlled health organisation
ARF/RHD	Acute rheumatic fever/rheumatic heart disease
BP	Blood pressure
CARPA	Central Australian Rural Practitioners Association
CQI	Continuous quality improvement
CRE-IQI	Centre for Research Excellence in Integrated Quality Improvement
CRE-STRIDE	Centre for Research Excellence: Strengthening Systems for Indigenous Health Care Equity
CVD	Cardiovascular disease
HbA1c	Glycated haemoglobin, blood glucose level
GP	General practitioner
HIV	Human immunodeficiency virus
NHMRC	National Health and Medical Research Council
PDSA	Plan-do-study-act
PHC	Primary health care
SEWB	Social and emotional wellbeing
STI	Sexually transmissible infection
WHO	World Health Organization

Part I

Core concepts in primary health care and continuous quality improvement

All people have the right to high-quality health care, delivered through high-quality health systems. High-quality health systems are those that consistently deliver care that improves or maintains health. They are equitable, valued and trusted by people and are responsive to changing population needs.[1] For most people, the first point of access to the health system is through primary health care (PHC).

Not all health care is high quality and one way of improving the quality of PHC is to use continuous quality improvement (CQI). CQI has been widely used in the healthcare system for more than two decades, and in 2005 the World Health Organization (WHO) identified quality improvement as one of the five core competencies needed by all of the healthcare workforce to meet the challenge of chronic illness care in the 21st century.[2] Despite considerable developments in the theory and practice of CQI,[3] there is no detailed explanation of how its concepts can be applied in the context of comprehensive PHC. This book aims to address this need and to support the PHC workforce, including policymakers, funders, health services and support organisations, in understanding and applying CQI.

Part I explains the concepts that underpin CQI approaches in PHC. We define comprehensive PHC and population health, and explain key concepts with reference to international and Australian contexts. Quality and CQI are defined and the origins of CQI are traced to explain some fundamental concepts and characteristics, how they translate in PHC settings and why CQI approaches in PHC differ from other parts of the health system. We focus on CQI research and practice in Aboriginal and Torres Strait Islander health settings in Australia to argue the importance of a comprehensive systems approach to CQI for improving PHC and healthcare equity.

References

Kruk, M., A. Gage, C. Arsenault, K. Jordan, H. Leslie, S. Roder-Dewan et al. (2018). High-quality health systems in the Sustainable Development Goals era: time for a revolution. *Lancet Global Health* 6(11): E1196–E252.

Sollecito, W. and J. Johnson (2019). *McLaughlin and Kaluzny's continuous quality improvement in health care*. Burlington, MA: Jones & Bartlett Learning.

World Health Organization (2005). *Preparing a health care workforce for the 21st century: the challenge of chronic conditions*. Geneva, Switzerland: WHO.

---

1   Kruk, Gage et al. 2018.
2   World Health Organization 2005.
3   Sollecito and Johnson 2019.

Primary health care

What is primary health care?

The fundamental premise of primary health care is that all people, everywhere, have the right to receive the right care in their community.[1] PHC attends to the majority of a person's health needs throughout their lifetime, including physical, mental and social wellbeing. PHC is people-centred rather than disease-centred. It is a whole-of-society approach that includes health promotion, disease prevention, treatment, rehabilitation and palliative care.[2]

> Primary health care attends to the majority of a person's health needs throughout their lifetime.

Primary health care was formally defined in 1978, in the landmark Declaration of Alma-Ata, but use of the terms "primary care" and "PHC" pre-date 1978, and approaches that we now call primary health care were being pioneered by progressive public health practitioners several decades earlier. The World Health Organization (WHO) Declaration endorsed an international definition of PHC in 1978 as follows:

> essential health care based on practical, scientifically sound and socially acceptable methods and technology made universally accessible to individuals and families in the community through their full participation and at a cost that the community and country can afford to maintain at every stage of their development in the spirit of self-reliance and self-determination. It forms an integral part both of the country's health system, and of the overall social and economic development of the community. It is the first level of contact of individuals, the family and community with the national health system bringing health care as close as possible to where people live and work, and constitutes the first element of a continuing health care process.[3]

1   World Health Organization 2018c.
2   World Health Organization 2018c.
3   World Health Organization 1978, 2–3.

The WHO declaration also established these key principles of primary health care:

- universal access to care
- health equity as part of social justice
- individual and community participation and empowerment
- multi-sectoral policy and action
- integrated health services that meet people's health needs throughout their lives
- health attainment through a fuller and better use of resources.

The 2018 Global Conference on Primary Health Care, held in Kazakhstan, affirmed these principles in a new declaration emphasising the critical role of PHC in meeting contemporary population health and health system challenges. The Declaration of Astana reinforces the ethical, political, social and economic imperative of achieving health equity and reducing disparities in health outcomes globally and for vulnerable populations. The declaration sets out this vision:

> PHC and health services that are high quality, safe, comprehensive, integrated, accessible, available and affordable for everyone and everywhere, provided with compassion, respect and dignity by health professionals who are well-trained, skilled, motivated and committed.[4]

"PHC" is a broader term than "primary care", which is used – mainly in the United Kingdom and northern America – to describe primary medical care or family practice.

A comprehensive approach

Comprehensive PHC is the most important part of the health system. Comprehensive PHC is vital to improving health outcomes and reducing health inequities – unnecessary, unfair and avoidable differences in health between groups within a population.[5] A comprehensive PHC approach, as described in the Alma-Ata and Astana declarations, provides care *in* and *through* the community. In addition to meeting health needs across a person's life span, comprehensive PHC attends to the broader social determinants of health through the involvement of other sectors in policy and action, such as food supply, education, housing, public infrastructure and communications.

In contrast, a selective PHC approach focuses on a disease or issue in isolation (for example, family planning, eradicating smallpox, reducing tuberculosis). After the Alma-Ata declaration, selective PHC was advocated as an interim strategy for improving health in low-income countries. A selective approach has had success in reducing diseases but has failed to promote community self-determination, equitable care and multi-sector action to improve and sustain health.[6]

Comprehensive PHC aims to empower individuals, families and communities to take charge of their own health and health care, and to tackle broader public health issues and risks to

---

4   World Health Organization 2018a, 1.
5   Starfield, Shi and Macinko 2005; Whitehead 1992.
6   Magnussen, Ehiri and Jolly 2004.

health. It also aims to meet the needs of defined populations, such as Indigenous peoples and those who, for various reasons, are missing out on services.[7]

> Comprehensive PHC is vital to improving health outcomes and reducing health inequities.

Comprehensive PHC has a rich heritage. We highlight two early examples from South Africa where, in the late 1930s, public health practitioners who understood the links between broad aspects of health and development laid the foundations for a comprehensive curative and preventive service characterised by intersectoral action. The group argued that clinical services must be brought within the sphere of a broader social health scheme, and that health policy and practice must be informed by evidence. With government support, Kark, Cassel and colleagues established a rural health centre and trained community health workers to conduct an annual household health census, using the results to argue for sanitation and food production planning, and to study epidemiology and the influence of various environmental factors on people. These steps were the basis for what later became known as "community-oriented primary care".[8] It influenced the work of other PHC pioneers, such as the epidemiologist Susser and colleagues, who in the 1940s highlighted the connections between social justice and health, and the family, community and societal influences on health and disease. Although related ideas originated in the environmental conditions and epidemic contexts created by mass urban immigration (for example, in 19th-century industrial Britain and Europe), the South African approach in the mid-20th century heralded the emergence of community-oriented PHC and was pivotal for establishing international principles of PHC: health as a human right, health equity between populations as an aim of public health and service delivery by multidisciplinary teams.[9] The right to health was institutionalised in the 1948 United Nations Universal Declaration of Human Rights.[10]

Health systems that are focused on PHC deliver better and more equitable outcomes at lower cost than other aspects of the health services delivery system. Studies by Starfield and colleagues found that countries with stronger and more comprehensive PHC generally had a healthier population and lower all-cause mortality, while countries with low PHC scores as a group had poorer health outcomes across various indicators. There was a positive association between adequate features of PHC (accessible, comprehensive, coordinated, continuous and accountable care) and the provision of preventive services, and between PHC and (in contrast to specialty care) greater health equity within populations.[11] High-quality PHC is also associated with strong PHC policy, lower hospitalisation rates for conditions managed by good clinical care, and lower healthcare costs.[12]

---

7   Keleher 2001; World Health Organization 2008, 2018b.
8   Kark and Cassel 1999-2005; Yach and Tollman 1993.
9   Susser 1993, 1999.
10   Susser 1993.
11   Starfield 1994, 2012; Starfield, Shi and Macinko 2005.
12   Starfield 2012.

Population health

What is population health?

Population health can be described as the study of health and disease in defined populations. It is an organised response to protect and improve the health outcomes of a population: for example, children, First Nations peoples, refugees, people with low incomes.

In population health there is a focus on populations as entities (rather than the individuals who make up the population), an emphasis on health promotion and disease prevention strategies at a population level, and concern with the underlying social, economic, biological, genetic, environmental and cultural determinants of health of whole population groups. For example, using a population health approach one would ask "why does this particular population have a high incidence of diabetes or renal disease?", whereas working at an individual level one might ask "why did this person develop diabetes or renal disease?"

Common principles

Population health shares many principles with comprehensive PHC, including a focus on holistic health and equity, community empowerment, intersectoral collaboration, health promotion, integrated services, multidisciplinary teams and evidence-based practice. These principles also align with the holistic definition of Aboriginal health (see below).

Population health responses often involve changes to policies, systems and structures to maintain and improve health and to prioritise health interventions for groups who are most in need. It is widely accepted that a comprehensive PHC approach can improve population health outcomes. It can link and strengthen health systems to meet population health needs.

> Population health responses often involve changes to policies, systems and structures.

A population health approach is fundamental in continuous quality improvement in primary health care. While CQI often uses data gathered from individual client records, these data are brought together to show trends in the population's health or in service delivery, and to inform population health improvement strategies.

The social, cultural, structural and environmental determinants of health

"Social determinants" is the commonly used term to describe the non-medical and behavioural influences on health: the conditions in which people are born, grow, live, work and age, and the wider forces and systems that shape daily life (for example, food and housing security). According to the WHO, these social conditions are the single most important determinant of good health or poor health.[13]

---

13   Commission on Social Determinants of Health 2008.

The social determinants of health identified by the WHO are social gradient, stress, early life, social exclusion, work, unemployment, social support, addiction, food and transport.[14] Education, gender and ethnicity also have a marked influence on how healthy a person is. Factors such as girls' access to schooling and the number of years of education have been shown to affect maternal, infant and child health.[15] Discrimination against ethnic and racial minorities shapes some people's access to services, employment and resources, with significant effects on health and wellbeing.[16] In these respects, the social determinants of health are shaped by political, social and economic structures – sometimes called "structural determinants of health" – that are largely beyond a person's control.

The social and structural determinants of health highlight the inequalities in health between and within countries. For example, the average life expectancy in low-income countries is 62 years compared with 81 years in high-income countries.[17] As a wealthy country with one of the highest life expectancies in the world and a universal health insurance system, Australia provides a telling example of how social and structural inequalities influence health and life expectancy within countries. There is an estimated 8-year gap in life expectancy between Aboriginal and Torres Strait Islander peoples and the Australian average, with two-thirds of the health gap attributed to preventable chronic conditions.[18] The social determinants of health and wellbeing for Aboriginal and Torres Strait Islander Australians are complex, multi-dimensional and bound in the history and legacy of colonisation. At least 34 per cent of the health gap is linked to education, employment, income, incarceration and housing quality.[19] Forty-four per cent of Indigenous peoples live in regional areas and 18 per cent in remote and very remote areas with poorer access to services and employment.[20] Framed from an Aboriginal and Torres Strait Islander viewpoint, social determinants include the history of health, racism and marginalisation, poverty, control over health, powerlessness, family separation, land and reconciliation.[21] Improving health involves genuine commitment to tackling these determinants and strengthening the cultural determinants of health and wellbeing, such as connection to Country and community, kinship, cultural expression, language and cultural leadership.

Environmental determinants, for example water and air quality and the impacts of extreme weather events, are also critical to health. The environmental effects of climate change pose an increasing risk to human health into the future.

A comprehensive approach to PHC takes intersectoral action on the various determinants of health.

---

14   Wilkinson and Marmot 2003.
15   Mensch, Chuang et al. 2019.
16   Anderson, Baum and Bentley 2004; Crear-Perry, Correa-de-Araujo et al. 2021.
17   World Health Organization 2018b.
18   Productivity Commission 2021.
19   Burns, Burrow et al. 2015.
20   Australian Institute of Health and Welfare 2020.
21   Anderson, Baum and Bentley 2004.

A comprehensive approach to PHC takes intersectoral action on the various determinants of health to improve health and reduce health inequalities. It aims to improve the circumstances in which people live and work, and complements efforts to control major diseases, improve health systems and reduce poverty.[22] This requires high-quality health systems that consistently deliver services to improve or maintain health, are valued and trusted, and respond to changing population needs.[23]

In Australia

In Australia, PHC encompasses a range of providers and services across the public, private and non-government sectors. PHC services include health promotion, prevention and screening, early intervention, treatment of acute conditions and management of chronic conditions. PHC services are delivered in settings such as general practices, community health centres, allied health practices and via communication technologies such as telehealth and video consultations. Use of these technologies increased during the Covid-19 pandemic. PHC professionals include, but are not limited to, general practitioners (GPs), nurses, nurse practitioners, allied health professionals, midwives, Aboriginal and Torres Strait Islander health practitioners and workers, pharmacists and dentists, and a broader network of community and social support workers. The Australian universal public health insurance scheme, Medicare, is funded to provide free or subsidised PHC, and approximately 35 per cent of total health funding is spent on PHC, similar to spending on hospital services.[24]

Despite Australia's comparatively well-funded and well-functioning health systems, many Australians experience inequitable access to PHC services and a lack of integration between PHC and other parts of the health system. Policy and system reforms have been implemented to reduce the fragmentation of services and to improve the efficiency and integration of local systems to meet client and population needs. Examples include the 2020–2025 National Health Reform Agreement;[25] the establishment of Primary Health Networks, which aim to streamline health services and improve care coordination; the trial of "Health Care Homes";[26] and MyMedicare,[27] a voluntary patient registration model to formalise relationships between clients and general practices or between clients and PHC providers or both. Improvement is most needed in regional and remote areas, where around one-third of all Australians live, and where health outcomes are generally poorer relative to metropolitan areas. In fact, the prevalence of health risk factors, levels of illness and mortality generally worsen with increased distance from major cities, while access to PHC is reduced. So, while Australia matches or outperforms many comparable countries on selected measures of health, there is a need for a more equitable distribution of health resources and better access to core PHC services (listed below) across the population.[28]

---

22   Marmot 2005.
23   Kruk, Gage et al 2018.
24   Australian Institute of Health and Welfare 2016.
25   Department of Health and Aged Care 2021.
26   Department of Health 2020; Jackson and Hambleton 2017.
27   Department of Health and Aged Care 2024.
28   Australian Institute of Health and Welfare 2018; Thomas, Wakerman and Humphreys 2015.

Despite Australia's comparatively well-funded and well-functioning health systems, many Australians experience inequitable access to PHC services.

A study conducted in 2012 found consensus among policymakers, academics, clinical practitioners and consumers on the essential PHC services that all Australians should expect to receive, regardless of where they live. These are the essential services:

- care of the sick and injured
- mental health and social and emotional wellbeing
- maternal and child health
- allied health
- sexual and reproductive health
- rehabilitation
- oral and dental health
- public health and illness prevention.

The essential PHC functions needed to support these services were identified as management (including governance and leadership), coordination, health infrastructure, quality systems, data systems, professional development and community participation.[29]

The Aboriginal and Torres Strait Islander approach

Aboriginal and Torres Strait Islander peoples are the first peoples of Australia, comprising hundreds of nations with distinct histories, languages and cultural traditions. Across diverse nations and communities, and shared with other Indigenous peoples, is a strong tradition of unity with the environment[30] (often expressed in Australia as connection to Country) and a holistic view of health incorporating the spiritual, intellectual, physical and emotional dimensions of life. Health and survival are viewed as both a collective and individual intergenerational continuum.[31] This concept underpins contemporary definitions of Aboriginal and Torres Strait Islander health and wellbeing. Seen through this lens, PHC is a holistic approach that is culturally embedded in a way that supports the social, emotional, physical and cultural wellbeing of Aboriginal and Torres Strait Islander peoples, families and communities.

Aboriginal and Torres Strait Islander Australians access PHC through Aboriginal community controlled and government-managed health services and through private general practices. Aboriginal community controlled health organisations emerged in the 1970s because mainstream services were not dealing adequately with the health needs of Aboriginal and Torres Strait Islander peoples who wanted to be able to provide care to their communities that was culturally appropriate, holistic and accessible. By the 1990s, these organisations were important providers of comprehensive PHC for Aboriginal and Torres Strait Islander peoples.[32]

---

29 Thomas, Wakerman and Humphreys 2014.
30 Durie 2004.
31 Committee on Indigenous Health 2002.
32 National Aboriginal Community Controlled Health Organisation 2022.

Because most Aboriginal and Torres Strait Islander PHC services deliver care to the communities that operate and control them (through elected boards), they are also important for employment, professional education, community empowerment and social action. Aboriginal and Torres Strait Islander PHC services (which can be government-run or community controlled) have close relationships with the people they serve, local knowledge of community, and increased cultural awareness.[33] The Aboriginal and Torres Strait Islander model of PHC delivery embodies comprehensive PHC as defined in the Declaration of Alma-Ata.

PHC complexity and systems approaches

PHC is complex in its scope and the way it is delivered. It requires the provision of holistic and client-centred care for people of all ages, for physical, psychological and social conditions, and for diseases affecting any body organ. It also needs to take account of complex health needs and personal and family circumstances. In terms of delivery, PHC providers are diverse, widely dispersed, relatively independent in their practice and work within a variety of funding and governance models with differing resources and infrastructure support. The PHC information systems available to providers are often relatively undeveloped and fragmented, yet PHC providers need to work closely with many other providers, funders, policymakers and their local communities to deliver effective care.[34] Furthermore, the balance between acute and chronic health problems continues to shift globally, with increases in chronic conditions and comorbidities, and a corresponding need for health promotion, prevention, referral to specialised services (sometimes distant), integration of care and support for self-management. This complexity has implications for the PHC workforce, who need knowledge of public and population health perspectives and skills in client-centred care, partnering, using information and communication technology, and continuous quality improvement.[35] The systems through which PHC is governed, managed and delivered need to respond effectively to these complexities.

> PHC is complex in its scope and the way it is delivered.

Health systems and systems thinking

Advances in systems thinking have helped in understanding and attending to complexity in PHC. A system is a set of interacting parts, which form an integrated whole. All systems are made up of multiple elements, links between elements (the processes and interrelationships that hold the elements together) and a boundary that determines what is inside and outside the system. Systems thinking is a way of thinking about health systems as holistic, dynamic and interconnected.

The WHO defines a health system as *"all organisations, people, and actions whose primary interest is to promote, restore, or maintain health"*. This includes efforts to influence determinants of health as well as direct health-improving activities. The goals of a health system are

---

33   Larkins, Woods et al. 2016.
34   Bailie, Matthews et al. 2013.
35   World Health Organization 2005.

"improving health and health equity in ways that are responsive, financially fair, and make the best, or most efficient, use of available resources".[36]

Six building blocks for strengthening health systems

To advance health system goals, the WHO identified "six building blocks" for strengthening health systems:

- service delivery
- health workforce
- information
- medical products, vaccines and technologies
- financing
- leadership and governance.[37]

Each building block represents an essential health system function and is interdependent with other parts of the system, highlighting the need for integrated responses to build overall health system capacity.

The WHO model has been criticised for excluding a community health element, which may be added when interpreting the building blocks.[38] Including "community" as a foundational building block recognises that health systems, through governments and policy leaders, need to respond to the effects of social and environmental determinants of health to design inclusive services tailored to community needs. It is also recognised that multi-sectoral approaches and community participation are needed to tackle underlying causes of poor health such as food insecurity, unsafe water and poor sanitation.[39]

Ten building blocks for high performance

Bodenheimer and colleagues studied exemplar PHC practices in the United States of America and used a similar building-blocks approach to describe key elements of high-performing, client-centred PHC. They propose engaged leadership, data-driven improvement, empanelment (patient registration) and team-based care as the foundation for implementing six other elements: client–team partnership; population management; continuity of care; prompt access to care; comprehensiveness and care coordination; and informing a template of the future (Figure 1.1).[40]

---

36   World Health Organization 2007, 2.
37   World Health Organization 2007.
38   Sacks, Morrow et al. 2019.
39   Sacks, Morrow et al. 2019.
40   Bodenheimer, Ghorob et al. 2014.

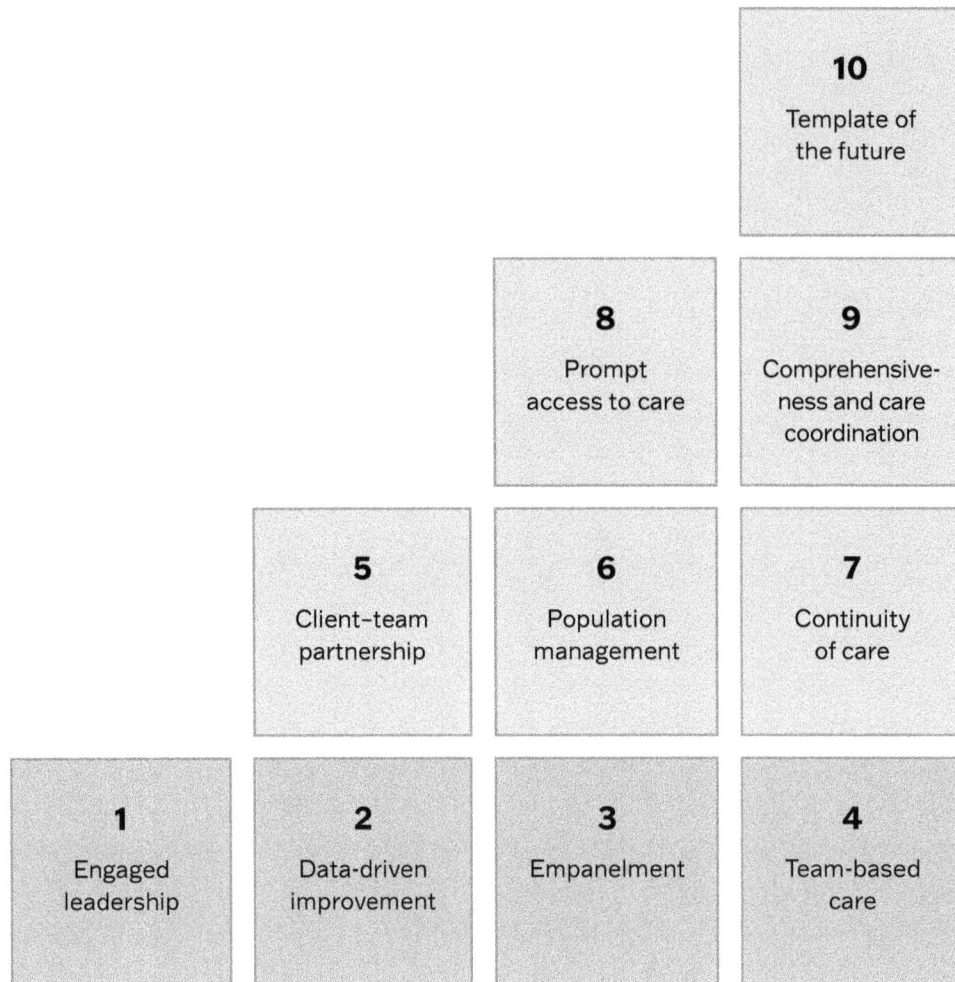

Figure 1.1 The 10 building blocks of high-performing primary health care. Adapted with permission from the Center for Excellence in Primary Care 2002. Source: 2012 UCSF Center for Excellence in Primary Care.

Innovative Care for Chronic Conditions Framework

The "Innovative Care for Chronic Conditions Framework" represents a systems approach to the prevention and management of chronic conditions in PHC settings. The Framework (Figure 1.2) presents the actions and interactions required at three levels of the healthcare system to achieve better outcomes for chronic conditions. Each part of the framework needs to function effectively, while interacting with and dynamically influencing actions and events at the other two levels.

1. A positive policy environment serves to strengthen partnerships, support legislative frameworks and integrate policies into care and provide leadership and advocacy. Consistent financing is promoted, and human resources are developed and allocated.
2. Healthcare organisations promote care continuity and coordination, encourage quality through leadership and incentives, organise and equip healthcare teams, use information systems, and support self-management and prevention.

Positive policy environment

Strengthen partnerships	Provide leadership and advocacy
Support legislative frameworks	Promote consistent financing
Integrate policies	Develop and allocate human resources

Community   **Links**   **Healthcare organisation**

Raise awareness and reduce stigma

Encourage better outcomes through leadership and support

Mobilise and coordinate resources

Provide complementary services

Community partners   Prepared   **Healthcare team**

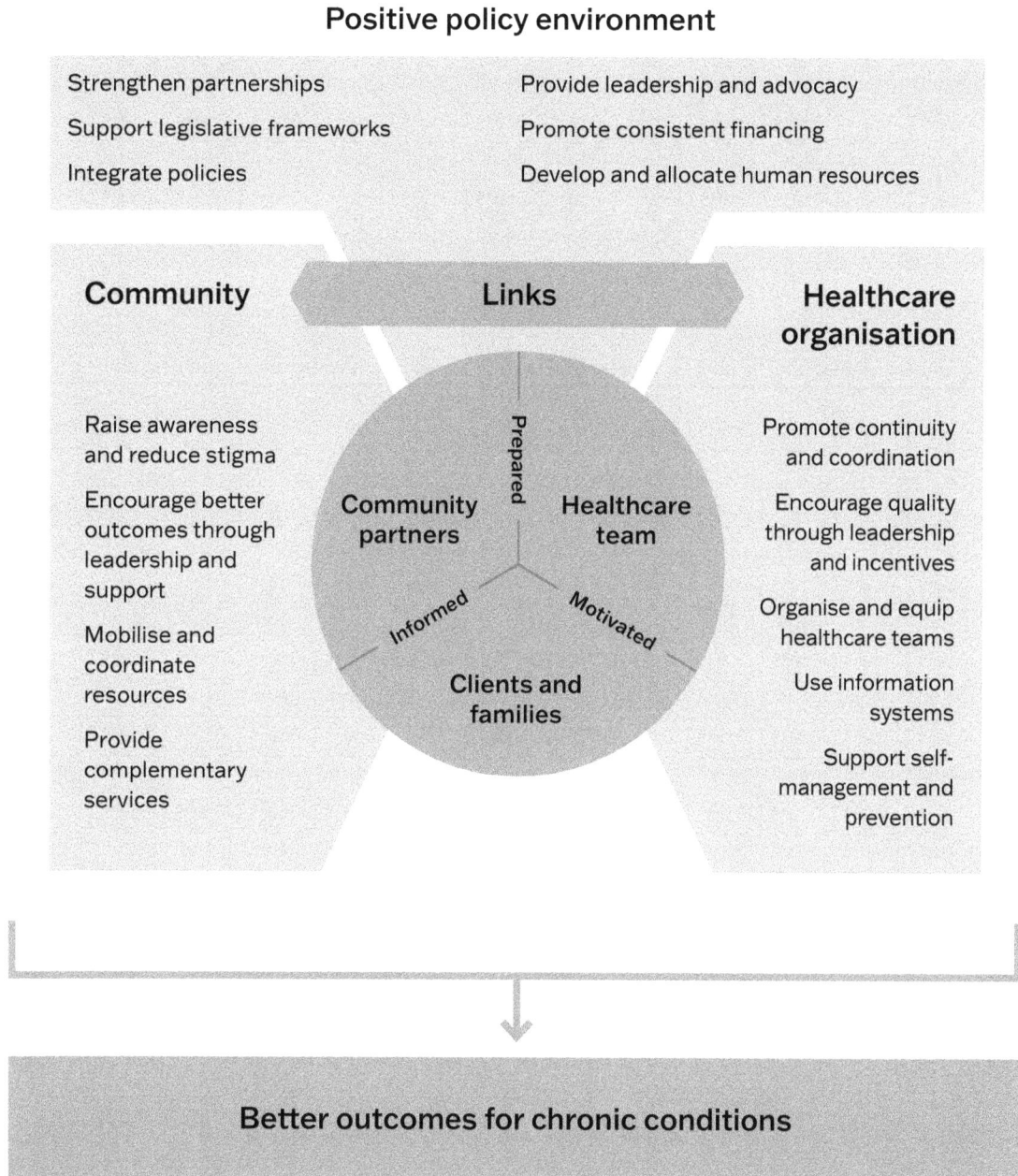

Informed   Motivated

Clients and families

Promote continuity and coordination

Encourage quality through leadership and incentives

Organise and equip healthcare teams

Use information systems

Support self-management and prevention

Better outcomes for chronic conditions

Figure 1.2 Innovative Care for Chronic Conditions Framework. World Health Organization 2002, 65.

3. Actions are taken at the community level to raise awareness and reduce stigma, encourage better outcomes through leadership and support, mobilise and coordinate resources, and provide complementary services. Informed community partners and motivated healthcare teams link patients and families.

In each of these concepts of health system frameworks, the individual elements (or building blocks) are important, and effective interactions between the building blocks are essential for effective system functioning. Both PHC frameworks highlight continuous, well-coordinated care and engaged clients and communities as important aspects of service performance.

Health services as complex adaptive systems

Health services are often described as complex adaptive systems. "Complexity" arises from a system's interconnected parts, and "adaptivity" from its ability to change based on what occurs.[41]

Each individual PHC service is a complex adaptive system within larger complex adaptive systems (for example, government, organisation, community). Consistent with other systems, PHC systems have these characteristics:

- self-organising, whereby parts of the system tend to organise into an ordered state
- dynamic, interdependent and tightly linked – they are constantly adapting to change and evolving over time, with effects that may differ in the short and long term
- driven by interactions between systems components and governed by feedback, with responses having a flow-on effect that may be positive, negative or neutral
- nonlinear and often unpredictable, with changes in one part of the system producing unexpected changes in other parts, and effects that may be greater or less than what was intended
- sometimes counterintuitive in the way they behave – for example, a simple intervention that works well in one setting may not work in a similar setting
- often resistant to policy change, because of these features.[42]

> Each individual PHC service is a complex adaptive system within larger complex adaptive systems.

Overall, a systems approach to PHC considers the many elements, dynamics and factors influencing health. By understanding how these elements operate independently, and how they depend on and influence one another, a systems approach can help with the design and integration of PHC staffing, processes, facilities, organisations and policies to promote better health and to improve client experiences and outcomes at lower cost.

Systems thinking is used to understand, analyse, learn from, manage and change how systems work. It is essential for improving the quality of PHC. We write about the skills and tools for systems thinking in Chapter 6.

Summary

This chapter has defined PHC and traced its development to understand how a comprehensive approach to PHC has evolved internationally and in Australia. We have explained important concepts in PHC, including population health, the social determinants of health, and systems approaches to care. These concepts also underpin quality improvement. In the next chapter, we define "quality" and CQI. We describe how CQI evolved in health care, before considering how conventional approaches to it need to be adapted for practical application in PHC in Chapter 3.

---

41   de Savigny and Adam 2009.
42   de Savigny and Adam 2009; Sterman 2006.

References

Anderson, I., F. Baum and M. Bentley, eds (2004). *Beyond bandaids: exploring the underlying social determinants of Aboriginal health*. Papers from the Social Determinants of Aboriginal Health Workshop, Adelaide, Darwin: Cooperative Research Centre for Aboriginal Health.

Australian Institute of Health and Welfare (2020). *Australia's health 2020 data insights*. Canberra: Australian Government. Australia's Health series no. 17. Cat. no. AUS 231.

Australian Institute of Health and Welfare (2018). *Australia's health 2018*. Canberra: AIHW. Cat. no. AUS 221.

Australian Institute of Health and Welfare (2016). *Primary health care in Australia*. Canberra: AIHW. Cat. No. WEB 132.

Bailie, R., V. Matthews, J. Brands and G. Schierhout (2013). A systems-based partnership learning model for strengthening primary healthcare. *Implementation Science* 8. DOI: 10.1186/1748-5908-8-143.

Bodenheimer, T., A. Ghorob, R. Willard-Grace and K. Grumbach (2014). The 10 building blocks of high-performing primary care. *Annals of Family Medicine* 12(2): 166–71. DOI: 10.1370/afm.1616.

Burns, J., S. Burrow, N. Drew, M. Elwell, C. Gray, M. Harford-Mills et al. (2015). *Overview of Australian Indigenous health status, 2014*. Perth, WA: Australian Indigenous HealthInfoNet.

Center for Excellence in Primary Care (2012). What are the building blocks? https://cepc.ucsf.edu/what-are-building-blocks.

Commission on Social Determinants of Health (2008). *Closing the gap in a generation: health equity through action on the social determinants of health*. Final report of the Commission on Social Determinants of Health. Geneva: World Health Organization.

Committee on Indigenous Health (2002). *The Geneva Declaration on the Health and Survival of Indigenous Peoples*. New York: United Nations Permanent Forum on Indigenous Issues.

Crear-Perry, J., R. Correa-de-Araujo, T. Lewis Johnson, M.R. McLemore, E. Neilson and M. Wallace (2021). Social and structural determinants of health inequities in maternal health. *Journal of Women's Health* 30(2): 230–5. DOI: 10.1089/jwh.2020.8882.

de Savigny, D. and T. Adam, eds (2009). *Systems thinking for health systems strengthening*. Geneva, Switzerland: Alliance for Health Policy and Systems Research, World Health Organization.

Department of Health (2020). Primary health networks. https://www.health.gov.au/our-work/phn.

Department of Health and Aged Care (2024). MyMedicare. https://www.health.gov.au/our-work/mymedicare.

Department of Health and Aged Care (2021). *National health reform agreement: long-term health reforms roadmap*. Canberra: Australian Government.

Durie, M. (2004) Understanding health and illness: research at the interface between science and indigenous knowledge. *International Journal of Epidemiology* 33(5) 1138–43. DOI 10.1093/ije/dyh250.

Jackson, C. and S. Hambleton (2017). Australia's Health Care Homes: laying the right foundations. *Medical Journal of Australia* 206(9): 380–1. DOI: 10.5694/mja16.01470.

Kark, S.l. and Cassel, J. (1999–2005). The Pholela Health Centre: A progress report. 1952. *Bulletin of the World Health Organization* 77 (5): 439–47.

Keleher, H. (2001). Why primary health care offers a more comprehensive approach to tackling health inequities than primary care. *Australian Journal of Primary Health* 7(2): 57–61. DOI: 10.1071/PY01035.

Kruk, M., A. Gage, C. Arsenault, K. Jordan, H. Leslie, S. Roder-Dewan et al. (2018). High-quality health systems in the Sustainable Development Goals era: time for a revolution. *Lancet Global Health* 6(11): E1196–E252.

Larkins, S., C.E. Woods, V. Matthews, S.C. Thompson, G. Schierhout, M. Mitropoulos et al. (2016). Responses of Aboriginal and Torres Strait Islander primary health-care services to continuous quality improvement initiatives. *Frontiers in Public Health* 3. DOI: 10.3389/fpubh.2015.00288.

Magnussen, L., J. Ehiri and P. Jolly (2004). Comprehensive versus selective primary health care: lessons for global health policy. *Health Affairs* 23(3): 167–76. DOI: 10.1377/hlthaff.23.3.167.

Marmot, M. (2005). Social determinants of health inequalities. *Lancet* 365: 1099–104.

Mensch, B., E. Chuang, A. Melnikas and S. Psaki (2019). Evidence for causal links between education and maternal and child health: systematic review. *Tropical Medicine and International Health* 24(5): 504–22. DOI: 10.1111/tmi.13218.

National Aboriginal Community Controlled Health Organisation (2022). Publications and resources. Key facts. https://www.naccho.org.au/publications-resources/.

Productivity Commission (2021). *Innovations in care for chronic health conditions*. Productivity Reform Case Study. Canberra: Commonwealth of Australia.

Sacks, E., M. Morrow, W. Story, K. Shelley, D. Shanklin, M. Rahimtoola et al. (2019). Beyond the building blocks: integrating community roles into health systems frameworks to achieve health for all. *BMJ Global Health* 3(Suppl 3): e001384. DOI: 10.1136/bmjgh-2018-001384.

Starfield, B. (2012). Primary care: an increasingly important contributor to effectiveness, equity, and efficiency of health services. SESPAS report 2012. *Gaceta Sanitaria* 26(S): 20–6. DOI: 10.1016/j.gaceta.2011.10.009.

Starfield, B. (1994). Is primary care essential? *Lancet* 344(8930): 1129–33. DOI: 10.1016/S0140-6736(94)90634-3.

Starfield, B., L. Shi and J. Macinko (2005). Contribution of primary care to health systems and health. *Milbank Quarterly* 83(3): 457–502.

Sterman, J. (2006). Learning from evidence in a complex world. *American Journal of Public Health* 96(3): 505–14. DOI: 10.2105/AJPH.2005.066043.

Susser, M. (1999). Pioneering community-oriented primary care. *World Health Organization. Bulletin of the World Health Organization* 77(5): 436–8.

Susser, M. (1993). Health as a human right: an epidemiologist's perspective on the public health. *American Journal of Public Health* 83(3): 418–26. DOI: 10.2105/AJPH.83.3.418.

Thomas, S., J. Wakerman and J. Humphreys (2015). Ensuring equity of access to primary health care in rural and remote Australia – what core services should be locally available? *International Journal for Equity in Health* 14(1): 111. DOI: 10.1186/s12939-015-0228-1.

Thomas, S.L., J. Wakerman and J.S. Humphreys (2014). What core primary health care services should be available to Australians living in rural and remote communities? *BMC Family Practice* 15: 143. DOI: 10.1186/1471-2296-15-143.

Whitehead, M. (1992). The concepts and principles of equity and health. *International Journal of Health Services* 22(3): 429–45. DOI: 10.2190/986L-LHQ6-2VTE-YRRN.

Wilkinson, R. and M. Marmot, eds (2003). *Social determinants of health: the solid facts*, 2nd edn. Copenhagan, Denmark: World Health Organization.

World Health Organization (2018a). *Declaration of Astana*. Global Conference on Primary Health Care: From Alma-Ata towards universal health coverage and the Sustainable Development Goals. Astana, Kazakhstan 25–26 October 2018: World Health Organization and the United Nations Children's Fund (UNICEF).

World Health Organization (2018b). Health inequities and their causes. https://www.who.int/news-room/facts-in-pictures/detail/health-inequities-and-their-causes.

World Health Organization (2018c). Primary health care. http://www.who.int/primary-health/en/.

World Health Organization (2008). *The world health report 2008: primary health care – now more than ever*. Geneva, Switzerland: WHO.

World Health Organization (2007). *Everybody's business: strengthening health systems to improve health outcomes: WHO's framework for action*. Geneva, Switzerland: WHO.

World Health Organization (2005). *Preparing a health care workforce for the 21st century: the challenge of chronic conditions*. Geneva, Switzerland: WHO.

World Health Organization (2002). *Innovative care for chronic conditions: building blocks for action: global report*. Geneva, Switzerland: WHO.

World Health Organization (1978). *Declaration of Alma-Ata*. International Conference on Primary Health Care, Alma-Ata, USSR: WHO.

Yach, D. and S. Tollman (1993). Public health initiatives in South Africa in the 1940s and 1950s: lessons for a post-apartheid era. *American Journal of Public Health* 83(7): 1043–50. DOI: 10.2105/AJPH.83.7.1043.

Continuous quality improvement

What is quality in health care?

The World Health Organization (WHO) defines quality in health care as "the extent to which health care services provided to individuals and patient populations improve desired health outcomes. In order to achieve this, health care must be safe, effective, timely, efficient, equitable and people centred."[1] Each of these terms is worth examining:

- *effective* – providing evidence-based healthcare services to those who need them
- *safe* – minimising risk and avoiding harm, which includes avoiding preventable injuries and reducing medical errors, and involves safe care systems and safe practices
- *people-centred* – providing care that responds to the preferences, needs and values of individuals and communities. Clients should be engaged in care decisions.

Realising the benefits of high-quality health care requires services that display the following characteristics:

- *timely* – reducing wait times and delays in providing and receiving health care
- *equitable* – providing care that does not differ in quality according to individual characteristics such as gender, sexuality, race, ethnicity, geographical location or socio-economic status
- *integrated* – making available the full range of health services, which work together to provide "joined up" care throughout the life course
- *efficient* – maximising resource use and avoiding waste of supplies, space, capital, time and opportunities.[2]

Other concepts closely linked to quality in health care are access, continuity of care and value.

Access and quality

Access to primary health care (PHC) is central to receiving care that is timely, efficient, equitable and people-centred. Access can be defined as the opportunity to identify healthcare needs, to seek healthcare services, to reach, to obtain or use healthcare services and to have service needs met.[3]

---

1   World Health Organization 2023.
2   Rakhmanova and Bouchet 2017; World Health Organization 2023.
3   Levesque, Harris and Russell 2013.

Providing access to PHC services continues to be a key issue in many low- and middle-income countries. Overcoming barriers to accessing care is also critical for improving health equity in wealthy countries where race, ethnicity, socio-economic status, disability status, age, gender, sexual orientation, gender identity or geographic location can influence access to care and social services. Indigenous peoples in colonised countries,[4] resettled refugees[5] and people experiencing homelessness[6] are among groups at risk of inequitable access to services.

Levesque and colleagues identified five dimensions of healthcare accessibility: approachability; acceptability; availability or accommodation; affordability; and appropriateness.[7] We found these dimensions to be useful criteria for analysing the complex range of factors influencing Aboriginal and Torres Strait Islander Australians' access to healthcare services.[8] Accessibility is both a precursor to providing high-quality health care and one measure of PHC quality.

Continuity of care and quality

Continuity of care is the ability to provide uninterrupted care across programs, practitioners and levels of service over time. Care continuity is a core value and major focus of both PHC and general practice, and is a crucial element of high-quality PHC. It is associated with greater client satisfaction, lower mortality, fewer hospital admissions and improved health and system outcomes.[9] Continuity of care is of growing importance as populations increasingly live with chronic and complex illnesses, and other health and social challenges (for example, food and housing insecurity, warming climates).

There are many aspects of care continuity, such as ongoing client–practitioner relationships, ongoing management of chronic illness or disability, teamwork for care coordination, cross-boundary care (for example, between PHC, specialist and hospital services), and transfer of information that follows the client.[10]

> Continuity of care is a crucial element of high-quality PHC.

PHC models in some countries are being reformed to promote continuity of care. These include the Patient-centred Medical Home (United States of America), Primary Care Home (United Kingdom) and Health Care Homes (Australia – see below).

Value and quality

The concepts of value and quality are closely connected in health care, with policy debate around value-based care gaining momentum.[11] The idea of value-based health care is not new. Promoting better health at lower cost is an identified benefit of using a systems approach, and definitions of quality care include efficiency and sustainability concepts. But, as the cost

---

4   Davy, Harfield et al. 2016.
5   Russell, Harris et al. 2013.
6   Davies and Wood 2018.
7   Levesque, Harris and Russell 2013.
8   Bailie, Schierhout et al. 2015.
9   Jackson and Ball 2018.
10   Al-Azri 2008.
11   Coulter 2017; European Commission 2019.

of health care is rising faster than economies are growing, there is increasing emphasis on the need for health systems to spend their resources in a cost-effective way. Value-related issues differ between low- and middle-income countries and high-income countries. In the former, improving access to essential PHC services is a "high-value" investment as countries aim for universal healthcare coverage. High-income countries aiming for more value-based models are likely to prioritise system integration and the strengthening of existing healthcare infrastructure and operations.

> Value and quality are closely connected in health care.

Four types of value are reflected in current thinking around a value-based approach: personal value (appropriate care to achieve client goals); technical value (best possible outcomes with available resources); allocative value (equitable resource distribution across population groups); and societal value (contribution to social participation and connectedness).[12]

The World Economic Forum's definition of value-based health care explicitly focuses on the value delivered to the client: "the health outcomes that matter to patients relative to the resources or costs required".[13] By focusing on health outcomes instead of the volume of services delivered, value-based care systems help providers to manage cost increases, make the best use of finite resources and deliver improved care. Value is measured with a dual focus on improving accountability and improving quality.

Domains of quality are often measured in terms of meeting expected standards: for example, with indicators that measure clinical outcomes, care processes or care structures. Indicators may or may not measure client perceptions of quality care. But measures of value-based care do include client perspectives of value while factoring in the cost (to providers, clients and their families or carers) of delivering care.[14] This development supports the increasing use of quality improvement tools that measure care outcomes and experiences from a client viewpoint (see Chapter 5). Importantly, the change in approach stimulates discussion around who decides what is valuable and valued in health care, and provides greater scope for consumer-led measures of quality and consumer involvement in service design. For example, communities may place high value on the availability of cultural healing practices through the PHC clinic, or in-home visits for new mothers, elderly or disabled clients. Value-based care aligns with the way we define PHC and "quality" in several ways: it is client-centred; recognises complexity; and depends on integrated work by providers. Value-based care allows for different perceptions of value (for example, cultural safety) and aims for equity and efficiency in care.

In Australia, projects trialling the use of client-centred outcomes to improve the value of care include the staged rollout of the Health Care Homes model. The model promotes continuity of care and provides PHC practices with monthly bundled payments to care for registered clients with chronic conditions.[15] Measures being used to evaluate the model include use of services (including potentially preventable hospitalisations), client and service experiences, and the cost of care for the government, providers and clients.

---

12   European Commission 2019.
13   World Economic Forum 2017, 8.
14   Woolcock 2019.
15   Woolcock 2019.

What is continuous quality improvement?

Quality improvement in health care is an interdisciplinary and participatory process designed to raise the standards of care to maintain, restore and improve outcomes for individuals and populations. Continuous quality improvement (CQI) is one method of quality improvement, in which data are systematically collected and used in cyclical learning processes, such as the plan-do-study-act model.[16] We favour CQI over other approaches because of its focus on continuous learning and improvement. Other terms used under the broad banner of quality management are "quality assurance", a process focused on determining standards, guidelines and procedures to prevent risks to quality, and "quality control", which focuses more on testing the quality of a service or product.

> CQI is about ongoing learning and improvement.

Batalden and Davidoff defined CQI as "the combined and unceasing efforts of everyone— healthcare professionals, patients and their families, researchers, payers, planners and educators—to make the changes that will lead to better patient outcomes (health), better system performance (care) and better professional development (learning)".[17] This definition is based on a conviction that health care would be able to realise its potential if making positive change was part of everyone's job, in all parts of the health system. This accurately defines CQI in a PHC context, where many stakeholders need to be involved in improving and, in some contexts, transforming care. The definition is also consistent with the concept of a learning health system, where evidence and experience are continually brought together and applied to deliver higher quality, safer, more efficient care.[18]

Another widely accepted definition comes from McLaughlin and Kaluzny, who defined CQI as "a structured organisational process for involving personnel in planning and executing a continuous flow of improvements to provide quality health care that meets or exceeds expectations".[19] CQI is therefore both an approach and a process to improve the quality of care. A common concept across these definitions is continuous, collective effort to improve care systems and health outcomes.

Features of CQI

The following features are guiding principles for implementing or strengthening CQI.[20]

Data-driven continuous cycles of learning and improvement

In general, CQI facilitates ongoing improvement by using objective data to analyse and improve processes. It involves an ongoing cycle of gathering data on how well organisational systems are functioning and developing and implementing improvements. A 2014 study found consensus among quality improvement researchers and practitioners that all CQI methods involve these elements:

---

16   Bailie, Matthews et al. 2013.
17   Batalden and Davidoff 2007, 2.
18   Agency for Healthcare Research and Quality 2019.
19   Sollecito and Johnson 2019, 4–5.
20   As numerous sources and CQI resources identify these features, specific sources are not cited.

- systematic data-guided activities
- design for local conditions
- iterative development and testing.[21]

An essential starting point is the systematic and objective assessment of performance, and of the systems that support good performance. Good-quality information is needed, so that goals can be set, and strategies developed for improving care. Changes are made and the effects are monitored, leading to further change. CQI assumes that the effort to improve processes is never-ending, and that organisational and individual learning is ongoing.

Until recently, CQI processes and data had a strong focus on elements of clinical care for particular conditions or population groups. There is increasing focus on using CQI to address the social, cultural, structural and environmental determinants of health.

Small, incremental improvements

CQI aims for small changes that are realistic and achievable. Incremental changes made over successive CQI cycles are more likely to be sustainable than major, one-off changes. It takes time for small, incremental improvements in care quality to be reflected in data, which reinforces the importance of implementing continuous cycles of improvement.

> CQI involves ongoing data-driven cycles of learning and improvement, aiming for small incremental changes that are realistic and achievable.

Systems focus

CQI places emphasis on the efficient and effective functioning of organisational systems, and how system factors influence quality. CQI processes assume that people engaged within systems are well placed to identify system deficiencies and options for improvement. The focus of CQI to date has largely been on care teams and processes (sometimes called "clinical micro-systems"), but increasing attention is being paid to the way higher level systems influence the effective functioning of clinical micro-systems. This development is expanding the focus of CQI to include the way "meso-level" systems (those at organisational or community level) and "macro-level" systems (health and other large-scale systems) influence quality and value in health care. CQI can be used to strengthen policy, managerial and professional processes for delivering high-quality care: that is, the entire "production system".

Use of systems thinking

As highlighted in Chapter 1, health systems are complex, typically including many providers, organisations of varying size, and providing care for diverse health conditions, clients and communities. Systems thinking is a way of thinking about systems as holistic, dynamic and interconnected. The use of systems thinking in CQI helps in analysing and understanding the complex interactions that occur between different parts of the healthcare system and predicting the effects of system adjustments (for example, on integration of care, on client experiences and outcomes).

---

21   Rubenstein, Khodyakov et al. 2014.

CQI uses systems thinking: a way of thinking about systems as holistic, dynamic and interconnected.

Client or "customer" focus

CQI focuses on the evidence-based processes and outcomes that matter to users and potential users of the service (for example, people who are unable to access PHC), including clients and families or carers, organisations that refer clients or receive referrals from the PHC service, funders, and those who interact with the service in other ways.

Data is used for learning and decision-making, not blame

The primary purpose of data and measurement in CQI is learning. CQI data should not be used for performance monitoring, reward or punishment. Use of data for such purposes may detract from the quality of the data and its use and potential for driving improvement.

Decentralised and participative

CQI places ownership of improvement processes in the hands of the people who implement these processes. This does not absolve management of fundamental responsibility. Where there are weaknesses in the service system, management and policymakers should bear responsibility for system improvement. But CQI encourages those directly involved in care processes to be part of solutions for overcoming system weaknesses.

Values the contribution of everyone who is involved in care

CQI increases the dignity of the people involved because it recognises the important role of each member of the team and involves them as partners and leaders in the design and implementation of an improvement process. It respects the knowledge and experience that each person brings to the process and assumes that all are intrinsically motivated to do good work. Organisations involved in CQI often experience improvements in morale and higher levels of staff engagement. CQI provides evidence of the quality of work being done, and justification for staff to take pride in their work.

Leadership for improvement

There is substantial CQI experience in the manufacturing, business and health sectors to show that improvement in performance is strongly linked to leadership and people management. It is not a top-down approach, but it requires commitment and leadership for improvement at all levels of an organisation to create a culture that drives out fear and blame, seeks truth, respects and inspires people, and continually strives for improvement.

Responsive to context

CQI is sensitive to context. Locally relevant data are analysed, and changes planned and implemented using contextual knowledge – which is why participatory processes are important. Improvement initiatives that are not sufficiently sensitive and responsive to context are bound to fall short of goals.

CQI is sensitive and responsive to context.

A strategic approach

As described above, CQI needs to be part of a strategic approach to improvement, reflected in organisational goals, principles and strategic plans.

Origins and development

CQI has its origins in the total quality management (TQM) philosophy and techniques developed in the manufacturing industries in the early 20th century. Core concepts have been adapted for use in health care. Table 2.1 tracks major developments and pioneers in the shift from a total quality management approach to a CQI approach in health care.

Table 2.1 Key developments in CQI in health care.

1930s	• Walter Shewhart found that defects in product quality were built into industrial production processes and developed statistical methods to control product variation and assure product quality.
	• Shewhart originated the plan-do-study-act cycle, later made popular by W. Edwards Deming.
1950s	• Deming and Joseph Juran worked with Japanese industrial manufacturers after World War II to improve product quality and advance TQM concepts.
	• Other pioneers of the quality improvement movement included Armand Feigenbaum, Philip Crosby and Genichi Taguchi.
1960s	• Kaoru Ishikawa advanced quality management techniques.
	• Avedis Donabedian proposed a quality improvement framework for systematically examining healthcare quality with three domains: structure, process and outcomes.[22] Recognising interrelationships between the domains, he applied systems thinking concepts.
	• John Williamson advocated for linking measurement and feedback to learning processes. Kerr White linked study of quality to study of epidemiology. Health services research emerged as a defined area of research incorporating the study of quality improvement.
1970s	• Advances in quality improvement theory and practice continued, including Philip Crosby's work around improvement culture within organisations.

22   Information about the framework is expanded in Chapter 4.

1980s	• W. Edwards Deming published a 14-point program for leading quality improvement based on organisational processes, a continuous improvement cycle and statistical data analysis. The program promoted organisation-wide commitment and common improvement purpose, leadership, teamwork, learning and self-improvement, lack of fear and innovative thinking for improvement.
	• Deming developed a quality management philosophy called "system of profound knowledge" that combined systems thinking, knowledge about variation, the psychology of change and the theory of knowledge.
	• Management experts in health care and manufacturing quality came together to explore ways to assess the quality-of-care processes and outcomes.
	• The quality improvement movement entered health care widely.
1990s	• Don Berwick argued that care is improved by learning from mistakes, and continuously improving systems so mistakes are not repeated.
	• Berwick founded the Institute for Healthcare Improvement in the United States of America. The institute advocated for resources and restructuring, respect for the knowledge and motivation of providers, provider–client dialogue, use of theoretically grounded tools and techniques, and training for quality improvement.[23]
	• CQI was promoted as a way of improving health system performance.
2000s onwards	• Awareness that conformity to evidence-based best practices varied widely focused the quality agenda on client safety and reducing variation in care.[24]
	• More organisations were established to support quality improvement in health care.
	• Improvement science emerged as a field of study aiming to produce generalisable knowledge about quality improvement within a scientific framework.[25]
	• SQUIRE (Standards for Quality Improvement Reporting Excellence) publication guidelines were developed to strengthen evidence for quality improvement.[26]

Source: Sollecito and Johnson 2019.

The shift from TQM to CQI reflected a major change in approach to health services management. Many organisations continue to adapt CQI to their healthcare contexts, and CQI processes have been integrated into clinical governance in many settings. The scope for adapting CQI is part

23   Berwick 1996.
24   Sollecito and Johnson 2019.
25   Nilsen, Thor et al. 2022.
26   Ogrinc, Mooney et al. 2008.

of its intuitive appeal, but it does present challenges for cross-organisational comparisons and learning, especially in PHC. We discuss some of these challenges and solutions in the following chapters.

Advancements in health care have enabled CQI uptake and implementation. These include the availability of evidence-based practice guidelines against which to measure health service performance, and the development of information technology systems. Increased knowledge about the factors that affect health have helped to define care priorities and focus improvement efforts.

Advancements in CQI have seen the development of a range of tools and techniques. Examples are tools for collecting and analysing data, for assessing systems and teamwork, and for measuring client experiences. There are techniques for identifying causes of variation in quality, for setting goals, planning improvements, managing change and other processes. Throughout these developments, the relevance of foundational quality improvement work, such as the plan-do-study-act cycle, has endured.

Quality improvement cycles

Plan-do-study-act cycle – the scientific method

We have described data-driven ongoing cycles of improvement as a feature of CQI. The plan-do-study-act (PDSA)[27] cycle is a widely used framework for this approach. PDSA cycles use a small-scale iterative approach to test changes in real work or community settings. They enable teams to make rapid assessment and provide flexibility to adjust a change according to feedback to ensure that the solutions developed are fit for purpose.[28]

The broad use of the PDSA cycle in health care responds to Deming's premise that organisational management needed to undergo transformation through deliberative learning, the "system of profound knowledge". By applying this cycle, teams can develop insights into systems, variations in care and psychology to build theory about how to achieve improvement. This theory is tested by making changes and learning from data whether the changes are improvements, and what further improvements are needed.

The plan-do-study-act cycle is widely used in CQI.

The simplicity of the PDSA cycle also contributes to its wide use. The four steps of the cycle (plan, do, study, act) provide a structure, a common language and an orderly process whereby workers can be engaged in improving organisational systems and outcomes. At the same time, it offers scope to use a variety of other tools to collect data, measure quality and drive improvement strategies.

The PDSA cycle has been used in high- and low-resource settings, in public health and traditional medical care.[29] It has been used to improve the quality of comprehensive PHC, including various aspects of clinical care, health promotion and food security.[30]

---

27   Deming 2018.
28   Taylor, McNicholas et al. 2014.
29   Sollecito and Johnson 2019.
30   Bailie, Si et al. 2007; Brimblecombe, Bailie et al. 2017; Percival, O'Donoghue et al. 2016.

Taylor and colleagues describe five features of any PDSA process:

- iterative cycles – lessons learnt from one cycle link and inform cycles that follow
- prediction-based test of change – the expected change should be in line with the target for improvement, as identified in the plan stage
- small-scale testing – with the expectation that changes may be scaled out as confidence grows, and that interventions will be adapting according to feedback and learning
- data – used over time to understand variation in the system and the effect of change
- documentation – to support and share learning.[31]

We suggest a need to modify "small-scale testing" in many PHC contexts. In a single PHC centre, it may not make sense to make a change to a specific process on a scale smaller than the whole centre. A change made across the whole centre may need to be tested for a short period of time – but long enough for the change to have a measurable effect on the target for improvement. Where a PHC service covers multiple PHC centres, the initial testing can be done in one or two centres before extending the change to other centres, based on what is learnt from the initial testing.

There are many adaptations and representations of the PDSA cycle. Figure 2.1 captures the fundamental elements.[32] We expand on how to use PDSA cycles in Chapter 6.

Improvement scientists Langley and colleagues combined the PDSA cycle with three questions to develop a framework they called the "Model for Improvement". The questions can be asked in any order.

- "What are we trying to accomplish?" This question clarifies the improvement aim.
- "How will we know that a change is an improvement?" This question guides the feedback that will be gathered.
- "What changes can we make that will result in improvement?" This question focuses the actions to be taken.[33]

These questions reflect the importance of careful study and reflection, described by Don Berwick as "inductive learning – the growth of knowledge through making changes and then reflecting on the consequences of those changes".[34]

Summary

This chapter has defined quality and CQI in health care and considered related concepts such as "access" and "value". We have described the key features of CQI and how it evolved in health care, and summarised how CQI cycles are used to improve care. In the next chapter, we discuss how conventional approaches to CQI need to be adapted for practical application in PHC settings.

---

31   Taylor, McNicholas et al. 2014.
32   Deming 2018, 91.
33   Langley, Moen et al. 2009.
34   Berwick 1996, 620.

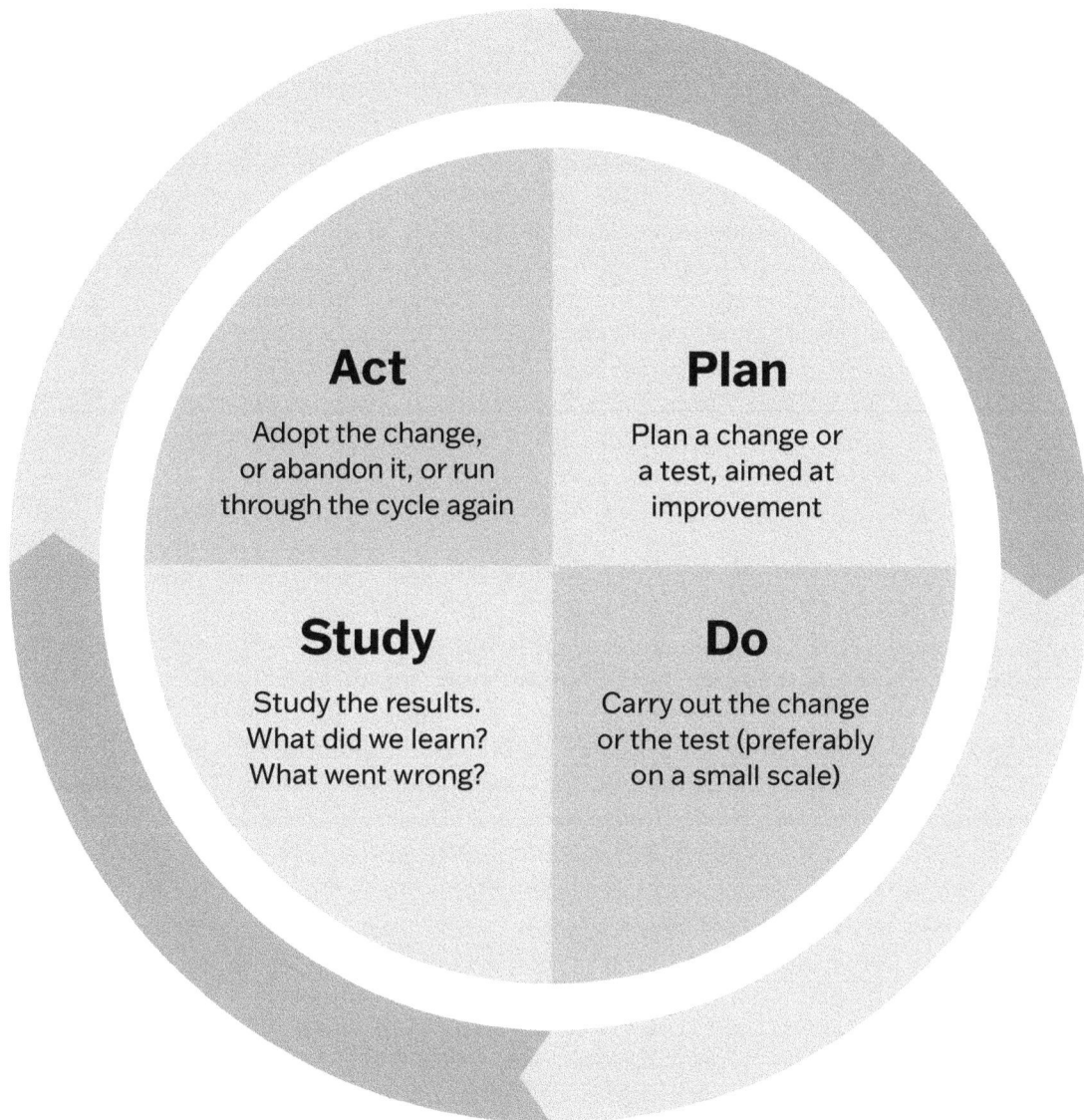

Act
Adopt the change, or abandon it, or run through the cycle again

Plan
Plan a change or a test, aimed at improvement

Study
Study the results. What did we learn? What went wrong?

Do
Carry out the change or the test (preferably on a small scale)

Figure 2.1 The PDSA Cycle. Adapted from: Deming, W. Edwards. foreword by Kevin Edwards Cahill, *The New Economics for Industry, Government, Education, third edition*, The PDSA Cycle, page 91 © 2018 Massachusetts Institute of Technology, by permission of The MIT Press.

References

Agency for Healthcare Research and Quality (2019). About learning health systems. https://www.ahrq.gov/learning-health-systems/about.html.

Al-Azri M. (2008). Continuity of care and quality of care – inseparable twin. *Oman Medical Journal* 23(3): 147–9 PMC3282321.

Bailie, J., G. Schierhout, A. Laycock, M. Kelaher, N. Percival, L. O'Donoghue et al. (2015). Determinants of access to chronic illness care: a mixed-methods evaluation of a national multifaceted chronic disease package for Indigenous Australians. *BMJ Open* 5(11): e008103. DOI: 10.1136/bmjopen-2015-008103.

Bailie, R., V. Matthews, J. Brands and G. Schierhout (2013). A systems-based partnership learning model for strengthening primary healthcare. *Implementation Science* 8: 143. DOI: 10.1186/1748-5908-8-143.

Bailie, R.S., D. Si, L. O'Donoghue and M. Dowden (2007). Indigenous health: effective and sustainable health services through continuous quality improvement. *Medical Journal of Australia* 186(10): 525–7.

Batalden, P.B. and F. Davidoff (2007). What is "quality improvement" and how can it transform healthcare? *Quality and Safety in Health Care* 16(1): 2–3. DOI: 10.1136/qshc.2006.022046.

Berwick, D.M. (1996). A primer on leading the improvement of systems. *BMJ* 312 (7031): 619–22. DOI: 10.1136/bmj.312.7031.619.

Brimblecombe, J., R. Bailie, C. van Den Boogaard, B. Wood, S. Liberato, M. Ferguson et al. (2017). Feasibility of a novel participatory multi-sector continuous improvement approach to enhance food security in remote Indigenous Australian communities. *SSM – Population Health* 3(C): 566–76. DOI: 10.1016/j.ssmph.2017.06.002.

Coulter, A. (2017). Measuring what matters to patients. *BMJ* 356: j816. DOI: 10.1136/bmj.j816.

Davies, A. and L. Wood (2018). Homeless health care: meeting the challenges of providing primary care. *Medical Journal of Australia* 209(5): 230–4. DOI: 10.5694/mja17.01264.

Davy, C., S. Harfield, A. McArthur, Z. Munn and A. Brown (2016). Access to primary health care services for Indigenous peoples: a framework synthesis. *International Journal for Equity in Health* 15(1): 163. DOI: 10.1186/s12939-016-0450-5.

Deming, W.E. (2018). *The new economics for industry, government, education, 3rd edn*. Cambridge, MA: MIT Press.

Cahill, K.E. (2018). Foreword. In W. Edwards Deming, *The New Economics for Industry, Government, Education, 3rd edition*: 19. Cambridge, MA: MIT Press.

European Commission (2019). Defining value in "value-based healthcare": report of the expert panel on effective ways of investing in health (EXPH). Luxembourg: European Union. DOI: 10.2875/872343.

Jackson, C. and L. Ball (2018). Continuity of care: vital, but how do we measure and promote it? *Australian Journal of General Practice* 47: 662–4. DOI: 10.31128/AJGP-05-18-4568.

Langley, G., R. Moen, K. Nolan, T. Nolan, C. Norman and L. Provost (2009). *The improvement guide: a practical approach to enhancing organisational performance*. San Franscisco, CA: Jossey-Bass.

Levesque, J.-F., M.F. Harris and G. Russell (2013). Patient-centred access to health care: conceptualising access at the interface of health systems and populations. *International Journal for Equity in Health* 12: 18. DOI: 10.1186/1475-9276-12-18.

Nilsen, P., J. Thor, M. Bender, J. Leeman, B. Andersson-Gäre and N. Sevdalis (2022). Bridging the silos: a comparative analysis of implementation science and improvement science. *Frontiers in Health Services* 1: 817750. DOI: 10.3389/frhs.2021.817750.

Ogrinc, G., S. Mooney, C. Estrada, T. Foster, D. Goldmann, L. Hall et al. (2008). The SQUIRE (Standards for QUality Improvement Reporting Excellence) guidelines for quality improvement reporting: explanation and elaboration. *Quality and Safety in Health Care* 17(Suppl 1): i13. DOI: 10.1136/qshc.2008.029058.

Percival, N., L. O'Donoghue, V. Lin, K. Tsey and R. Bailie (2016). Improving health promotion using quality improvement techniques in Australian Indigenous primary health care. *Frontiers in Public Health* 4: 53. DOI: 10.3389/fpubh.2016.00053.

Rakhmanova, N. and B. Bouchet (2017). *Quality improvement handbook: a guide for enhancing the performance of health care systems*. Durham, NC: FHI 360.

Rubenstein, L., D. Khodyakov, S. Hempel, M. Danz, S. Salem-Schatz, R. Foy et al. (2014). How can we recognize continuous quality improvement? *International Journal for Quality in Health Care* 26(1): 6–15. DOI: 10.1093/intqhc/mzt085.

Russell G., M. Harris, I.-H. Cheng, M. Kay, S. Vasi, C. Joshi et al. (2013). *Coordinated primary health care for refugees: a best practice framework for Australia*. Report to the Australian Primary Health Care Research Institute. Melbourne: Southern Academic Primary Care Research Unit.

Sollecito, W. and J. Johnson (2019). *McLaughlin and Kaluzny's continuous quality improvement in health care*. Burlington, MA: Jones & Bartlett Learning.

Taylor, M., C. McNicholas, C. Nicolay, A. Darzi, D. Bell and J. Reed (2014). Systematic review of the application of the plan–do–study–act method to improve quality in healthcare. *BMJ Quality & Safety* 23: 290–8. DOI: 10.1136/bmjqs-2013-001862.

Woolcock, K. (2019). *Value based health care: setting the scene for Australia*. Deeble Institute for Health Policy Research. Canberra: Australian Healthcare and Hospital Association.

World Economic Forum (2017). *Value in healthcare: laying the foundation for health system transformation*. Geneva, Switzerland: World Economic Forum.

World Health Organization (2023). Quality of care. https://www.who.int/health-topics/quality-of-care#tab=tab_1.

Adapting continuous quality improvement for primary health care

Why is adaption needed?

The CQI approach to health care has been dominated by the hospital sector, where a relatively controlled environment and relatively routine models of care have some similarities with the industrial sector from which CQI evolved. The standard characteristics of CQI, as described in McLaughlin and Kaluzny's seminal text[1] and cited by Sollecito,[2] reflect these features: links to the organisation's strategic plan; a quality council made up of the organisation's top leadership; staff training; mechanisms for selecting improvement opportunities; and the formation of process improvement teams. Staff support for process analysis and redesign, policies that motivate and support staff participation in process improvement, and application of the most rigorous techniques of the scientific method and statistical process control are also specified. Lacking in the list of features is client or consumer involvement in CQI, an aspect of quality receiving increased attention. While the CQI structures and processes identified are feasible in medium-size or large hospitals, or for managing networks of community-based health services through centralised organisational structures, they do not reflect the way most PHC is delivered. CQI needs to be modified for application in PHC.

PHC delivery models

As highlighted earlier, PHC services tend to have these characteristics:

- are widely dispersed across diverse contexts
- are of varied size – some delivery models include multiple sites and clinicians (for example, nurses, doctors, health workers), some have only a few clinicians (in some cases one) and administration staff
- are of varied composition (for example, a medical practice, a group of medical and allied professionals or a community-based organisation)
- are governed through a variety of small business, corporate or government structures
- are relatively independent or autonomous, and reliant on professionalism for ensuring quality.

---

1   McLaughlin and Kaluzny 1994.
2   Sollecito and Johnson 2019.

Compared with hospitals and corporate networks, individual PHC services and practices are less likely to have a shared (or any) strategic plan that local staff can identify with, or a quality council to which most staff feel accountable. Where efforts to establish the types of structures and processes described by McLaughlin and Kaluzny have been made in PHC, the participation or engagement by individual PHC services and practices has varied greatly, with limited effect across the PHC service system or at a population level. Despite these challenges, strategic and systemic approaches to improvement are necessary for dealing with the complexity of PHC delivery and for improving care quality.

> Strategic and systemic approaches to improvement are necessary for dealing with the complexity of PHC.

Traditions in healthcare delivery also challenge systemic approaches to PHC and CQI. Up to the 1970s, PHC was largely perceived as a cottage industry, in which "healthcare was seen as a craft or art delivered by individual professionals who had learned by apprenticeship and who worked independently in a decentralised system".[3] Practitioners generally developed their own systems for recording the care they provided and were individually accountable, with no mechanisms for linking records with other providers and limited opportunities to share learning. While some policy debate continues to focus on the weaknesses of the professional system for improving quality (due to excessive professional autonomy and protectionist practices by "guilds" of practitioners), this historical reliance on the professionalism of health practitioners for self-regulation and quality of care is changing. The development of clinical guidelines and of more standardised clinical information systems are examples. A systems approach to CQI is one way of sharing ownership for quality improvement and mobilising change.

Timing and scope of care

In PHC, items of service need to be delivered to members of the service population at relatively infrequent intervals, when people present for care. For example, blood pressure checks for generally healthy adults may be recommended once a year, or once every two years, as a preventive health strategy. Glycated haemoglobin (HbA1c) tests are recommended once every three or six months for people with diabetes. Care delivery for these service items relies on people accessing care for checks (or for acute care that may or may not be related) or being accessible through outreach services. The measurements need to be taken over a sufficiently long period (sometimes years) for changes in the level of care delivery to be observed.

> Measurements need to be taken over a sufficiently long period for changes in the level of care delivery to be observed.

In addition, a very broad scope of care is delivered through PHC maternal, child and preventive health care, care and management of chronic conditions, mental health, sexual health and

---

3   Sollecito and Johnson 2019, 18.

so on. Within each of these areas of PHC, there are essential items of care to be delivered in order to meet expected standards of care.

Quality improvement challenges and responses

For the reasons we have identified, the gains made in the hospital sector during the 1980s and 1990s (re-engineering care delivery, improving care processes and adopting CQI techniques) have been slower and more challenging to implement in the PHC sector. The effects of poor-quality PHC may not be as immediate and dramatic as safety incidents in hospital care, where patients are generally sicker and treatments more intensive. But poor access to care, unacceptable (for example, disrespectful) care, missed opportunities, missed diagnoses, inappropriate investigations or treatment, and adverse events related to poor quality of PHC can all contribute to unnecessary human suffering and waste on a massive scale at the population level.

PHC teams and practices have the challenge of identifying which areas and which items of care should be the focus of their improvement efforts. This requires knowledge of what is being done relatively well and not so well by the service or practice, which in turn requires complete client records that accurately reflect the care delivered. Individual practitioners and teams also require knowledge about what is a reasonable level of care delivery in a population group: clear standards and measures of care quality established through quality assurance processes. While striving for 100 per cent delivery of "essential" care items is the ideal, it is rarely achievable, and is often much less than 100 per cent for a range of reasons. Teams need to prioritise improvements that are achievable and that offer the most benefit to clients.

> PHC teams need to prioritise improvements that are achievable and that offer the most benefit to clients.

In addition, CQI requires comparable data from other PHC services and practices, to help benchmark quality of care. Local and regional variability in health care has long been known to exist, but there is a lack of evidence of this variability across PHC services on a wide scale and across the broad scope of clinical PHC. This is largely for reasons related to the diverse and dispersed nature of PHC services, and associated challenges in coordination, planning, delivery, monitoring and evaluation of PHC systems.

Substantial progress has been made in important areas, including the development, implementation and increased acceptability of clinical best-practice guidelines,[4] the development of data systems that can support CQI and the use of "collaboratives" as a means of improving quality[5] (see Chapter 7). Health practitioners and services have also embraced the concept of "client-centredness" to address the care needs and values of individual clients. Designing services that are appropriate and responsive to clients' needs and the local context is especially important in PHC, to ensure easy and timely access to preventive care and treatment of health conditions throughout the life course. These PHC principles are strong motivators for staff to engage in CQI. PHC and CQI also have core concepts in common: both emphasise the

---

4   National Health and Medical Research Council 2018; World Health Organization 2023.
5   de Silva 2014; Lindenauer 2008; Schouten, Hulscher et al. 2008; Wells, Tamir et al. 2018.

importance of teamwork, and both PHC and CQI advocate systems approaches and systems thinking as a way of achieving better client outcomes.

> PHC and CQI have core concepts in common.

The integrated nature of PHC can extend the benefits of improvement interventions, because system changes targeting one group of clients frequently flow on to benefit other groups. For example, changes made to a clinical information system to generate automated reminders when child health checks are due can be used to schedule other items of care for other groups; skills developed to provide brief interventions for smoking have application for other behavioural health risk factors.

Applying CQI

Consistent with the features of PHC delivery, CQI approaches need to allow practitioners and managers a high degree of autonomy to respond to local circumstances and population needs, and time to observe improvement.

Effective CQI in PHC has these characteristics:

- use of adaptable tools and processes
- use of clinical practice guidelines
- preparedness to begin in at least some areas
- use of local data and benchmarking
- active management
- "no blame" culture
- leadership by primary healthcare teams and communities
- participatory interpretation of data
- design of interventions to suit local conditions
- sharing of learning across teams
- investment by the health service and region
- improvement initiatives in four categories.

We will look at each of these in more detail.

Use of adaptable tools and processes

One size does not fit all: CQI tools and processes need to be readily adaptable to suit the context and capacity of each local PHC team or practice.

Use of clinical practice guidelines

Regardless of the tools used, CQI in a clinical context is guided by locally relevant clinical practice guidelines.

Preparedness to begin in at least some areas

It is important to start CQI from where the service is at. PHC services and practices have different levels of readiness for CQI. Where accurate data on care processes are not consistently available, this is often due to poor or fragmented clinical information systems. It is important not to wait for perfect data, but to focus efforts on where the biggest gains can be made – such as improving systems for accessible and reliable clinical records. Staff use of data in CQI cycles can act as a catalyst for improving data quality.[6]

Use of local data and benchmarking

Access to local data enables PHC teams to target improvement efforts where they will most benefit their service population. It is useful and important to have data from other PHC services for comparison, with the greatest value of benchmarking being in how data are used to gain deeper understanding of the influence of local contexts and service systems.

Active management

CQI needs to be actively managed and facilitated as part of core business. Active management can take various forms, and may involve dedicated CQI facilitators or coaches, regular progress reviews, the identification of CQI leaders who are not necessarily in management roles, and regional support structures.[7]

"No blame" culture

As in other healthcare settings, a "no blame" culture is essential for PHC staff to embrace CQI. To establish and sustain this culture within an organisation, managers at all levels need to understand and be committed to CQI, and have a relationship of trust with practitioners.[8] Clear distinction needs to be made between collecting data for reporting purposes and using data to drive improvement.[9]

Leadership by PHC teams and communities

PHC teams need to be able to selectively monitor items of care (or indicators) in locally identified priority areas for improvement (for example, diabetes management, childhood anaemia). Priorities are typically selected based on comparing performance between areas of care within the local health service or practice, as well as comparing performance with other services (for benchmarking). Priorities may also be informed by client groups. Local ownership of CQI contrasts with top-down quality improvement programs that focus on a small number of indicators that are prescribed by senior policymakers. Such top-down approaches tend to rely on data systems of questionable quality and insufficient detail, and the top-down approach creates perverse incentives for accuracy in reporting of data.

---

6   Gardner, Dowden et al. 2010; Wise, Angus et al. 2013.
7   Best, Greenhalgh et al. 2012; Powell, Rushmer and Davies 2009; Wise, Angus et al. 2013.
8   Shojania and Grimshaw 2005; Wensing, Wollersheim and Grol 2006.
9   Allen and Clarke Consulting 2013; Wise, Angus et al. 2013.

> Local ownership of CQI contrasts with top-down quality improvement programs.

Related to ownership, staff members need to value the use of data for improvement purposes and believe they can influence change.[10] This comes from demonstrated improvements in care and clinical outcomes for clients, and increased confidence and skills as teams implement CQI.

Participatory interpretation of data

The meaningful interpretation of CQI data and the development of improvement strategies requires insight into the complex interactions between practitioners and clients, cultural and contextual factors, the nuanced decision-making that occurs, clinical system design and how all of these factors interact.[11] Depending on the service context and structure, CQI may involve input from people in a range of PHC delivery roles: for example, clinicians, administration staff, cleaners, drivers, managers, visiting staff who provide specialised services, clients, families or carers and communities.[12]

Design of improvement interventions to suit local conditions

There is strong evidence that improving the quality of care requires a good match between the conditions or context for care delivery, and the strategies used to achieve improvement.[13] Often, cultural and social influences need to be considered, emphasising the importance of local knowledge for ensuring that improvement strategies have practical relevance and address systemic problems.[14]

> Improvement interventions should be designed or adapted to suit local conditions.

Sharing of learning across teams

Sharing knowledge about CQI and learning practical information from others about what works is particularly valuable for PHC teams, because of the dispersed location and relatively small scale of many PHC services.[15]

---

10   Schierhout, Hains et al. 2013.
11   MacIsaac, Tam et al. 2019.
12   Bailie, Si et al. 2007.
13   Greenhalgh, Robert et al. 2004; Kaplan, Provost et al. 2012.
14   Gardner, Dowden et al. 2010; Larkins, Carlisle et al. 2019; Turner, Taylor et al. 2019; Wise, Angus et al. 2013.
15   Riley, Parsons et al. 2010; Schierhout, Hains et al. 2013.

Investment by the health service and region

CQI requires clinical leadership and administrative support. It also requires specific investment to support the development of staff capability and systems, and the ongoing use of quality improvement tools and techniques to enhance health services for communities and individual clients. Regional CQI support systems can be important for supporting and coordinating these functions, due to the limited resources of PHC practices and smaller services. Such systems reflect supportive CQI policies at regional or national levels of the healthcare system.[16] CQI approaches are most effective when the external environment is supportive.[17]

Improvement initiatives in four categories

Most CQI initiatives in PHC aim to improve the delivery of recommended care processes, as specified in practice guidelines. CQI approaches and activities are likely to involve localised improvement efforts; organisational learning; process re-engineering; or evidence-based practice and management.[18]

- Localised improvement efforts: CQI processes are used by PHC teams to identify and address improvement needs or opportunities (for example, the use of audit and feedback processes as a basis for planning improvement interventions).
- Organisational learning: this occurs when improvement processes result in changes to policies and procedures, such as changes to clinical protocols, client follow-up and recall procedures, adjustment in staff roles or community engagement strategies.
- Process re-engineering: this category covers changes or investments that affect organisational processes. These may be initiated within a PHC practice or service, or result from external or partnered investment (for example, the upgrade of a client information system or the introduction of a system-wide electronic health record).
- Evidence-based practice and management: improvements are classified in this category when approaches and practices are adjusted to reflect up-to-date health, management and systems research, clinical guidelines and the real-world knowledge and experience of staff, clients and communities.

An Indigenous context

Key features of CQI approaches make them well suited to Indigenous healthcare settings. The participatory approach and client focus of CQI, and the combination of scientific and humanistic professional values,[19] align with the principles and values expressed in ethics guidelines for Aboriginal and Torres Strait Islander and other health research with First Nations peoples.[20] Ethics guidelines emphasise the need for Indigenous health research to tackle underlying causes of poor health (for example, social and economic conditions), to

---

16   Bailie, Matthews et al. 2017.

17   Shojania and Grimshaw 2005; Wensing, Wollersheim and Grol 2006.

18   Sollecito and Johnson 2019.

19   Wensing, Wollersheim and Grol 2006.

20   For example, Gachupin, Lameman and Molina 2019; National Health and Medical Research Council 2018; Ryerson University Research Ethics Board 2017; The Pūtaiora Writing Group 2010.

build capacity (including community capacity to use data), and to improve outcomes. These concepts are central to CQI. Strengths-based approaches and a culture of self-evaluation that affirm the capabilities within Indigenous communities are also central. In addition, CQI provides a structure to refine and reinvigorate programs to promote sustainability.[21]

> Strengths-based approaches that affirm the capabilities within Indigenous communities are central.

Factors that lead to the successful use of CQI in Aboriginal and Torres Strait Islander settings reflect those in other settings, but high-improving Aboriginal and Torres Strait Islander health services also have unique features. A multi-site study found services that showed a high level of improvement were embedded in the cultural and historical context of their communities. Staff in these health services understood how history (for example, cultural knowledge, colonisation) had shaped ways of seeing, being and doing, and how to act and communicate in culturally appropriate and respectful ways. Trusting, respectful and caring relationships were established between the clients and health service staff, who had a deep knowledge of their communities and PHC. There was cross-cultural learning for CQI, and improvement strategies tended to be driven by the community.[22] Our CQI research in Aboriginal and Torres Strait Islander PHC has also shown that Indigenous staff in these contexts are crucial to improving the delivery of evidence-based care,[23] including access to culturally safe and continuous care and informing and implementing CQI initiatives.[24]

Health equity

Health equity is a key principle of PHC. Inequalities in health and life expectancy between countries, and between population groups within countries and communities (for example, ethnic groups, socio-economic groups), draw attention to the need to improve PHC for groups with poorer health outcomes. Recent health frameworks targeting low- and middle-income countries have focused on improving processes of PHC delivery and strengthening the systems that provide client- and community-centred care.[25] This is the core business of CQI.

> The links between CQI and equitable health care are indisputable.

Quality improvement leaders have claimed that for care to be considered high quality, it must be equitable, and conversely, there cannot be health equity without high-quality care.[26] The links between CQI and equitable health care are indisputable. The natural fit between CQI and efforts to improve health equity is evident in several ways:

---

21   Bailie, Si et al. 2007.
22   Larkins, Carlisle et al. 2019; Redman-MacLaren, Turner et al. 2021; Turner, Taylor et al. 2019.
23   Bailie, Laycock et al. 2019; de Witt, Cunningham et al. 2018.
24   Larkins, Carlisle et al. 2019; Smith, Kirkham et al. 2018; Turner, Taylor et al. 2019.
25   World Health Organization 2015.
26   Dzau, Mate and O'Kane 2022.

- Equity is one of the seven domains of quality in health care (effective, safe, people-centred, timely, equitable, integrated and efficient).
- Health disparities are a marker of poor health system performance – CQI aims to strengthen care systems and processes to reduce variation in care delivery and improve the overall quality of care.
- The type of data collected for CQI (for example, demographic, service delivery and clinical indicators) is suitable for measuring health disparities. Data can show which groups are missing out on services or experiencing poorer health outcomes within a service population.
- CQI processes enable PHC services and teams to identify evidence-based priorities for improvement, and to design strategies targeting groups with greater needs.
- Use of CQI tools over consecutive CQI cycles can show progress in achieving equitable service delivery or health outcomes over time.

A system-wide approach to CQI enables system improvements to target issues associated with inequity, such as access to services by under-served populations (for example, people living in rural and remote areas), diseases of poverty (for example, tuberculosis and rheumatic heart disease) and improving the health of particular groups within populations (for example, refugees, Indigenous peoples, people living with disabilities). There is evidence that a system-wide approach to CQI can lead to large-scale improvements in care.[27] In Australia, sustained use of CQI in Indigenous community settings has improved the delivery of PHC in many Aboriginal and Torres Strait Islander communities, as later chapters detail. There is a long way to go to close the gap in health equity for Aboriginal and Torres Strait Islander Australians, but CQI is an important part of the process.

> CQI data can show variation in standards of care.

CQI data can show variation in standards of care. Variation is a measure of equity in care delivery: it shows the range in the quality of care delivered to clients. When CQI data from more than 270 PHC centres serving Aboriginal and Torres Strait Islander Australians were aggregated at a national level, it was evident that delivery of important items of care (for example, follow-up of clients with abnormal pathology results) varied widely between health centres. Trend data showed that the variation between health centre performance persisted over several audit cycles, and also that repeated CQI cycles decreased variation over time. Such evidence can help policymakers and managers to improve systems and allocate resources for more equitable service delivery.

---

27   Bailie, Matthews et al. 2017; Tricco, Ivers et al. 2012.

Comprehensive PHC

As highlighted earlier, adapting conventional CQI approaches to PHC can be challenging. The comprehensive nature of high-quality PHC is a significant part of the challenge: the broad scope and complexity of care, the need to take account of the many influences on people's health across the life course and to respond to individual, family and community health needs. Comprehensive care needs a comprehensive approach to identify and solve problems of quality across the scope of best practice.

> Comprehensive care needs a comprehensive approach to identify and solve problems of quality across the scope of best practice.

Despite the use of systems thinking in quality improvement, CQI processes used do not intrinsically take a big-picture approach. CQI processes generally aim to improve performance in specific areas of clinical care (for example, cardiovascular health) and may focus on improving specific indicators for a client cohort (for example, blood pressure control). These areas of focus are likely to be defined by data reporting requirements, such as clinical and service delivery data collected for reporting against key performance indicators. There is a risk that implementing CQI processes in this way can reinforce "siloed" care, missing opportunities for synergy when making changes to care systems or missing opportunities to develop new indicators that are important to clients.

Evidence also shows that improvement of healthcare performance alone is not enough to improve health outcomes. The relative contribution of health care to health outcomes is estimated to account for only between 10 and 20 per cent of gain,[28] which illustrates the importance of considering social, cultural and environmental circumstances when planning improvement interventions.

A comprehensive systems approach to CQI can enable PHC services to make evidence-based, locally responsive improvement decisions. To work in this way, CQI processes need to link with, and integrate, various stakeholders, influences and processes. McCalman, Bailie and colleagues have developed a framework to guide this approach.[29] The framework depicts the integration of CQI efforts in two dimensions: vertically across the health system and horizontally across sectors (Figure 3.1). Vertical integration applies CQI processes across all levels of health systems, from community engagement and client care through to various levels of policy. Horizontal integration extends CQI from clinical guideline adherence at PHC service sites through to linkages and advocacy for the social and cultural determinants of health. In the context of Aboriginal and Torres Strait islander PHC, these determinants might include connections to land and spirituality, family and culture, housing, education, employment, criminal justice, and other sectors that affect health. Equally central to a service's CQI approach are engaged service users, trained and supportive staff, strong management structures, systems and a culture of CQI, and resourcing and cost-effectiveness. Examples of the framework in action are provided in Chapter 20.

---

28   Booske, Athens et al. 2010; McGinnis, Williams-Russo and Knickman 2002.
29   McCalman, Bailie et al. 2018.

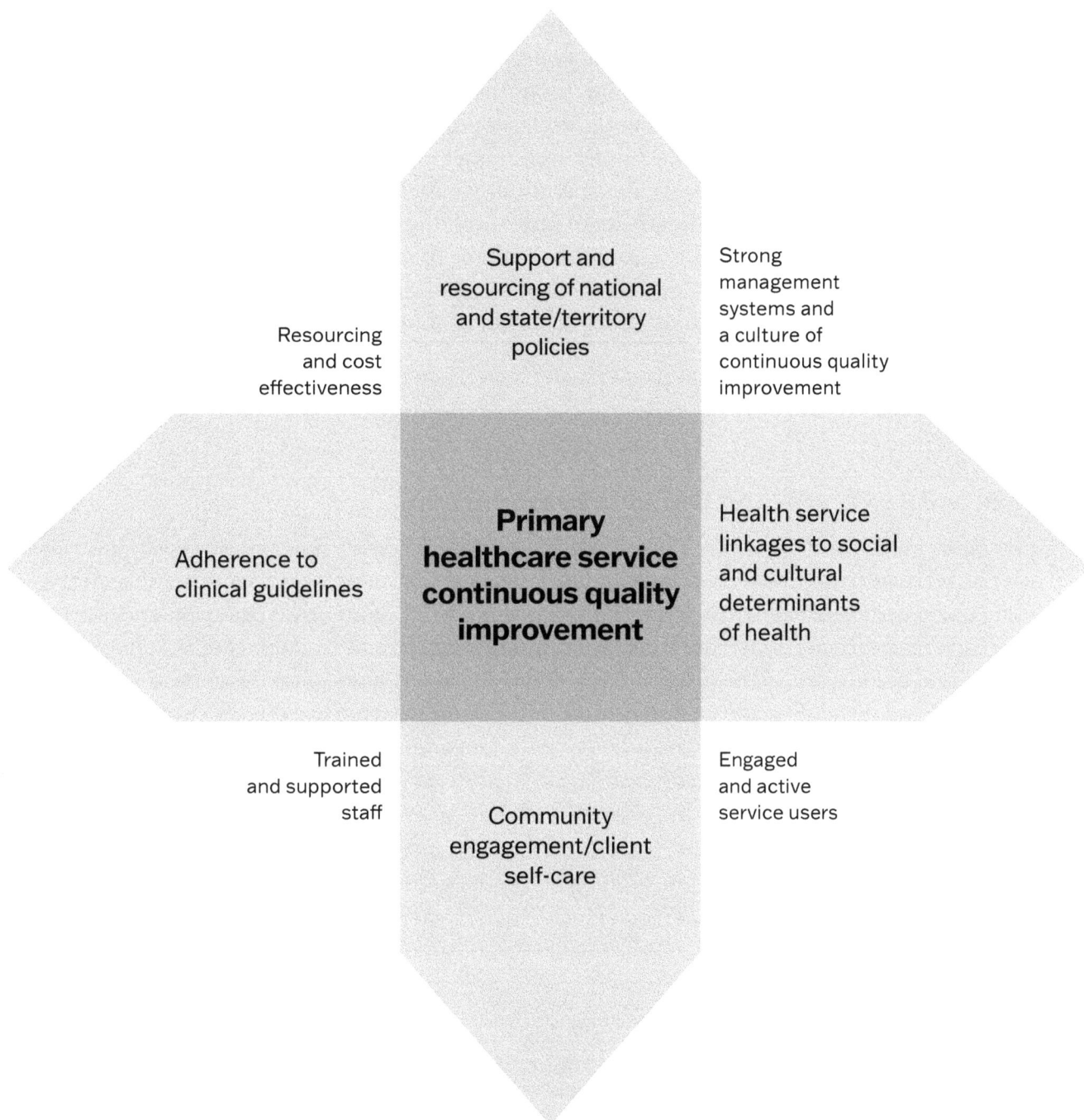

Figure 3.1 The vertical and horizontal enhancement of continuous quality improvement. Source: McCalman, Bailie et al. 2018.

Evidence of impact of CQI in comprehensive PHC

There is evidence that CQI works to improve the quality of PHC. Our research network has completed many studies investigating the effect of CQI and found that sustained use of CQI has improved the delivery of recommended care across complex and diverse PHC settings. Improvements in clinical care have resulted in improvements in maternal and women's health,[30] children's health,[31] preventive health,[32] social and emotional wellbeing,[33] diabetes,[34] sexual health[35] and rheumatic heart disease care.[36] CQI interventions have also had positive effects on the delivery of health promotion programs.[37] Research shows that a CQI approach is feasible and promising for improving programs that focus on the social determinants of health, including food security,[38] family wellbeing empowerment programs,[39] manager development programs in PHC services,[40] student wellbeing in school settings[41] and child protection processes.[42] While the effects of implementing CQI in clinical PHC appear to be relatively under-researched internationally, examples of research in other settings include improvement in diabetes care,[43] reduced hospital admissions among people with chronic conditions and among older clients[44] and improved PHC team functioning.[45]

> There is evidence that CQI works to improve the quality of PHC.

Audit and Best Practice for Chronic Disease program

The Audit and Best Practice for Chronic Disease (ABCD) research program developed and supported quality improvement tools and processes in PHC centres across Australia, with a focus on comprehensive PHC and services that serve predominantly Aboriginal and Torres Strait Islander populations. The tools are described in Part II. In Part III of this book, we summarise the history of the program and how PHC teams have used the clinical CQI tools and processes developed through this research. The approach described is supported by a strong evidence base of over 180 studies to date (several are cited above). The evidence is stronger than for any other approach to CQI in PHC as far as we are aware.

The knowledge gained from this work in Australia has wider relevance for implementing CQI in PHC. Internationally accepted principles for the effective implementation of CQI underpin the ABCD approach and, while PHC settings, characteristics and resources differ, similar improvement challenges prevail across countries. Part IV describes the ongoing system strengthening work of the quality improvement research network to help meet these challenges.

---

30   Diaz, Vo et al. 2019; Gibson-Helm, Rumbold et al. 2016; Gibson-Helm, Teede et al. 2015.
31   Edmond, Tung et al. 2018; McAullay, McAuley et al. 2018.
32   Bailie, Laycock et al. 2019.
33   Langham, McCalman et al. 2017.
34   Matthews, Schierhout et al. 2014; Schierhout, Matthews et al. 2016.
35   Gunaratnam, Schierhout et al. 2019; Nattabi, Matthews et al. 2017.
36   Read, Mitchell et al. 2018.
37   Percival, O'Donoghue et al. 2016.
38   Brimblecombe, Bailie et al. 2017.
39   McCalman, Bainbridge et al. 2018.
40   Onnis, Hakendorf et al. 2019.
41   McCalman, Bainbridge et al. 2016.
42   Zuchowski, Miles et al. 2017.
43   Tricco, Ivers et al. 2012.
44   Tricco, Antony et al. 2014.
45   Harris, Green et al. 2015.

Summary

This chapter has identified characteristics of PHC that influence the implementation of CQI and discussed how conventional approaches to CQI can be adapted for practical application in PHC. We referred to CQI research in Australian Indigenous PHC settings to argue that a comprehensive systems approach to CQI can have a positive impact on health care and health equity.

References

Allen and Clarke Consulting (2013). *Evaluation of the Northern Territory Continuous Quality Improvement Investment Strategy: Final report*. Canberra: Department of Health.

Bailie, J., A. Laycock, V. Matthews, D. Peiris and R. Bailie (2019). Emerging evidence of the value of health assessments for Aboriginal and Torres Strait Islander people in the primary healthcare setting. *Australian Journal of Primary Health* 25(1): 1–5. DOI: 10.1071/PY18088.

Bailie, R., V. Matthews, S. Larkins, S. Thompson, P. Burgess, T. Weeramanthri et al. (2017). Impact of policy support on uptake of evidence-based continuous quality improvement activities and the quality of care for Indigenous Australians: a comparative case study. *BMJ Open* 7. DOI: 10.1136/bmjopen-2017-016626.

Bailie, R.S., D. Si, L. O'Donoghue and M. Dowden (2007). Indigenous health: effective and sustainable health services through continuous quality improvement. *Medical Journal of Australia* 186(10): 525–7.

Best, A., T. Greenhalgh, S. Lewis, J. Saul, S. Carroll and J. Bitz (2012). Large-system transformation in health care: a realist review. *Milbank Quarterly* 90(3): 421–56. DOI: 10.1111/j.1468-0009.2012.00670.x.

Booske, B., J. Athens, D. Kindig, H. Park and P. Remington (2010). *Different perspectives for assigning weights to determinants of health*. County Health Rankings Working Paper. Madison, WI: University of Wisconsin, Population Health Institute.

Brimblecombe, J., R. Bailie, C. van Den Boogaard, B. Wood, S. Liberato, M. Ferguson et al. (2017). Feasibility of a novel participatory multi-sector continuous improvement approach to enhance food security in remote Indigenous Australian communities. *SSM – Population Health* 3(C): 566–76. DOI: 10.1016/j.ssmph.2017.06.002.

de Silva, D. (2014). *Improvement collaboratives in health care. Evidence scan No. 21*. London: Health Foundation.

de Witt, A., F. Cunningham, R. Bailie, N. Percival, J. Adams and P. Valery (2018). "It's just presence", the contributions of Aboriginal and Torres Strait Islander health professionals in cancer care in Queensland. *Frontiers in Public Health* 6: 344. DOI: 10.3389/fpubh.2018.00344.

Diaz, A., B. Vo, P.D. Baade, V. Matthews, B. Nattabi, J. Bailie et al. (2019). Service level factors associated with cervical screening in Aboriginal and Torres Strait Islander primary health care centres in Australia. *International Journal of Environmental Research and Public Health* 16(19): 3630. DOI: 10.3390/ijerph16193630.

Dzau, V.J., K. Mate and M. O'Kane (2022). Equity and quality—improving health care delivery requires both. *JAMA* 327(6): 519–20. DOI: 10.1001/jama.2022.0283. DOI: 10.1001/jama.2022.0283

Edmond, K., S. Tung, K. McAuley, N. Strobel and D. McAullay (2018). Improving developmental care in primary practice for disadvantaged children. *Archives of Disease in Childhood* 104: 372–80. DOI: 10.1136/archdischild-2018-315164.

Gachupin, F.C., B. Lameman and F. Molina (2019). *Guideline for researchers: a guide to establishing effective mutually-beneficial research partnerships with American Indian tribes, families and individuals*. Tucson, AZ: University of Arizona, Department of Family and Community Medicine, College of Medicine.

Gardner, K.L., M. Dowden, S. Togni and R. Bailie (2010). Understanding uptake of continuous quality improvement in Indigenous primary health care: lessons from a multi-site case study of the Audit and Best Practice for Chronic Disease project. *Implementation Science* 5: 21. DOI: 10.1186/1748-5908-5-21.

Gibson-Helm, M., A. Rumbold, H. Teede, S. Ranasinha, R. Bailie and J. Boyle (2016). Improving the provision of pregnancy care for Aboriginal and Torres Strait Islander women: a continuous quality improvement initiative. *BMC Pregnancy and Childbirth* 16: 118. DOI: 10.1186/s12884-016-0892-1.

Gibson-Helm, M., H. Teede, A. Rumbold, S. Ranasinha, R. Bailie and J. Boyle (2015). Continuous quality improvement and metabolic screening during pregnancy at primary health centres attended by Aboriginal and Torres Strait Islander women. *Medical Journal of Australia* 203(9): e1–7. DOI: 10.5694/mja14.01660.

Greenhalgh, T., G. Robert, F. Macfarlane, P. Bate and O. Kyriakidou (2004). Diffusion of innovations in service organizations: systematic review and recommendations. *Milbank Quarterly* 82(4): 581–629. DOI: 10.1111/j.0887-378X.2004.00325.x.

Guidelines International Network (2024). GIN international guideline library. https://g-i-n.net/international-guidelines-library.

Gunaratnam, P., G. Schierhout, J. Brands, L. Maher, R. Bailie, J. Ward et al. (2019). Qualitative perspectives on the sustainability of sexual health continuous quality improvement in clinics serving remote Aboriginal communities in Australia. *BMJ Open* 9(5): e026679. DOI: 10.1136/bmjopen-2018-026679.

Harris, S., M. Green, J. Brown, S. Roberts, G. Russell, M. Fournie et al. (2015). Impact of a quality improvement program on primary healthcare in Canada: a mixed-method evaluation. *Health Policy* 119(4): 405–16. DOI: 10.1016/j.healthpol.2014.10.019.

Kaplan, H., L. Provost, C. Froehle and P. Margolis (2012). The model for understanding success in quality (MUSIQ): building a theory of context in healthcare quality improvement. *BMJ Quality and Safety* 21: 13–20. DOI: 10.1136/bmjqs-2011-000010.

Langham, E., J. McCalman, V. Matthews, R.G. Bainbridge, B. Nattabi, I. Kinchin et al. (2017). Social and emotional wellbeing screening for Aboriginal and Torres Strait Islanders within primary health care: a series of missed opportunities? *Frontiers in Public Health* 5: 159. DOI: 10.3389/fpubh.2017.00159.

Larkins, S., K. Carlisle, N. Turner, J. Taylor, K. Copley, S. Cooney et al. (2019). "At the grass roots level it's about sitting down and talking": exploring quality improvement through case studies with high-improving Aboriginal and Torres Strait Islander primary healthcare services. *BMJ Open* 9(5): e027568DOI: 10.1136/bmjopen-2018-027568.

Lindenauer, P.K. (2008). Effects of quality improvement collaboratives. *BMJ* 336(7659): 1448–9. DOI: 10.1136/bmj.a216.

MacIsaac, M.B., M. Tam, K. McLean, M. Morgan, F. Jones and M. Saito (2019). We need to talk about quality in general practice. *Medical Journal of Australia*(28), *Insight+* 28, 22 July 2019. https://insightplus.mja.com.au/2019/28/.

Matthews, V., G. Schierhout, J. McBroom, C. Connors, C. Kennedy, R. Kwedza et al. (2014). Duration of participation in continuous quality improvement: a key factor explaining improved delivery of type 2 diabetes services. *BMC Health Services Research* 14(1): 578. DOI: 10.1186/s12913-014-0578-1.

McAullay, D., K. McAuley, R. Bailie, V. Mathews, P. Jacoby, K. Gardner et al. (2018). Sustained participation in annual continuous quality improvement activities improves quality of care for Aboriginal and Torres Strait Islander children. *Journal of Paediatrics and Child Health* 54(2): 132–40. DOI: 10.1111/jpc.13673.

McCalman, J., R. Bailie, R. Bainbridge, K. McPhail-Bell, N. Percival, D. Askew et al. (2018). Continuous quality improvement and comprehensive primary health care: a systems framework to improve service quality and health outcomes. *Frontiers in Public Health* 6: 76. DOI: 10.3389/fpubh.2018.00076.

McCalman, J., R. Bainbridge, C. Brown, K. Tsey and A. Clarke (2018). The Aboriginal Australian Family Wellbeing Program: a historical analysis of the conditions that enabled its spread. *Frontiers in Public Health* 6. DOI: 10.3389/fpubh.2018.00026.

McCalman, J., R. Bainbridge, S. Russo, K. Rutherford, K. Tsey, M. Wenitong et al. (2016). Psycho-social resilience, vulnerability and suicide prevention: impact evaluation of a mentoring approach to modify suicide risk for remote Indigenous Australian students at boarding school. Report. *BMC Public Health* 16: 98. DOI: 10.1186/s12889-016-2762-1.

McGinnis, J., P. Williams-Russo and J. Knickman (2002). The case for more active policy attention to health promotion. *Health Affairs* 21(2): 78–93. DOI: 10.1377/ hlthaff.21.2.78.

McLaughlin, C. and A. Kaluzny, eds (1994). *Continuous quality improvement in health care: theory, implementation, and applications*. Gaithersburg, MD: Aspen Publications.

National Health and Medical Research Council (2018). *Ethical conduct in research with Aboriginal and Torres Strait Islander Peoples and communities: guidelines for researchers and stakeholders*. Canberra: Commonwealth of Australia.

Nattabi, B., V. Matthews, J. Bailie, A. Rumbold, D. Scrimgeour, J. Ward et al. (2017). Wide variation in sexually transmitted infection testing and counselling at Aboriginal primary health care centres in Australia: analysis of longitudinal continuous quality improvement data. *BMC Infectious Diseases* 17: 148. DOI: 10.1186/s12879-017-2241-z.

Onnis, L.-A., M. Hakendorf, M. Diamond and K. Tsey (2019). CQI approaches for evaluating management development programs: a case study with health service managers from geographically remote settings. *Evaluation and Program Planning* 74: 91–101. DOI: https://doi.org/10.1016/j. evalprogplan.2019.03.003.

Percival, N., L. O'Donoghue, V. Lin, K. Tsey and R. Bailie (2016). Improving health promotion using quality improvement techniques in Australian Indigenous primary health care. *Front Public Health* 4: 53. DOI: 10.3389/fpubh.2016.00053.

Powell, A., R. Rushmer and H. Davies (2009). A systematic narrative review of quality improvement models in health care. Edinburgh, UK: NHS Quality Improvement Scotland.

Read, C., A. Mitchell, J. de Dassel, C. Scrine, D. Hendrickx, R. Bailie et al. (2018). Qualitative evaluation of a complex intervention to improve rheumatic heart disease secondary prophylaxis. *Journal of the American Heart Association* 7(14). DOI: 10.1161/JAHA.118.009376.

Redman-MacLaren, M., N.N. Turner, J. Taylor, A. Laycock, K. Vine, Q. Thompson et al. (2021). Respect is central: a critical review of implementation frameworks for continuous quality improvement in Aboriginal and Torres Strait Islander primary health care services. *Frontiers in Public Health* 16: 9. DOI: 10.3389/fpubh.2021.630611.

Riley, W., H. Parsons, G. Duffy, J. Moran and B. Henry (2010). Realizing transformational change through quality improvement in public health. *Journal of Public Health Management Practice* 16(1): 72–8. DOI: 10.1097/PHH.0b013e3181c2c7e0.

Ryerson University Research Ethics Board (2017). *Guidelines for research involving Indigenous peoples in Canada*. Toronto, Canada: Toronto Metropolitan University.

Schierhout, G., J. Hains, D. Si, C. Kennedy, R. Cox, R. Kwedza et al. (2013). Evaluating the effectiveness of a multifaceted, multilevel continuous quality improvement program in primary health care: developing a realist theory of change. *Implementation Science* 8: 119. DOI: 10.1186/1748-5908-8-119.

Schierhout, G., V. Matthews, C. Connors, S. Thompson, R. Kwedza, C. Kennedy et al. (2016). Improvement in delivery of type 2 diabetes services differs by mode of care: a retrospective longitudinal analysis in the Aboriginal and Torres Strait Islander primary health care setting. *BMC Health Services Research* 16: 560. DOI: 10.1186/s12913-016-1812-9.

Schouten, L., M. Hulscher, J. van Everdingen, R. Huijsman and R. Grol (2008). Evidence for the impact of quality improvement collaboratives: systematic review. *BMJ* 336(7659): 1491–4. DOI: 10.1136/ bmj.39570.749884.BE.

Shojania, K. and J. Grimshaw (2005). Evidence-based quality improvement: the state of the science. *Health Affairs* 24(1): 138–50. DOI: 10.1377/hlthaff.24.1.138.

Smith, G., R. Kirkham, C. Gunabarra, V. Bokmakarray and C.P. Burgess (2018). "We can work together, talk together": an Aboriginal Health Care Home. *Australian Health Review* 43(5): 486–91. DOI: 10.1071/ah18107.

Sollecito, W. and J. Johnson (2019). *McLaughlin and Kaluzny's continuous quality improvement in health care*. Burlington, MA: Jones & Bartlett Learning.

The Pūtaiora Writing Group (2010). *Te Ara Tika. Guidelines for Māori research ethics: a framework for researchers and ethics committee members*. Auckland, New Zealand: Health Research Council of New Zealand.

Tricco A., J. Antony, N. Ivers, H. Ashoor, P. Khan, E. Blondal et al. (2014). Effectiveness of quality improvement strategies for coordination of care to reduce use of health care services: a systematic review and meta-analysis. *Canadian Medical Association Journal* 186(15): E568–78. DOI: 10.1503/cmaj.140289.

Tricco, A., N. Ivers, J. Grimshaw, D. Moher, L. Turner, J. Galipeau et al. (2012). Effectiveness of quality improvement strategies on the management of diabetes: a systematic review and meta-analysis. *Lancet* 379(9833): 2252–61. DOI: 10.1016/S01406736(12)60480-2.

Turner, N., J. Taylor, S. Larkins, K. Carlisle, S. Thompson, M. Carter et al. (2019). Conceptualizing the association between community participation and CQI in Aboriginal and Torres Strait Islander PHC Services. *Qualitative Health Research* 29(13): 1904–15. DOI: 10.1177/1049732319843107.

Wells, S., O. Tamir, J. Gray, D. Naidoo, M. Bekhit and D. Goldmann (2018). Are quality improvement collaboratives effective? A systematic review. *BMJ Quality and Safety* 27(3): 226–40. DOI: 10.1136/bmjqs-2017-006926.

Wensing, M., H. Wollersheim and R. Grol (2006). Organizational interventions to implement improvements in patient care: a structured review of reviews. *Implementation Science* 1: 2. DOI: 10.1186/1748-5908-1-2.

Wise, M., S. Angus, E. Harris and S. Parker (2013). *National appraisal of continuous quality improvement initiatives in Aboriginal and Torres Strait Islander primary health care: final report.* Melbourne: Lowitja Institute.

World Health Organization (2023). *WHO guidelines.* https://www.who.int/publications/guidelines/en/.

World Health Organization (2015). *Primary Health Care Performance Initiative.* https://improvingphc.org/.

Zuchowski, I., D. Miles, C. Woods and K. Tsey (2017). Continuous quality improvement processes in child protection: a systematic literature review. *Research on Social Work Practice* 29(4). DOI: 10.1177/1049731517743337.

Part II

Continuous quality improvement data, tools and processes for primary health care

Quality improvement is now a driving force in health care, and an essential aspect of primary healthcare service organisation and management at all levels. Put simply, CQI is everyone's business.

In PHC, this principle is put into action through participatory and inclusive CQI processes (see Part I, Chapter 3). Our approach to CQI in PHC engages all members of the PHC workforce, not just clinicians and their managers. Administrators, receptionists, staff who transport clients, cleaners and others in healthcare support roles may be the key to identifying weaknesses in care systems and the driving force in making positive change. The involvement of clients, their families and carers and community agencies is also key to identifying issues that matter, and harnessing community strengths and resources to improve health.[1]

PHC organisations with a genuine culture of CQI provide opportunities for all staff to learn and be involved in CQI. They engage clients and communities in improving care. They work with researchers, planners and educators to improve system performance and professional learning.[2]

In Part I, we defined key concepts in PHC and CQI, and how they come together in efforts to improve health. In this second part of the book, we explain how CQI can be used in a comprehensive approach to PHC. We consider the purpose of CQI data. We describe the quality indicators used in CQI tools and how evidence is used to guide clinical practice, the types and sources of data for CQI, and the principles that guide decisions about generating information to measure care quality. We present a modified CQI cycle for PHC, based on the PDSA cycle, and discuss CQI facilitation. Tools, techniques and tips for facilitating CQI cycles are illustrated with examples and stories from PHC settings, particularly Aboriginal and Torres Strait Islander settings in Australia. The final chapter in Part II discusses what PHC services can do to embed and sustain a culture of CQI.

References

Bailie, R.S., D. Si, L. O'Donoghue and M. Dowden (2007). Indigenous health: effective and sustainable health services through continuous quality improvement. *Medical Journal of Australia* 186(10): 525–7. DOI: 10.5694/j.1326-5377.2007.tb01028.x.

Batalden, P.B. and F. Davidoff (2007). What is "quality improvement" and how can it transform healthcare? *Quality and Safety in Health Care* 16(1): 2–3. DOI: 10.1136/qshc.2006.022046.

---

1   Bailie, Si et al. 2007.
2   Batalden and Davidoff 2007.

Evidence to guide and improve care

Decisions about care quality need to be based on the best available evidence. This chapter discusses the purpose of CQI data, and the evidence commonly used in continuous quality improvement (CQI), focusing mainly on evidence for improving clinical care. We introduce the concept of quality indicators and the role of best-practice guidelines in relation to measures of quality. Types and sources of CQI data, and common challenges and strategies relating to data quality, are also discussed. The chapter includes practical tips for generating information to assess quality of care in primary healthcare (PHC) settings.

The purpose of CQI data

CQI cycles (see Chapters 2, 6) provide a systematic approach to collecting and using data. Data are essential for guiding improvement efforts by identifying quality problems, knowledge gaps and improvement opportunities. You and your PHC team may accurately identify improvement needs based on your experience and observation, but these decisions are likely to be influenced by your individual interests, and different colleagues will have different opinions. Sometimes the focus of improvement is determined by external experts rather than data or evidence on performance of local primary healthcare services; this approach may divert quality improvement efforts from actual priorities. Data provide evidence to confirm priority issues that should be addressed through CQI at the local service level. Data also have an ongoing role in helping to monitor service performance and sustain improvement. Without appropriate data of suitable quality, it is difficult to determine the effect of change initiatives or demonstrate success. Most data used in CQI should already be routinely collected for client or organisation management purposes. This is an important principle: CQI should be part of routine business and as efficient as possible.

> Most data used in CQI should already be routinely collected for client or organisation management purposes.

Quality indicators

Data collected for CQI are organised around various indicators of healthcare quality. In general terms, a health indicator is a measure that summarises information about a topic or organises information from data collected through health practice systems. This information is used to inform health system performance and research in population health. Healthcare indicators transform data on healthcare encounters between providers and clients into numbers and metrics to allow for monitoring of healthcare practices and quality, and for making (non-descriptive) comparisons: for example, between age groups in a population. Examples of health indicators are the proportion of children with up-to-date immunisation records and the percentage of clients satisfied with their care experience.

Indicators expressed in this way are useful in CQI because they can track changes over time. They enable comparison across geographic, administrative or organisational boundaries. It is important to be aware that numbers and metrics are merely that; they don't provide comprehensive information for understanding people's experiences of care or caregiving, the quality of relationships between service providers and clients or communities, or the nuanced factors that influence health outcomes. Qualitative data are needed for these purposes.

Indicators of healthcare quality generally focus on the structure, processes and outcomes of care: the quality improvement framework developed by Donabedian (see Chapter 2). Table 4.1 summarises how the structure-process-outcome quality framework is applied in PHC. Data on care structure, processes and outcomes are all potentially important for effective CQI. Furthermore, these data need to be brought together for an accurate assessment of care quality. Most of the CQI tools described in the next chapter collect and bring together data for different types of indicators, as determined by the focus of the CQI activity, the purpose of the tool and contextual factors. In Indigenous PHC contexts, for example, questions are raised about who decides what and how indicators of quality are used.[1] More generally, there are calls for Indigenous community control of data about Indigenous peoples, to ensure that data reflect Indigenous values and concepts of health and have meaning for improving Indigenous health and wellbeing (see Chapters 21 and 22).

> Data on care structures, processes and outcomes are all potentially important for CQI.

---

1   Darr, Franklin et al. 2021.

Table 4.1 Applying a structure-process-outcome quality framework in primary health care.

Health care: general		Primary health care: considerations
Structure	Facilities, equipment, finances	Health governance arrangements
	Human resources (e.g., mix and availability of practitioners, training)	Size and characteristics of the service population (e.g., languages spoken, groups represented, average income)
	Organisational structures (e.g., policies, care guidelines, how services are paid for)[2]	Geographical setting and access to hospital/ specialist care and community resources
Processes	Care delivery processes (e.g., obtaining information, therapeutic procedures, care coordination and continuity, interactions)	Care processes include preventive care and health promotion; client/family education; diagnosis, treatment and management of health conditions including client self-management; health-related interactions between service providers, families and communities
	Organisational processes (e.g., processes and systems for managing information, staff, facilities and other resources)[3]	Processes and pathways by which needs are assessed, care is provided and therapeutic relationships are developed; leadership and teamwork; use of client information systems and decision support; links and collaboration with other services/agencies and integration of systems for meeting the healthcare needs of clients and communities or population groups
Outcomes	Effects of care on the health of clients and populations (e.g., changes in clinical outcomes, behaviours, knowledge)	Social, cultural and environmental wellbeing outcomes are included as measures of care quality
	Client satisfaction/ experience	
	Physical rehabilitation	
	Health-related quality of life[4]	

---

2   Donabedian 2003, 2005.
3   Donabedian 2003, 2005.
4   Donabedian 2003, 2005.

Clinical guidelines for best practice

Indicators or measures of quality in clinical care are based on knowledge of what comprises best practice. There has been a widespread move towards developing and implementing clinical practice guidelines for best-practice clinical care, and their use is well established in many PHC settings. Intended as recommendations to optimise client care, clinical practice guidelines help practitioners to make decisions about appropriate health care for specific clinical circumstances, and support clinicians and clients in shared decision-making. Guidelines are available across the scope of clinical PHC relevant to various settings. Some examples are referenced in Part III.

> Measures of quality in clinical care are based on knowledge of what comprises best practice.

Clinical practice guidelines should be informed by systematic reviews of the best available evidence and expert consensus. They should be collaboratively developed and updated by unbiased experts from relevant medical and health disciplines, researchers, health practitioners who will be end users, and clients. Guidelines are often developed under the auspices of a professional college or association, with approval by a high-level health governing body such as the World Health Organization (WHO) or, in Australia, the National Health and Medical Research Council (NHMRC). International online repositories make clinical guidelines widely accessible.[5] In addition to international and national guidelines, local guidelines or specific guidelines for working with population groups (such as Indigenous peoples) are available.

Most published guidelines aid diagnosis and treatment of a single disease or condition, such as diabetes, or a specific aspect of care (such as blood sugar level or blood pressure). Some clinical resources for PHC practitioners bring guidelines together to promote coordinated, standardised client-centred care. This is appropriate to PHC, where it is vital that practitioners take a holistic approach, and where care of specific conditions needs to be considered in the context of other immediate and longer-term care needs and risks to health. These types of resources are also of practical value where service populations have particular health, social and cultural needs, where resources are limited, or where factors such as high staff turnover or location mean that strategic, coordinated and locally appropriate approaches to care are particularly important. An Australian example is the suite of PHC manuals for practitioners working in geographically remote and Aboriginal and Torres Strait Islander settings. The PHC manuals cover clinical presentations that are common and significant, that have different presentations and management issues to those in "mainstream" Australian general practice, are life threatening and need emergency care, and are important for public health. For example, the *Standard Treatment Manual*[6] covers (among other conditions) the prevention and management of diabetes, cardiovascular and renal disease, which occur at high rates among Aboriginal and Torres Strait Islander

---

5   Examples are the WHO guidelines portal (https://www.who.int/publications/ guidelines/en/) and the International Guidelines Library (https://g-i-n.net/ international-guidelines-library).

6   Remote Primary Health Care Manuals 2022a.

peoples and can be challenging to manage under remote living conditions. A *Women's Business Manual*[7] is a culturally respectful resource that keeps women's health confidential and separate from other health issues. Preventive health assessment guidelines have also been developed for Aboriginal and Torres Strait Islander PHC by the National Aboriginal Community Controlled Health Organisation and the Royal Australian College of General Practitioners (2018).[8]

> Clinical practice guidelines are important resources for CQI.

Clinical practice guidelines are important resources for CQI in clinical care. They provide a reference point or standard for PHC teams and services to compare the care they provide with the best available evidence on recommended care. Clinical practice guidelines generally form the foundations of the clinical audit tools used to generate data on clinical performance, and which in turn can be used for CQI. The focus on best-practice guidelines in developing and using audit tools raises awareness of contemporary evidence-based care and is an important educational and professional development element of the CQI process.

It is important to note that gathering data on clinical performance in relation to best-practice guidelines does not in itself constitute CQI, even when it includes a process for feeding back data to staff – but these are important steps in the CQI process. The CQI process (or cycle) includes gathering data, reporting, analysis and interpretation, and then using that information to identify priorities for improvement and to plan and implement improvement strategies.

> Generating and feeding back data on clinical performance in relation to best-practice guidelines does not constitute CQI. It is only part of the CQI process or cycle.

Regardless of how clinical practice guidelines are presented, they are just one element informing good medical decision-making. Decisions about care should take account of factors such as clients' preferences and values, clinicians' experience and values, the context in which care is provided, and the availability and distribution of resources. These factors are relevant for assessing care quality. As a resource for informing value-based care, clinical practice guidelines are also being used to develop incentives (such as pay for performance) and standards for PHC. (See "Value and quality" in Chapter 2.)

Guidelines for best-practice health promotion

By conventional measures of evidence quality, the evidence base guiding best practice in non-clinical areas of PHC, such as health promotion, is generally not as strong as the evidence

---

7   Remote Primary Health Care Manuals 2022b.
8   National Aboriginal Community Controlled Health Organisation and Royal Australian College 2024.

base for clinical care for medical conditions. Step-by-step guides, packages, frameworks and resources are available to help with evidence-informed health promotion practice and tend to be designed around specific topics such as smoking, alcohol use, heart health, cancer symptom awareness or mental health. Some resources are designed for use with specific populations, such as Indigenous populations. We note that there is limited information about the effectiveness of health promotion tools designed for use with Aboriginal and Torres Strait Islander populations.[9]

Knowledge for developing and implementing effective health promotion interventions is growing. We expect the availability of CQI tools and processes in health promotion and other areas of comprehensive PHC to increase as the evidence base for improving the cultural, social and environmental determinants of health grows in quality and in scope.

Types and sources of data

Different types of data are brought together to build meaningful information about the quality of PHC. These are some common types:

- clinical indicator and service delivery data derived from client health records – for example, data about care processes, clinical measures/results, client health behaviours (such as smoking) and medications prescribed
- demographic and health status data recorded in client health records, which can be used to define population groups – for example, by age, gender, diagnosis of a chronic condition
- health service and community data, collected to understand the PHC service's operating environment – for example, size of service population, geographic location, governance arrangements
- data about the range of health professionals providing client care, which are needed to understand how the PHC service operates – for example, staff numbers and skill mix, team structure and function, health infrastructure and resources
- data about client perceptions of care quality and experiences of service delivery – for example, client-reported experience and outcome surveys, complaints data
- staff perceptions of care quality and experiences of delivering care.

Incident-reporting and risk-management data, claims data (for example, claims made through a health insurance or medication subsidy scheme), and key performance indicator data collected for higher level policy purposes (such as to measure progress on health equity between population groups) may also be useful for CQI.

---

9   McCalman, Tsey et al. 2014.

Other types of data relevant to improving comprehensive PHC may include:

- data about changes in client knowledge and behaviours recorded in client records or health promotion program records
- data about community health program activities and outcomes
- data from research and evaluation reports – for example, health outcomes, health literacy, client and staff perceptions, community actions, system responses
- community stories/narratives about actions taken for improving health and wellbeing
- other data relevant to the social, cultural and environmental determinants of health – for example, demographic, education, child care, child protection, recreation, housing, aged care, emergency services, food security, employment, income, community governance, criminal justice data.

CQI tends to use data on structures, processes and outputs, which are relatively short term and feasible to collect and monitor locally, rather than outcomes and effect. Outcome and effect data require longer timeframes, may not be readily available at a service or local level, and could be more affected by factors outside the direct control of the PHC service or team.

> CQI tends to use data on structures, processes and outputs, which are relatively short term and feasible to collect and monitor.

With so much data to choose from, the key question is "Which data fit our CQI purpose and question?" Where data do not exist, you also need to ask, "What data do we need to collect to fill in our gap in knowledge and understanding?"

> Which data fit our CQI purpose and question? What data do we need to collect to fill in our gap in knowledge and understanding?

Data quality

No matter which data sources are used in CQI, the reality is that decisions will be as good as the quality of the data they are based on. Accurate and more complete data enables more precise identification of problems, the prioritisation of improvement initiatives and objective assessment of whether change and improvement have occurred. Conversely, inaccurate or incomplete data can undermine the credibility and value of the CQI process.[10]

Overcoming common challenges to data quality

Complete and accurate recording of client information is vital for providing high-quality PHC. Some characteristics of PHC (as described in Part I) present challenges to data quality and some gaps in quality occur because PHC is provided by multiple health professionals, through different services and locations. Furthermore, PHC services generally have regular clients and

---

10   Gardner, Dowden et al. 2010; Wise, Angus et al. 2013.

long-term responsibility for providing care (for example, to manage chronic conditions), and for responding to needs across the life cycle. Clinical information systems need the ability to hold, generate, link and share information for the purposes of ongoing care and for CQI. Attention to data quality and consistency improves the effectiveness of CQI. Some tips for improving data quality are listed in Box 4.1.

> Attention to data quality and consistency improves the effectiveness of CQI.

Box 4.1: Strategies for improving data quality

- Ensure clinical information systems are easy to use and accessible to all staff who provide client care.

- Offer regular staff training in the use of clinical information systems and correct documentation of care in client files. Depending on the service structure, this may involve staff based at the PHC centre or practice, locum staff and visiting practitioners (for example, vision services, dietitians).

- Ensure timely data entry into clinical information systems, so that clinical decisions and CQI priorities are based on current circumstances.

- Establish systems for efficient transfer of client care information between providers (for example, between specialists and general practitioners, between hospitals and PHC services, between PHC program teams).

- Use the same clinical information system across PHC services where possible. This enables benchmarking of CQI data between similar services/practices, aggregation of data and efficient information transfer.

- Use CQI techniques to assess and improve data quality.

The use of data in CQI cycles can be a catalyst for improving data quality.[11] Undertaking CQI can demonstrate the type of information that is useful for improving care and expose gaps in client records and data entry that may negatively affect continuing care. So, a message for readers with concerns about the quality of available data is not to wait until you have perfect data for CQI. Remember, CQI is about continuous learning and improvement. By starting where your PHC service or program data are at, you will see how to improve data to support CQI and improve care for clients. You will be able to reflect, over successive CQI cycles, on how far the team or service has come in CQI learning and implementation.

---

11   Allen and Clarke Consulting 2013; Schierhout, Hains et al. 2013; Wise, Angus et al. 2013.

> **Example: participating in CQI can improve data quality**
>
> An evaluation of the Northern Territory's CQI investment strategy was untaken after five years of implementation. The evaluation found that the quality of clinical data at the PHC service level had improved due to staff participation in clinical audits:
>
>> PHC staff participation in file audits as part of the CQI process has been a key reason behind the increase in data quality. Several clinicians spoke of a 'light bulb moment' when they realised the importance of accurate data entry. Going through audit processes was also seen as supporting improved patient care, for example, by increasing understanding of how to use the recall system correctly, meaning patients are being more actively followed up.[12]

Don't wait until you have perfect data for CQI. Undertaking CQI improves data quality.

Generating information to assess the quality of clinical care

There are links between the quality of systems for managing clients' health records, the integration of those records with information technology systems (for example, to recall clients) and service quality.[13]

Functional clinical information systems are crucial for generating information to assess care quality. PHC services may have an electronic clinical information system, a mix of electronic information systems and paper-based systems, or a fully paper-based record system in use. All are suitable for generating data for use in CQI.

Generating data from electronic clinical information systems

There is widespread adoption of electronic clinical information systems in PHC. These computer systems capture, store and display current client data to inform clinical decision-making and care planning. Client data may include clinical notes, medication history, laboratory reports, images and reports. In addition to supporting evidence-based and client-centred care, the use of electronic clinical information systems has the potential to overcome some of the challenges of gathering data to support CQI in PHC settings.

It is important that the data captured are reliable: that is, complete and accurate. We need to be able to trust that the data we use for CQI can provide the information we require, free from duplicates and errors. In general, research shows poor reliability of client data extracted from electronic clinical information systems,[14] with critical gaps in the recording of client data (for example, missing data on diagnoses) and inconsistent recording of different

---

12   Allen and Clarke Consulting 2013, 53.
13   Larkins, Carlisle et al. 2019; Woods, Carlisle et al. 2017.
14   Barkhuysen, de Grauw et al. 2014.

indicators.[15] Many electronic information systems currently in use in Australia, for example, are not designed for detailed data analysis: the information extracted may be too generalised for a CQI process at the PHC service level. Further, the use of various software systems and data extraction tools makes it difficult to link and aggregate data across services to identify common improvement priorities.

When starting to extract CQI data from electronic data systems, it is likely that the first few cycles will be around improving data quality and building confidence in data: agreeing on what and how client diagnoses and items of care will be captured in the system, and where they need to be recorded so they can be extracted. For example, if a client's blood pressure record is entered in the wrong place in the system (for example, in progress notes instead of as a service item), it will not be captured in data reports. As electronic clinical information systems in PHC continue to be developed and improved, the ability to extract detailed, high-quality data about client care is increasing.

Generating data for clinical auditing

Clinical auditing is widely used as a step in the CQI process. A clinical audit is used to find out if health care is being provided in line with clinical practice guidelines. Audit results let providers and clients know where their service is doing well, and where there could be improvements. Our approach to CQI has been to develop and use audit tools to collect information that has been recorded in clinical client records about a particular area of health care (for example, maternal health care, preventive cardiovascular disease care). These audit tools are based on evidence-based best-practice guidelines or other protocols or both, and their use provides information on the extent to which care recorded in client records reflects best practice across the range of items of care in relevant guidelines (including commonly used and important indicators, such as blood pressure and blood glucose levels for adult clients with chronic illnesses). This approach provides data on aspects of care that are being delivered relatively well or not so well at the local service level, thus providing a basis for local healthcare teams to identify locally relevant priorities for improvement. The benefits of using this approach are summarised in Box 4.2.

Box 4.2 Six benefits of using evidence-based clinical audit tools

- Supports implementation of best-practice guidelines or protocols

- Focuses on the most important items of care within the guidelines or protocols

- Collects information already recorded in client clinical records

- Measures the extent to which care recorded reflects best practice

- Provides data on aspects of care that are being delivered relatively well or not so well

- Helps PHC teams to identify locally relevant priorities for improvement

---

15   R. Bailie, J. Bailie et al. 2015.

There are two ways to generate client data for clinical auditing: by electronically generating all relevant client records from your service; or by selecting a representative sample of client records for more detailed (perhaps manual) auditing. Manual extraction of data is necessary where the required indicators cannot be generated automatically from electronic systems with sufficient reliability for the CQI purpose. Both approaches are valid. The approach that should be used will depend on the focus of the CQI audit, the level of detail required about client care, the resources available to carry out the audit, and the capability of the electronic information system to generate data of adequate quality. Using both electronic data extraction and sampling is often ideal, because an electronic system download can provide an overview of an entire group of service users (for example, all children without a major health anomaly aged 3 months to 15 years), while sampling provides detailed information about the quality of care delivered to clients with specific characteristics, including the way care is documented in client records.

Practical tips for generating data

There are several practical issues to consider when generating data for clinical auditing.

What is the CQI question?

The focus of the clinical audit and the CQI question will determine the data that are needed. If the question relates to the whole service population, or to a subgroup of clients who can be identified in the electronic information system, electronic data extraction may be feasible. For example, electronic data extraction may be feasible if the CQI question relates to services received by women enrolled for antenatal and postnatal care. Otherwise, sampling of client records is necessary.

The size of the service population is also a factor in decision-making. If doing an audit of adolescent care in a service with 30 adolescent clients, then an audit of all 30 records would be feasible. In contrast, sampling would be appropriate when auditing social and emotional wellbeing care for all adult clients of a large health service if the data cannot be electronically generated.

Does the electronic record system contain the data needed? AND are the data complete and reliable?

These are critical questions when deciding the most appropriate data source. The electronic information system may be able to generate data for laboratory results and clinical measurements, for example, but not data about counselling and follow-up provided to clients who are at risk for social and emotional wellbeing, or data about smoking status.

A related issue is that deficiencies in the quality of information held in client health records may not be readily evident in electronic system downloads. Manual audits, in comparison, are likely to highlight incomplete and poor documentation in client records, even when the audit is only done on a sample of records. The need to improve the accuracy and quality of data in client records is evident in many CQI studies.[16]

---

16 Bailie, Laycock et al. 2016; Bailie, Matthews et al. 2014; D'Aprano, Silburn et al. 2016; de Witt, Cunningham et al. 2017.

Is it possible to extract data for all the required population?

The capability of the health service information system (and the capability of health service staff to use the system) also determines whether it is possible to electronically extract data for all the required population, or whether sampling is the best approach for meeting auditing needs.

We have brought these questions together in a decision flowchart (Figure 4.1). When the electronic clinical information system contains the data needed to answer the CQI question, when the data are complete and reliable, and when it is possible to extract data for all the required population, electronic data can be extracted for analysis. When there is doubt about any of these criteria, the reliability of data for CQI is likely to be compromised. In these circumstances, drawing a sample of clients' records and auditing each clinical record to identify relevant clients is the recommended approach.

Sampling client records to generate data

A well-functioning electronic clinical information system can usually generate a sample of client records for auditing. Otherwise, a sample of client records can be drawn from a client list. Whatever method of sampling is used must result in an unbiased representation of clients. The sampling method used should also be consistent between audit cycles, so that audit results can be reliably compared over time. There are two commonly used approaches to generating a sample:

- Systematic sampling is a probability sampling method. It involves sampling members from a larger client population (for example, all children aged 3 months to 15 years), selected according to a random starting point but with a fixed, periodic interval. This interval, called the "sampling interval", is calculated by dividing the population size by the desired sample size.
- Random sampling selects clients by chance from a complete list (for example, a list of all clients diagnosed with coronary heart disease). Each client record has an equal probability of being selected and the selection must occur in a random way.

The number of client records audited needs to be sufficient to provide a snapshot of whether processes are being followed in line with clinical practice guidelines, but not so large that the audit takes more time and resources than necessary. If a high degree of accuracy and confidence is required, a sample size that is representative of the entire client population can be calculated in a scientific way (for example, using free epidemiology and statistical software).

An additional consideration will be whether to stratify your sample. Stratification is an important concept in sampling. A stratified sample includes equal numbers of clients from each of a number of specified groups. In your random sample, you may want equal numbers of male and female clients, or equal numbers of clients in different age ranges.

The sample needs a clear timeframe and should include current or recent clients. Clearly specified inclusion and exclusion criteria are required but, when drawing a sample of client records for auditing, discussion may be needed to include or exclude individual client records. At this point, local knowledge is important. For example, you may decide not to include the record of a client you know has moved away and therefore not attended for scheduled care, or a client who has passed away.

**Focus
of audit**

What is the continuous quality
improvement question?

Does the continuous quality
improvement question relate to the
whole service population?

YES · NO

Which subgroup
of clients does the
question relate to?

Does the electronic
record system contain
the data to answer the
CQI question AND is it
complete and reliable?

YES

Can you identify these
clients in the electronic
information system?

NO

NO

Is it possible to extract
data for all of the
required population?

NO →

Draw a sample of client
records

—

See
information
on sampling

YES

Electronic data
extraction for analysis

Audit each clinical
record to identify
relevant clients. Extract
data for analysis

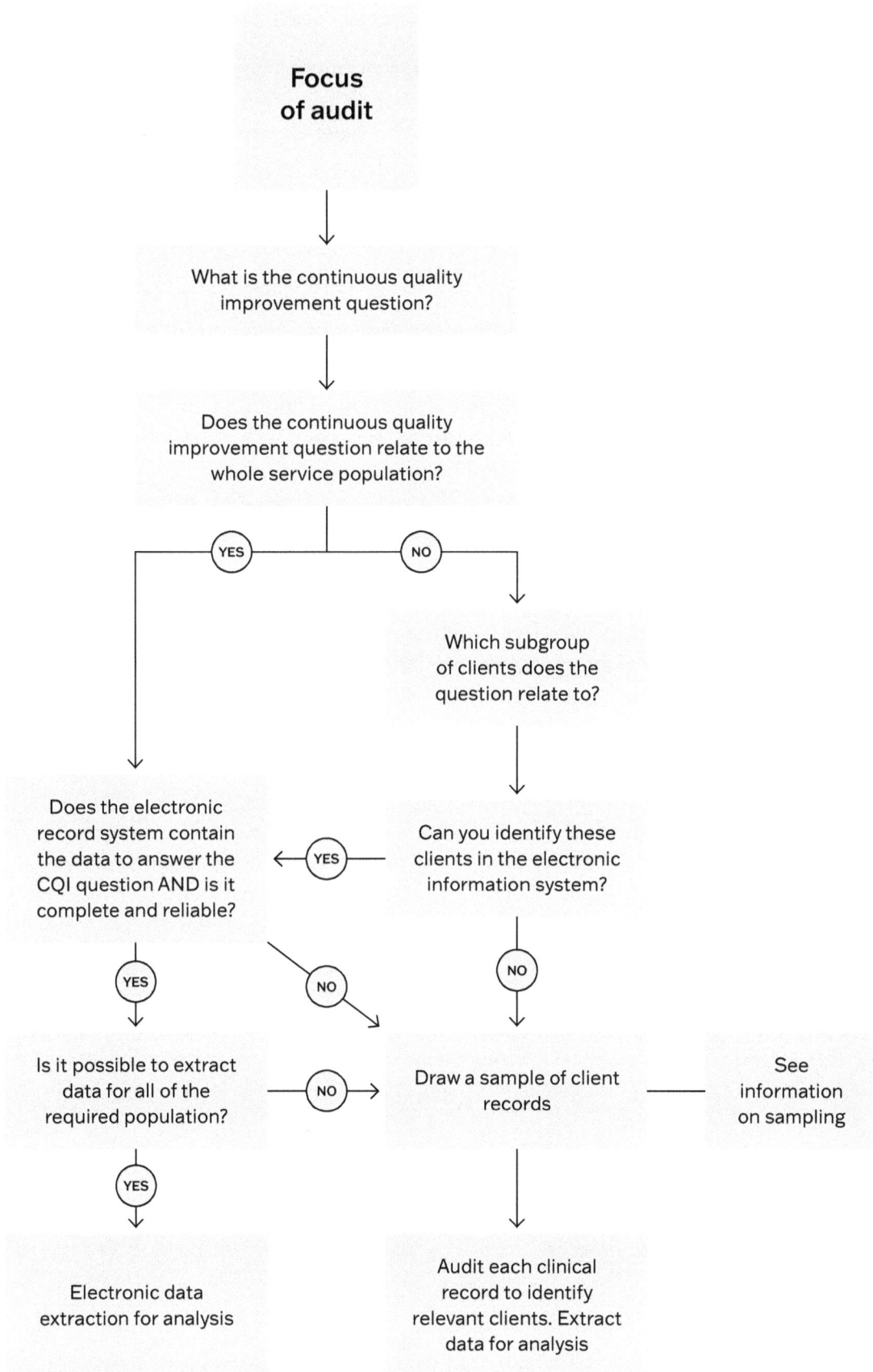

Figure 4.1 Decision flowchart: generating data for analysis in a clinical audit.

Denominators – an important concept in clinical auditing

Denominator data are very important in clinical auditing, because they allow us to measure (quantify) the extent to which care is being delivered in line with best-practice guidelines. The denominator is the total number of clients who meet the inclusion criteria for auditing. In a diabetes care audit, for example, the denominator is the total number of adult clients with diabetes who use the health service for their diabetes care.

> Denominator data allow us to measure the extent to which care is being delivered in line with best-practice guidelines.

Denominators need to be reliable to provide an accurate picture of the percentage of clients who have received the recommended standard of care, and to assess trends in care quality over time. Consistent definitions for denominators are essential for clarity about which clients are included in or excluded from an audit (for example, based on disease diagnosis, age, regular or recent attendance).

Reliable denominator data can be difficult to achieve for various reasons. These reasons include not applying client definitions consistently (for example, the definition of a "regular client"), or not having a record archiving system in place to remove the files of clients who cease attending the service or practice. Denominator data can be compromised by inconsistent use of electronic clinical information systems by staff, by data being entered incorrectly, by difficulty with using filters to extract data, by difficulty migrating client data from old to new software systems and other factors.[17] It is important not only to accurately enter, manage and extract data, but also to scrutinise electronically extracted data for possible errors before using the information to prioritise improvements. The following example illustrates the need for scrutiny and the value of involving staff with local knowledge in analysing audit data.

Table 4.2 shows that at one health centre in 2023, 40 out of 42 (95 per cent) clients with diabetes had received a glycated haemoglobin (blood glucose) check within the past 6 months. This appears to be a significant improvement on 75 per cent recorded in the previous audit. But a denominator of 42 clients with diabetes in 2023, compared with 56 in 2022 and 58 in the following audit would suggest the denominator was incorrect. Staff members should be able to confirm whether an error had been made when extracting data for auditing – for example, whether they had selected a function that removed all clients without a recent blood glucose record.

Table 4.2 Clients with diabetes who received a blood glucose (HbA1c) check in the past 6 months, over three consecutive audits.

Audit year	Number	Denominator	%
2022	42	56	75
2023	40	42	95
2024	46	58	79

17   R. Bailie, J.Bailie et al. 2015.

One way of overcoming the poor reliability of denominator data is to audit samples of clinical records. For example, a sample of 50 eligible client records in consecutive audits (a consistent denominator of 50) would yield more accurate data about changes in quality indicators over time. We also need to consider the size of the denominator. When denominators are low numbers, a large percentage change in indicators may have less significance for identifying priorities for improvement.

Generating information

The characteristics of PHC services that set them apart from other healthcare settings extend beyond the type of client and the need for continuity of care. They include a range of PHC service models and a strong community focus. For CQI to be effective, PHC teams need knowledge of the service population, features of the health service, the historical, cultural, social and environmental influences on the community's health and healthcare priorities, and the resources available to improve health and wellbeing.

Various techniques can be used to record this information, such as surveys, gathering stories, and community or systems mapping techniques using various media. A range of sources might include health service data, central data repositories, data from other service agencies (for example, schools, police, local government, places of worship, charities) and from community leaders and groups. It is most important that the information is regularly updated and is available for use in CQI. It should include these types of data:

- demographic information about the community, such as population size, age and gender breakdown, ethnic and other identified population groups
- information about the health service, including governance arrangements, accreditation status if relevant, staffing including whether any regular visiting staff contribute to PHC delivery, location, outlying clinics, and number of clients (also broken down into demographic groups)
- information about other services and resources located in the community or accessible to residents
- evidence about factors affecting community and population health and wellbeing: relevant positive factors such as strong social supports and strong cultural identity, practices and values; negative measures such as recent catastrophic weather events, poor living conditions, extent of poverty, exposure to racism.

This information is considered when interpreting data and when benchmarking a service's CQI results against other services. It helps teams to consider the factors that contribute to results, and ways to overcome or manage barriers to providing high-quality care and supporting community wellbeing. It also helps PHC teams to harness available resources to plan improvement.

Data on care coordination

Care coordination in PHC involves organising care activities and sharing information between care providers to achieve effective and safe care for clients. It may involve structural arrangements or communication and support. The effective coordination of care is important for achieving high-quality PHC and quality of life for clients (for example, by avoiding duplication of services and long wait times) but can be challenging given the fragmented and siloed care that often occurs in health systems.

It can be difficult to systematically assess the quality of care coordination, because it requires data across service providers, healthcare sites and levels of care to be accessed and compared, while adhering to confidentiality and privacy principles. Clinical information systems rarely have the required compatibility or functionality for this purpose. In addition, client and staff experiences are a valuable measure of effective care coordination and may not be reflected in these data. PHC services with dedicated care coordinators may have more complete records. Care coordinators' knowledge of systems, patient histories, coordination protocols and lines of communication may also have a positive effect on quality of care (see also Chapter 2, "Continuity of care and quality").[18]

Clinical audit tools usually include indicators relating to care coordination (for example, records of a team care plan); systems assessment tools should evaluate care coordination or continuity of care or both. Data from use of these tools can be combined to assess and set priorities for improving care coordination.

Summary

In this chapter, we have focused on the evidence commonly used in CQI, particularly for improving clinical PHC. Quality indicators, the role of best-practice guidelines and issues relating to data quality have been discussed. Key strategies for generating clinical data to measure care quality have been described. In the next chapter, we focus on practical tools that enable teams to use these data for improving clinical care and health systems.

References

Allen and Clarke Consulting (2013). *Evaluation of the Northern Territory Continuous Quality Improvement Investment Strategy: final report*. Canberra: Department of Health.

Bailie, J., A. Laycock, V. Matthews and R. Bailie (2016). System-level action required for wide-scale improvement in quality of primary health care: synthesis of feedback from an interactive process to promote dissemination and use of aggregated quality of care data. *Frontiers in Public Health* 4: 86. DOI: 10.3389/fpubh.2016.00086.

Bailie, R., J. Bailie, A. Chakraborty and K. Swift (2015). Consistency of denominator data in electronic health records in Australian primary healthcare services: enhancing data quality. *Australian Journal of Primary Health* 21(4): 450–9. DOI: 10.1071/PY14071.

Bailie, R., V. Matthews, J. Bailie and A. Laycock (2014). *Primary health care for Aboriginal and Torres Strait Islander children: priority evidence-practice gaps and stakeholder views on barriers and strategies for improvement: final report*. Brisbane: Menzies School of Health Research.

Barkhuysen, P., W. de Grauw, R. Akkermans, J. Donkers, H. Schers and M. Biermans (2014). Is the quality of data in an electronic medical record sufficient for assessing the quality of primary care? *Journal of the American Medical Informatics Association: JAMIA* 21(4): 692–8. DOI: 10.1136/amiajnl-2012-001479.

D'Aprano, A., S. Silburn, V. Johnston, R. Bailie, F. Mensah, F. Oberklaid et al. (2016). Challenges in monitoring the development of young children in remote Aboriginal health services: clinical audit findings and recommendations for improving practice. *Rural and Remote Health* 16(3852): 1–10.

---

18   Misra, Sedig et al. 2020.

Darr, J., R. Franklin, K. McBain-Rigg, S. Larkins, Y. Roe, K. Panaretto et al. (2021). Quality management systems in Aboriginal community controlled health services: a review of the literature. *BMJ Open Quality* 10(3): e001091. DOI: 10.1136/bmjoq-2020-001091.

de Witt, A., F.C. Cunningham, R. Bailie, C.M. Bernardes, V. Matthews, B. Arley et al. (2017). Identification of Australian Aboriginal and Torres Strait Islander cancer patients in the primary health care setting. *Frontiers in Public Health* 5(199). DOI: 10.3389/fpubh.2017.00199.

Donabedian, A. (2005). Evaluating the quality of medical care. *Milbank Quarterly* 83(4): 691–729. DOI: 10.1111/j.1468-0009.2005.00397.x.

Donabedian, A. (2003). *An introduction to quality assurance in health care.* New York, NY: Oxford University Press.

Gardner, K.L., M. Dowden, S. Togni and R. Bailie (2010). Understanding uptake of continuous quality improvement in Indigenous primary health care: lessons from a multi-site case study of the Audit and Best Practice for Chronic Disease project. *Implementation Science* 5: 21. DOI: 10.1186/1748-5908-5-21.

Larkins, S., K. Carlisle, N. Turner, J. Taylor, K. Copley, S. Cooney et al. (2019). "At the grass roots level it's about sitting down and talking": exploring quality improvement through case studies with high-improving Aboriginal and Torres Strait Islander primary healthcare services. *BMJ Open* 9(5): e027568. DOI: 10.1136/bmjopen-2018-027568.

McCalman, J., K. Tsey, R. Bainbridge, K. Rowley, N. Percival, L. O'Donoghue et al. (2014). The characteristics, implementation and effects of Aboriginal and Torres Strait Islander health promotion tools: a systematic literature search. *BMC Public Health* 14: 712.

Misra, V., K. Sedig, D. Dixon and S. Sibbald (2020). Prioritizing coordination of primary health care. *Canadian Family Physician* 66(6): 399–403. Erratum in: *Canadian Family Physician* 66(8): 554.

National Aboriginal Community Controlled Health Organisation and Royal Australian College of General Practitioners (2018). *National Guide to a Preventative Health Assessment for Aboriginal and Torres Strait Islander People*, 3rd edn. Melbourne: RACGP.

Remote Primary Health Care Manuals, ed. (2022a). *CARPA standard treatment manual for remote and rural practice.* Alice Springs, NT: Flinders University.

Remote Primary Health Care Manuals (2022b). *Minymaku kutju tjukurpa – women's business manual.* Alice Springs, NT: Flinders University.

Schierhout, G., J. Hains, D. Si, C. Kennedy, R. Cox, R. Kwedza et al. (2013). Evaluating the effectiveness of a multifaceted, multilevel continuous quality improvement program in primary health care: developing a realist theory of change. *Implementation Science* 8: 119. DOI: 10.1186/1748-5908-8-119.

Wise, M., S. Angus, E. Harris and S. Parker (2013). *National appraisal of continuous quality improvement initiatives in Aboriginal and Torres Strait Islander primary health care: final report.* Melbourne: Lowitja Institute.

Woods, C., K. Carlisle, S. Larkins, S.C. Thompson, K. Tsey, V. Matthews et al. (2017). Exploring systems that support good clinical care in Indigenous primary health-care services: a retrospective analysis of longitudinal systems assessment tool data from high-improving services. *Frontiers in Public Health* 5: 45. DOI: 10.3389/fpubh.2017.00045.

World Health Organization (2023). *WHO guidelines.* https://www.who.int/publications/guidelines/en/.

Practical tools for CQI in primary health care

Many tools have been developed for implementing CQI in health care. Selecting or adapting the best tools to suit the quality improvement needs of your primary healthcare (PHC) practice or service and your client population can be challenging. This chapter describes some practical tools that have been found to be useful at the health centre level for examining variation in clinical care and identifying priority areas for improvement. We introduce tools for assessing PHC structures, clinical auditing, assessing and improving PHC systems, measuring client experiences of care, and improving the quality of health promotion activities. These CQI tools were developed with PHC stakeholders using participatory action research. They may help your team to draw on the sources of data and best-practice guidelines discussed in Chapter 4 to improve the quality of PHC provided by your service or practice.

We then describe some other widely used CQI tools that, while designed mainly for hospital settings, are suitable for use in PHC. We explain how CQI methods and tools relate to each other and offer tips for selecting the best methods or tools for your PHC setting and CQI purpose. We begin the chapter with an overview of the included tools and their uses.

Different tools are used for different purposes

The different tools described in this chapter are used to collect data, to organise information, to understand variation in quality, to understand relationships between processes and outcomes, to identify causes of quality problems, and to strategically and systematically set improvement goals and develop plans for improvement. Tables 5.1, 5.2 and 5.3 provide an overview of the CQI tools and techniques described in this chapter, their purpose and how they are used.

Table 5.1 CQI tools assessing care structures, processes and outcomes.

Tool	Purpose	Use in primary health care
Health centre and community survey	Gather information about the context of PHC delivery.	Typically administered before using other tools, to understand the operating environment and structural context for PHC. Enables team to make sense of other data and plan context-specific improvement strategies.

Tool	Purpose	Use in primary health care
Clinical audit tools	Assess quality of care processes and clinical outcomes	Retrospectively measure quality of care documented in client records. Enable teams to identify priorities for improving clinical care. Used iteratively to monitor changes in quality over time.
Systems assessment tool	Assess strengths and weaknesses of PHC systems	Used in conjunction with clinical audit and other tools. Helps teams to understand the relationships between PHC systems and care provision; to identify priorities; and to integrate strategies for system improvement.
Surveys of clients' perspectives of the quality of care	Gather information about client experiences and satisfaction with care	Administered routinely to help teams understand how clients and families/carers experience care. Used to inform changes for improving experiences and satisfaction.

Table 5.2 Tools for health promotion.

Tool	Purpose	Use in primary health care
Health promotion audit and systems assessment tools	Assess the quality of health promotion activities/programs	Teams preferably use both tools to build a picture of health promotion quality and inform system changes that support health promotion activities. Can be used concurrently (and iteratively) with clinical audit tools to support a comprehensive PHC approach.
Tobacco control audit tool	Assess prevalence of smoking, support and actions for reducing tobacco-related harm	Provides a snapshot of clients' tobacco use and health promotion strategies relating to smoking. Enables teams to monitor change, improve responses and plan policies targeting tobacco control.
Good food planning tool	Engage communities in planning and improving local food systems	Brings food supply and consumer stakeholders together annually to assess food security and community nutrition, set improvement goals and plan actions to strengthen local food systems.

Table 5.3 Tools and techniques to visualise the systems and processes.

Tool	Purpose	Use in primary health care
Flowchart (process map)	Visualise systems and processes	Displays connected steps in a process, enabling teams to see interconnections, where processes work well and where flow breaks down. Used for improving and standardising a system or process.
Checklist	Identify persisting gaps and changes in routine care	Can be collated and analysed to help teams to implement care routines in line with best-practice guidelines.
Cause-and-effect (Ishikawa or fishbone) diagrams	Organise information and understand causes of variation	Organises and displays causes contributing to a quality effect or outcome. Enables the team to identify main factors contributing to gaps in care and priority areas for improvement.
Driver diagram	Identify causes of variation and plan change strategies	Visualises team theory of the key drivers or contributors to achieving a project aim. Sets out causal pathways for achieving the overall project aim.
Pareto diagram	Understand variation and prioritise improvement action	Identifies the vital few contributors to a problem. Enables teams to target improvement efforts that will lead to the greatest effect.
Run chart	Understand variation over time	Enables teams to observe variation in data over time, track and analyse the effect of change strategies on performance.

The tools described on the following pages collect data on quality indicators that relate to the structure, processes and outcomes of care.

Tools assessing care structures, processes and outcomes

Health centre and community survey

CQI data need to be analysed in relation to the operating environment for delivering care. Accurate information about care structures, available resources and the service population helps to make meaning of the data and set realistic improvement goals. It can identify operational barriers and strengths to build on when planning change.

Care structures can be systematically assessed using a simple survey tool. Administering the same survey at the start of each audit cycle enables a team to track changes in the operating environment over time.

The Health Centre and Community Survey[1] developed by the Audit and Best Practice for Chronic Disease (ABCD) CQI research group (introduced in Chapter 3) is an example. The tool collects data about the health centre location (for example, urban, rural or remote setting), the population size and number of regular clients, governance arrangement, staff numbers and roles including regular visiting staff, and accreditation status.

Clinical audit tools

Measuring the quality of clinical care

Clinical audit tools focus mainly on processes for delivering and receiving care and are useful for assessing variation in care. Clinical audit tools are used to retrospectively measure the quality of care documented in client records, using indicators based on the best available evidence and the service items listed in relevant best-practice clinical guidelines.

The tools are mainly used in "audit and feedback", in which data gathered are fed back to practitioners and used to improve service delivery. Clinical audit tools are designed to measure the quality of care for specific conditions, such as diabetes, or for important areas of PHC, such as maternal and child health. Data are collected on selected items of care that are important indicators of care quality.

> Data are collected on selected items of care that are important indicators of care quality.

Some indicators are more important than others for this purpose. Blood glucose level (HbA1c), for example, is a key indicator of the overall quality of diabetes care and would always be included in an audit tool for assessing diabetes care. The audit tool would also be expected to collect data about client self-management goals, blood pressure monitoring, prescribing of medications, body weight, vision testing, interventions for smoking and alcohol use, and other important indicators in diabetes care and management. The audit tool would not usually collect data about clinical events or care processes that are uncommon for clients with diabetes: this would be onerous and time consuming for auditors and would not add valuable evidence for assessing the quality of diabetes care for a service population.[2]

The information collected in a clinical audit can be used in these ways:

- assess the quality of health care received by patients in line with best-practice guidelines
- identify and prioritise areas of service delivery that should be improved as part of a CQI cycle
- track changes over time in the quality of care provided (through audits that measure delivery of care in different time periods), showing whether planned improvements to care systems have resulted in better care.

---

1   Menzies School of Health Research and One21seventy 2014.
2   For an example of a diabetes audit tool, see Menzies School of Health Research and One21seventy 2013.

Assessing care quality in areas of care where best practice is not well defined

In some areas of PHC, standards of care are not clearly articulated: evidence-based guidelines on which to base the quality indicators are limited. Where this is the case, it is possible to develop an audit process, drawing on the identification of relevant items from a review of other relevant guidelines and an expert consensus process – for example, experts in delivering clinical care to specific population groups. An example of this approach to clinical audit tool development is the Youth Health Clinical Audit Tool.[3] The tool was developed by service providers and researchers for use in Australian Indigenous PHC settings, through processes described in Chapter 14.

Benefits of auditing

Participating in clinical audits has benefits for PHC staff. Team members have opportunities to learn about the importance of keeping good client records, the standards of care regarded as best practice and the evidence that underpins best practice.

> Participating in clinical audits gives team members opportunities to learn about the importance of keeping good client records, the standards of care regarded as best practice and the evidence that underpins best practice.

Available tools

Many clinical audit tools have been developed for use in PHC. The audit tools that are available, related training and support, and data feedback systems are generally determined by government or health service policy, commercial agreements, available information technology and other factors. Whatever the arrangements, the interpretation of clinical audit data and improvement planning should occur at the level of the PHC team, using participatory group processes that involve as many people as possible. This is essential for PHC teams to own, drive and sustain improvement.

The following clinical audit tools were developed by the ABCD CQI research group and can be downloaded free of charge:[4]

- preventive services clinical audit
- child health clinical audit
- youth health clinical audit tool
- maternal health clinical audit
- mental health clinical audit
- sexual health (sexually transmissible infection/blood borne virus – STI/BBV) clinical audit tool
- vascular and metabolic syndrome management
- acute rheumatic fever/rheumatic heart disease (ARF/RHD) clinical audit.

---

3   Puszka, Nagel et al. 2015. The tool is available at https://www.menzies.edu.au/page/Resources/.

4   Download clinical audit tools and protocols from https://www.menzies.edu.au/page/Resources/.

Systems assessment tools

A systems assessment tool allows PHC teams to undertake a structured self-assessment of the strengths and weaknesses of their local health centre systems for supporting client care.

The ABCD Systems Assessment Tool[5] was designed to be used in conjunction with the clinical audit tools. The tool was developed collaboratively and is based on internationally accepted models that reflect the way health systems work and interact at organisation, practice, client and community levels[6] – namely the Chronic Care Model developed in the United States,[7] and the World Health Organization's Innovative Care for Chronic Conditions Framework (described in Chapter 1).[8]

The tool is used to measure the degree of support provided through the systems that relate to five key components of PHC. Each component comprises items that are scored and justified by the PHC team to reach an overall component score (Table 5.4).

Table 5.4 Components and items assessed using the ABCD Systems Assessment Tool.

System components	Items scored
Delivery system design	Team structure and function
	Clinical leadership
	Appointments and scheduling
	Care planning
	Systematic approach and follow-up
	Continuity of care
	Client access/cultural competence
	Physical infrastructure
Information systems and decision support	Maintenance and use of electronic client list
	Evidence-based guidelines
	Specialist and generalist collaborations
Self-management support	Assessment and documentation
	Self-management education and support
	Behavioural risk reduction and peer support

5   Menzies School of Health Research and One21seventy 2012.
6   Cunningham, Ferguson-Hill et al. 2016.
7   Bonomi, Wagner et al. 2002.
8   World Health Organization 2002.

System components	Items scored
Links with community, other health services and resources	Communication and cooperation on governance and operation of the health centre and other community-based organisations and programs
	Linking health centre clients to outside resources
	Working out in the community
	Communication and cooperation on regional health planning and development of health resources
Organisational influence and system integration	Organisational commitment
	Quality improvement strategies
	Integration of health system components

The interpretation of systems assessment data should be done in the context of clinical audit data, as measured by one or more clinical audit tools. This is because results from the systems assessment need to be compared to data on the quality of care delivered, in order to understand the relationships between PHC systems and the quality of care provided by PHC teams.

PHC systems need to be well integrated to provide holistic care, and use of a systems assessment tool can help teams to improve systems of care for clients with complex care needs. Together with the results of clinical auditing, a systems assessment can be used for these purposes:

- identifying strengths and weaknesses of the health centre system
- identifying priorities for improvement
- informing development of strategies to address those priorities
- informing development of action plans for implementation of those strategies.

The ABCD Systems Assessment Tool has proven useful for learning and improvement (Box 5.1), and also proven adaptable across programs and PHC settings. It has been adapted for assessing how well organisational systems are functioning to support health promotion activities[9] (as described later in this chapter). The tool was adapted for studying staff members' views on factors needed to improve chronic care systems in Aboriginal medical services in Australia, using these domains: health service governance and cultural safety; workforce issues and professional standards; experiences of CQI activities and supports; and navigation of care including access to hospital and specialist services.[10] It has also been adapted to assess the status of sexual health service delivery in Australian Indigenous communities,[11] and for developing community-driven PHC models for enhancing chronic disease management in First Nations communities across Canada.[12] The original tool is available for download.[13]

---

9   Percival, O'Donoghue et al. 2016.
10   Peiris, Brown et al. 2012.
11   Ward, McGregor et al. 2013.
12   Naqshbandi Hayward, Paquette-Warren et al. 2016.
13   From https://www.menzies.edu.au/page/Resources/Systems_Assessment_Tool_SAT/.

Box 5.1 Using the ABCD Systems Assessment Tool – a user survey

The ABCD Systems Assessment Tool (SAT) was reviewed after 12 years of implementation and refinement. A user survey found that systems assessments helped teams to learn about how PHC systems were functioning, and how to apply best practice and work together. Survey respondents made these comments:

> The SAT allowed the health centre to reflect on systems and system utilisation, identify differences between programs in system utilisation, and to identify barriers or issues in systems.

> The SAT supported clinic staff to discuss challenges within a safe space with management to help guide planning. It helped guide planning … Many clinic managers conveyed that they felt more in control of all the various challenges and could see the linkages and a map to help move forward.

> [The systems assessment] facilitated group discussion and decision-making; enabled staff to identify the things that they were doing well.[14]

A majority of the people surveyed wrote that using the tool had led to changes to their health centre structures and processes. Some commented that it could be challenging to find time to get all staff and service representatives together to complete the systems assessment unless time was allocated for CQI processes. Many thought it was important to have a skilled, external facilitator with a good understanding of the service delivery context: "This makes it easier for staff to participate openly in the process."[15]

Key message

Use CQI tools and participatory processes together to support learning and improvement. Allocate time to enable staff to participate in CQI processes.

Surveys of clients' perspectives of the quality of care

Client experience is an important measure of quality in health care[16] and links between client experiences of health care and clinical safety and effectiveness are well established.[17] CQI tools that measure client-centred care are essential for providing PHC that respects and responds to individual preferences, needs and values. There are two types of person-centred measures of care quality:

- Client experiences are people's interactions with the health system. Measures of client experience include effective communication, being treated with respect and dignity, and feeling emotionally supported.

---

14   Cunningham, Ferguson-Hill et al. 2016, 7.
15   Cunningham, Ferguson-Hill et al. 2016, 7.
16   Institute of Medicine 2001.
17   Doyle, Lennox and Bell 2013.

- Client satisfaction is evaluation of the care provided relative to clients' needs and expectations. Measures of client satisfaction include a client's experience of care, together with health outcomes and their confidence in the health system. [18]

CQI tools need to collect data about both aspects and should be designed to ensure that the data collected can be acted upon for improving care.

> There are two types of person-centred measures of care quality: client experiences and client satisfaction. Tools need to collect data about both aspects.

CQI processes involving clients can take different formats (for example, collecting stories from clients and family members or carers; client-reported experience or outcome surveys or both; focus groups; one-off community forums; advisory committees). Client participation can occur at different levels of the health system (for example, as individuals, as client representatives on governing boards). Populations with access to the internet and other media are better informed about health, illness and care options than ever before, increasing the potential benefits of client input into quality improvement. But there is a risk that inequities in access to the internet, inequities in information technology systems that support care and varying skills and confidence in using technology may further contribute to health inequities.

Client participation in CQI is determined by factors such as health literacy and numeracy, health status, confidence, perceptions about the ability to influence change, perceived power imbalances between clients and clinicians, and social status. It is essential that groups with generally poorer access to PHC, such as young people, people with disabilities, refugees and Indigenous populations, are included and feel safe contributing to CQI processes. Therefore, client satisfaction surveys and other tools for measuring client experiences and perceived outcomes of care should be developed with input from clients and tested prior to use.

Available tools

The ABCD Consumer's Perspective of the Quality of Care Survey[19] was designed to get feedback from clients about their perceptions of the quality of care they receive for their ongoing health condition. The tool was designed for use in remote primary health care in Australia but is easily adapted to suit other PHC settings. It captures general perceptions of health and care, access to care, participation in care, care design, care planning and self-management, respectful care, care coordination and follow-up, and recommendations for improving care.

The Royal Australian College of General Practitioners has developed several tools for collecting feedback about clients' experiences, and a toolkit for developing questionnaires.[20] Professional bodies in other countries, and government health services and health support organisations, offer similar resources for use in PHC. Many examples of client experience and satisfaction surveys, and survey templates, are available online. Some have been designed for PHC settings and can be adapted to meet your needs. Others, such as the tool described in the box below, are designed to meet the needs of identified groups.

---

18   Larson, Sharma et al. 2019.
19   Menzies School of Health Research and One21seventy 2015.
20   The feedback tools and toolkit can be downloaded: https://www.racgp.org.au/.

Developing an Indigenous-specific client-reported experience measure for Aboriginal and Torres Strait Islander peoples accessing PHC

Culturally secure and positive care experiences are critical for improving the health outcomes of Aboriginal and Torres Strait Islander peoples in Australia. PHC services are required to gather client feedback to meet accreditation requirements. But the currently available and endorsed tools have not been developed or validated with Aboriginal and Torres Strait Islander peoples, and do not reflect their values, beliefs and world views. Consequently, existing tools do not adequately capture important experiences of care in Indigenous PHC settings, and do not return information that is useful for improving health service delivery.

A collaborative research project is enabling health services, researchers and communities to develop and validate a culturally appropriate client-reported experience measure for urban, rural and remote PHC settings. The research integrates Indigenous and Western knowledge systems and research approaches with participatory action research to develop a product that meets accreditation standards and is acceptable and feasible for use with Aboriginal and Torres Strait Islander clients.

This tool will enable PHC services to respond to priorities and perspectives of the people in their communities, to improve the quality of care they provide, improve health outcomes and reduce inequities in health and wellbeing experienced by Indigenous Australians.[21]

Information about this work is available from the VOICE Project.[22]

Tools for health promotion

CQI in health promotion is less developed than in clinical health care. The shortage of CQI tools for health promotion reflects the relatively limited evidence about effective health promotion activities, compared with the evidence available about best-practice clinical care for specific health conditions. Consequently, developing a tool to audit clinical care may be relatively straightforward compared with developing a tool to measure the quality of a health promotion initiative and whether there has been behaviour change in a population.

> CQI in health promotion is less developed than CQI in clinical health care.

The lack of evidence about effective health promotion is often perpetuated by the limited documentation of health promotion activities (successful or otherwise). This also provides challenges for improving health promotion practice through CQI: it can lead to duplication

---

21   Chakraborty, Walke et al. 2023.
22   CRE-STRIDE n.d.

of effort and repetition of activities that may have little or no positive effect, and an inability to scale up effective health promotion interventions.[23]

The following strategies for addressing the limited availability of tools and processes for CQI in health promotion are suggested:

- Design your own process based on core CQI principles and concepts. Involve PHC team members, leaders and health service users; use a systematic process guided by data; use systems thinking to design improvement strategies around the local context; use repeated cycles of development and testing. CQI is about ongoing learning and improvement – and aspirations – so start with the health promotion data you have available (see "Types and sources of data" in Chapter 4).
- Seek out resources that have been developed for evaluating health promotion programs. Evaluation design, tools and methods may be adaptable for CQI.
- Link with others who have an interest in improving health promotion practice to share CQI resources, ideas and learning.
- Check international and local developments in this emerging area of PHC quality improvement, particularly innovations in health promotion CQI that are specific to your program setting or population.

Several CQI tools based on evidence about best-practice health promotion are described below. All of the tools, with accompanying protocols, can be downloaded and used for no cost.

Health promotion audit tool

The health promotion audit tool was developed through a research project investigating the acceptability and feasibility of using an audit-and-feedback technique to improve the quality of health promotion activities in Indigenous PHC. The tool development process included reviewing relevant guidelines, using expert consensus and testing CQI processes with PHC teams. The resulting health promotion audit tool was designed to capture information about five best-practice criteria:

- comprehensive planning
- systematic targeting
- community participation
- partnerships
- evaluation.[24]

These best-practice criteria apply across specific health promotion topics, making this a versatile tool for assessing the quality of health promotion activities.

The documentation of health promotion activities is often less systematic than the documentation of clinical care, so it is useful to complete a pre-audit information sheet to list the type of records and sources of information that can be used to complete an audit of health promotion activities. The health promotion audit tool, audit tool protocol and supporting resources are available to download.[25]

---

23   Percival, O'Donoghue et al. 2016.
24   O'Donoghue, Percival et al. 2014.
25   Download from https://www.menzies.edu.au/page/Resources/Health_Promotion_CQI_Tools/.

Health promotion systems assessment tool

The health promotion systems assessment tool[26] is designed to assess how the systems that support health promotion are working in a PHC service. The tool captures information about these areas: the service delivery system; information systems and decision support; the organisational environment; and the adaptability and integration of systems for health promotion. Items within these four system components (see Table 5.5) are scored and justified using a consensus approach to reach an overall score for each component. The scores are used to map system capacity for health promotion. This information is used by PHC teams to set goals and plan strategies to improve the quality of health promotion practice.

Table 5.5 Components and items assessed using the health promotion systems assessment tool.

System components	Items scored
Service delivery system	Access and cultural competence Programs and services Team structure and function
Information systems and decision support	Community links and participation Evidence-based tools and guidelines Maintenance and use of health information systems Systematic planning and monitoring
Organisational environment	Organisational commitment Organisational culture Organisational leadership
Adaptability and integration of systems for health promotion	Adaptability of systems Integration of systems

A health promotion systems assessment information sheet, systems assessment tool and systems assessment scoring form are available to download.[27]

Tobacco control audit tool

The tobacco control audit tool[28] is an example of a health promotion CQI tool developed to address a specific health risk factor. As with clinical auditing, this approach works well when the evidence for addressing a specific risk factor is well documented, as is the case for tobacco use. The tool can assist with data collection and monitoring, and improve responses to targeted public health policy initiatives.

---

26   One21seventy and Menzies School of Health Research 2012.
27   Download from https://www.menzies.edu.au/page/Resources/Health_Promotion_CQI_Tools/.
28   One21seventy and Heart Foundation 2016.

The tobacco control audit tool captures information on these factors:

- current and past smokers registered with the primary healthcare service
- smoking cessation support
- smoke-free policies
- smoke-free spaces
- social marketing
- systems and processes for staff and community involvement in tobacco control.

PHC teams and community groups can use the information to inform local improvement strategies.

The tobacco control audit tool, audit tool protocol and supporting resources are available to download.[29] A further tobacco control guide and supporting evidence were developed for Aboriginal and Torres Strait Islander communities in Australia's Northern Territory, as described in the box.[30]

Developing a comprehensive CQI approach for tobacco control

Reducing smoking and the harm it causes is one of Australia's public health success stories. Smoking rates have consistently declined among the Aboriginal and Torres Strait Islander community for over two decades, but smoking is still nearly three times as common compared with other Australians, and improvements in smoking rates have mainly occurred in urban areas. However, Aboriginal and Torres Strait Islander peoples who live in remote communities also now smoke fewer cigarettes. Fewer young people are taking up smoking and more children are living in smoke-free homes.

The Tobacco Working Group of the Northern Territory Aboriginal Health Forum in Australia is developing a system-wide, comprehensive approach to tobacco control to build on these successes. The group drew on evidence of what is working to help smokers to quit and consultations with health staff to develop a CQI guide underpinned by seven key principles. The principles relate to Aboriginal involvement; engagement of leadership; staff capacity building; making sure activities reach as many people as possible; making sure activities are at sufficient intensity to support behaviour change; the use of CQI processes; and the need for activities to focus mainly on three factors:

- marketing and messaging
- smoke-free spaces
- tobacco control as part of routine clinical care.

---

29   Download from https://www.menzies.edu.au/page/Resources/Tobacco_Control_Audit_Tool/.
30   Northern Territory Aboriginal Health Forum 2021; Thomas 2020. Download from http://amsant.org.au/tobacco-control/.

Local PHC teams innovate and adapt improvement activities to suit their communities. In the Katherine region, four PHC services came together to develop a collaborative regional CQI approach, the Big Rivers Early Action on Tobacco for Health, or BREATH. At the initial workshop, staff from each service used the guide to develop plan-do-study-act cycles in the three main areas of focus. Since then, representatives from the services have met monthly to reflect on progress, share resources, set their goals and plan improvement tasks for the next month.

Momentum is maintained in several ways. Tasks reflect what is achievable in each PHC service, their priorities and capacity: for example, around outbreak, epidemic or pandemic management. Monthly meetings keep members engaged and have flexible formats, including video conferencing. Improvement processes are supported by CQI facilitators, and the tobacco project officer and researcher based at the central PHC support organisation (Aboriginal Medical Services Alliance Northern Territory). Peers provide support and inspiration. For example, the discussions of work on smoke-free signage, spaces and events initiated by one service might inspire ideas used in planning at another service, which eventually lead to different locally relevant smoke-free activities by the second service. These are shared and the cycle continues.

– David Thomas and Theresa Paterson, Aboriginal Medical Services Alliance Northern Territory.

Download the Tobacco Control Guide at http://amsant.org.au/tobacco-control/.

Good Food Systems Planning Tool

Food insecurity is complex. It has many determinants and is experienced differently in different countries and contexts. Generally, food security can be increased and sustained by attending to the determinants of food insecurity at the community and population level. Social and economic inequalities result in food insecurity being a health and wellbeing issue for many Aboriginal and Torres Strait Islander peoples. The Good Food Systems Planning Tool[31] was developed to engage remote Australian communities in collectively planning and improving local food systems.

The Good Food Systems Planning Tool is designed to include food supply stakeholders in annual cycles of continuous improvement to move towards agreed nutrition and food security goals. Consistent with principles of comprehensive PHC, these stakeholders might include food wholesalers and retailers, freight companies, the health service, the community school, aged care and disability services, local government and community members.

The components of the tool were informed by best available evidence and local knowledge.

---

31   Brimblecombe 2014.

They encompass five domains:

- buildings, public places and transport
- community and services
- food businesses
- leadership and partnerships
- traditional food and local food production.[32]

The good food planning tool and supporting resources are available to download.[33]

Developing the Good Food Systems Planning Tool

The Good Food Systems Planning Tool was developed and tested using a participatory action research approach with four Aboriginal and Torres Strait Islander communities in northern and central Australia.

At annual planning meetings in the participating communities, facilitators used participatory methods with groups of people who had different interests in the food supply: families, store managers and staff, and health, education and other service providers. The carefully structured process had these aims:

- create a vision for the community food system
- map the food system and identify food-related activities, services and programs
- appraise the performance of these against improvement goals, using a good food planning tool
- consider current food purchasing using store sales data
- develop an action plan to improve food security and community nutrition.

Quarterly meetings were held to update activities and monitor progress in each community.

This CQI approach has shown potential to shift community diet. Links with high-level policy- and decision-makers, clear stakeholder roles and responsibilities, and processes to prioritise and communicate actions across sectors are needed.[34] Further work is developing a benchmarking approach to support healthy food stores in remote communities.

---

32   Brimblecombe, van den Boogaard et al. 2015.
33   Download from https://www.menzies.edu.au/page/Resources/Good_food_planning_tool/ and https://www.menzies.edu.au/page/Resources/Good_Food_Systems_Information_Sheets/.
34   Brimblecombe, Bailie et al. 2017.

Tools and techniques to visualise the systems and processes

In the rest of this chapter, we describe more CQI tools that are likely to be effective for engaging PHC teams with data to develop improvement initiatives. They are particularly useful for visualising systems and processes.

Flowcharts (process mapping)

A flowchart is developed through process mapping and provides a systematic, visual display of how a process works. It is a map of steps and decisions made in a process, the order in which these steps and decisions happen, who is involved and the connections between steps. This makes a flowchart useful for systems thinking. It shows staff how complex and interrelated their work is, and how their part in a process affects others.[35]

Flowcharts may be simple or complex, depending on the improvement purpose. A simple flowchart may provide an overview, for example, of how clients move through care processes at the PHC centre (Figure 5.1). A more detailed flowchart may specify who and what processes are involved at each step in the client's journey, how processes are completed and where each step occurs.

The process of collectively developing a flowchart (for example, using sticky notes and discussing scenarios) can provide insight into how clients experience care and can also support teamwork. Input from staff in different roles and from clients is more likely to produce a realistic flowchart and support client-centred changes in care processes.[36]

The flowchart may reveal that a process does not operate the way staff or management think it does. Arriving at a common understanding helps the group to identify where there may be opportunities to improve care systems, and what needs to change.

Checklists

For CQI purposes, a checklist is usually a time-ordered list of process activities, often developed from a flowchart. Checklists are frequently used in routine care to support the delivery of comprehensive care routines. Each listed process activity or task is checked off by a team member when it is complete, making it easier to track and coordinate care processes between different practitioners and to see when a task has been missed. Examples in PHC are checklists of care items that need to be completed as part of an antenatal check, a well-baby check, and triage checklists used for determining the degree of urgency of wounds or illnesses when a client presents at the health centre.

Checklists can help teams to implement care routines in line with best-practice guidelines. They specify each task that needs to be completed, promote communication within and between teams in the same PHC setting, and reinforce the importance of everyone's role in providing care. Use of checklists can reduce potential for errors and potentially lead to better care experiences and outcomes for clients.

Where records are kept of completed care for clients and then collated and analysed for CQI purposes, checklists can help teams to identify persisting gaps in routine care and to see whether changes made as part of a CQI program have improved workflow and team coordination.

---

35   Point of Care Foundation n.d.
36   Grazia, Laura et al. 2021.

Cause-and-effect (Ishikawa or fishbone) diagrams

A cause-and-effect diagram, also called an Ishikawa or fishbone diagram, is a simple graphic tool used to explore and display the possible causes of variation in quality of care, or a quality problem. It was first devised in the 1960s by Kaoru Ishikawa, a Japanese quality management pioneer.

A cause-and-effect diagram is used for these purposes:

- helping teams understand that there are many causes that contribute to an effect
- graphically displaying the relationship of the causes to the effect and to each other
- identifying the main factors that are contributing to gaps in care
- identifying priority areas for improvement.[37]

The primary axis or "spine" of a cause-and-effect diagram is an arrow leading to the effect – the variation in care or the quality problem to be addressed. The problem is written on the right-hand side of the diagram, representing the head of the fish. After a team has brainstormed the possible causes for the variation or problem, the facilitator helps the group to sort ideas into categories of contributing causes. These categories form the main ribs of the fish, which branch off the central spine. Commonly used categories to clarify quality problems in health care include client, provider, policies and procedures, physical environment/equipment, system and organisational culture.[38] Figure 5.2 is a simple cause-and-effect diagram exploring possible causes for low rates of foot screening among clients with diabetes.[39]

Another level of analysis could be added to this diagram, asking "why does this happen?" for each identified cause. This would help to establish the root causes or "drivers" of a problem. This diagram could also be expanded to include further detail about steps in the care process or protocol (for example, client recall) and possible barriers to completing each step to a high-quality standard (for example, an outdated contact list is a possible barrier to client recall).

> The process of developing the cause-and-effect diagram allows everyone in the PHC team to be involved.

While this simple tool has limitations for illustrating and understanding the complex interactions within PHC systems, the process of developing the cause-and-effect diagram allows everyone in the PHC team to be involved. It promotes the use of systems thinking before planning change. Once a diagram is completed, the team uses focus questions to make sense of the information. For example, are there causes identified for each rib on the fish? What do gaps tell us about care delivery systems and how we view them? Which causes are or are not supported by evidence? Which causes have most effect on clients? Other CQI tools may be used to answer some of these questions and to focus improvement efforts, such as Pareto diagrams (described below).

---

37   Institute for Healthcare Improvement 2017.
38   Halperin, Gilmour et al. 2019.
39   Halperin, Gilmour et al. 2019.

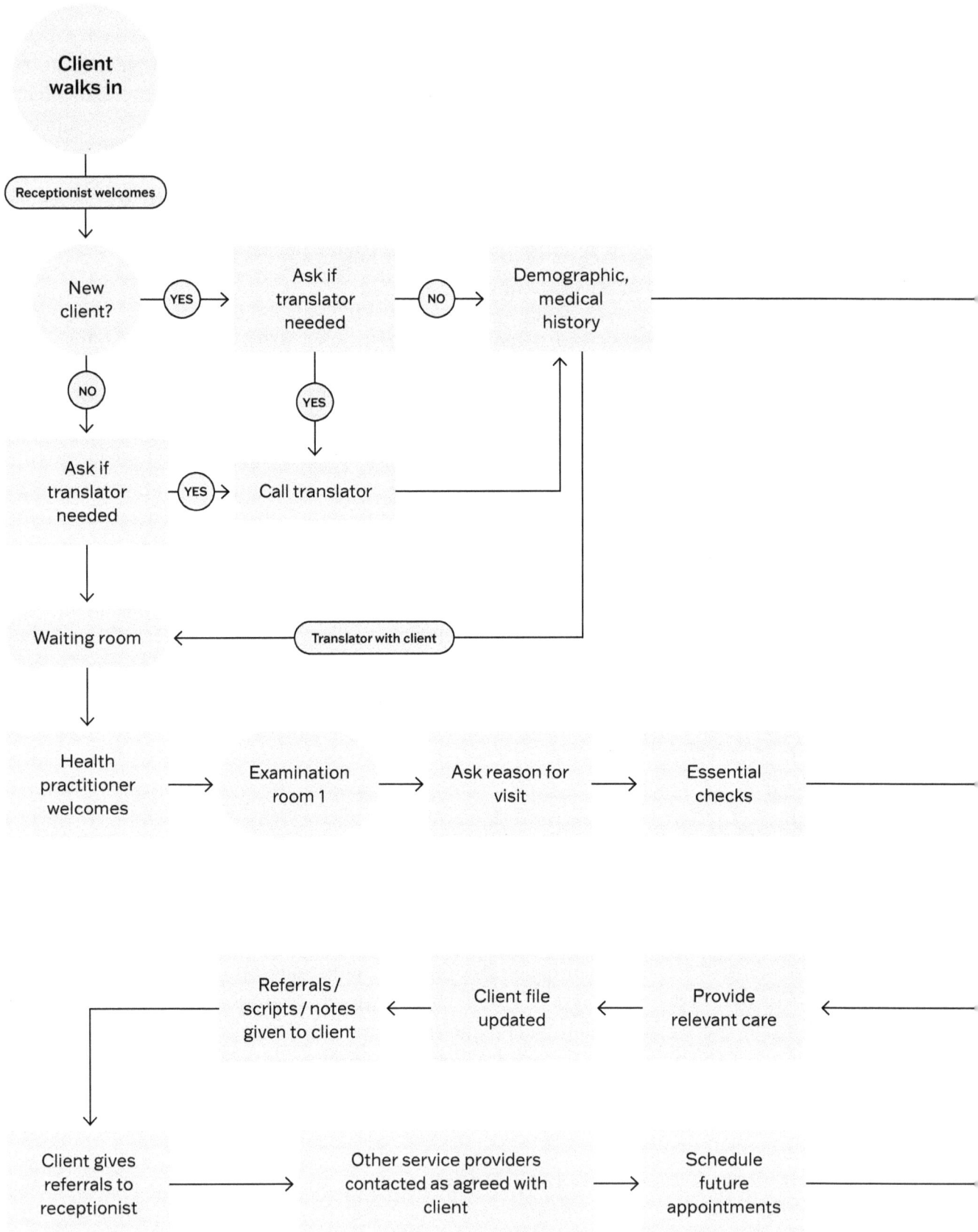

Figure 5.1 Example of client flow through a PHC centre.

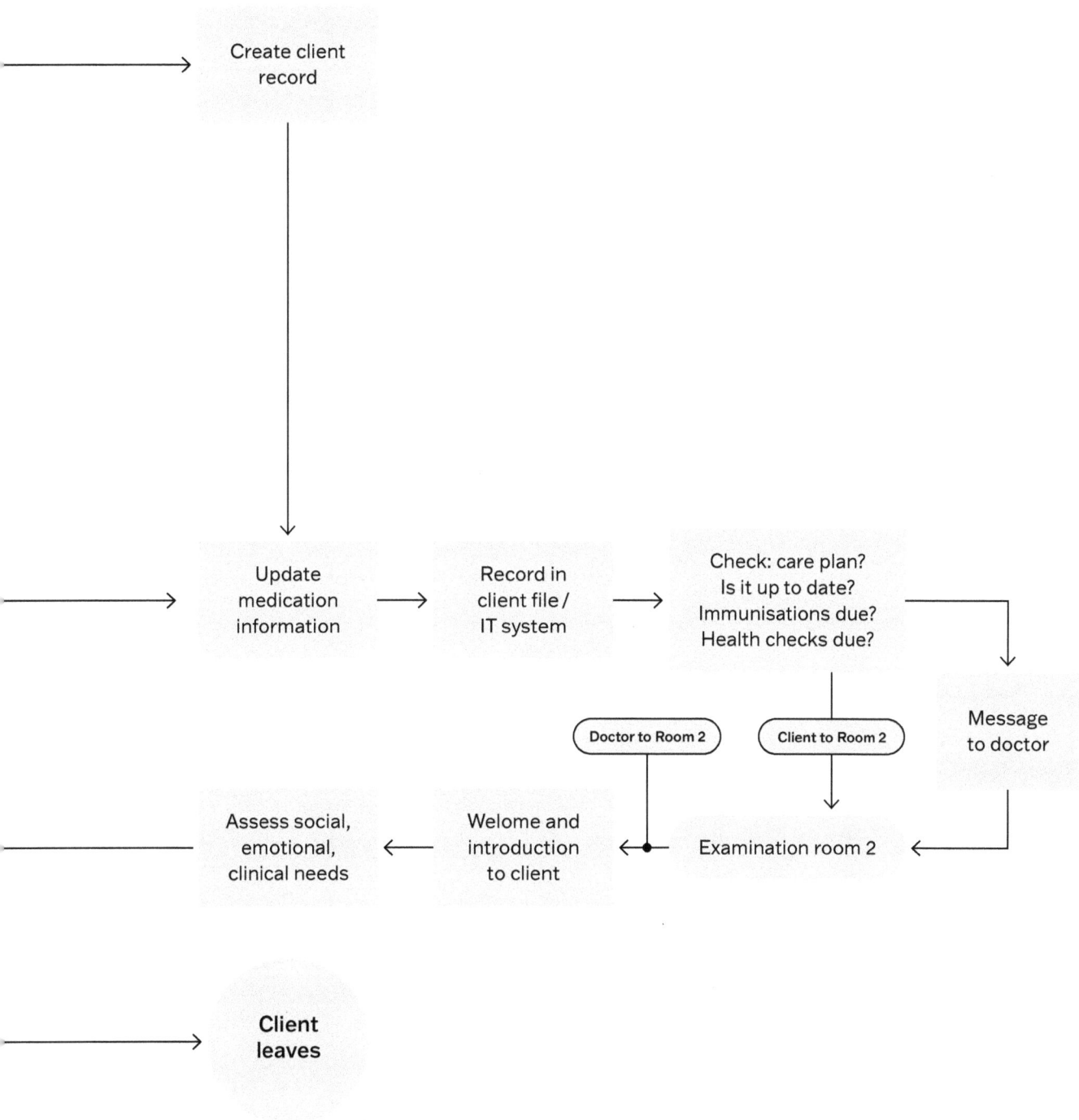

Create client record

Update medication information

Record in client file / IT system

Check: care plan?
Is it up to date?
Immunisations due?
Health checks due?

Message to doctor

Doctor to Room 2

Client to Room 2

Assess social, emotional, clinical needs

Welome and introduction to client

Examination room 2

Client leaves

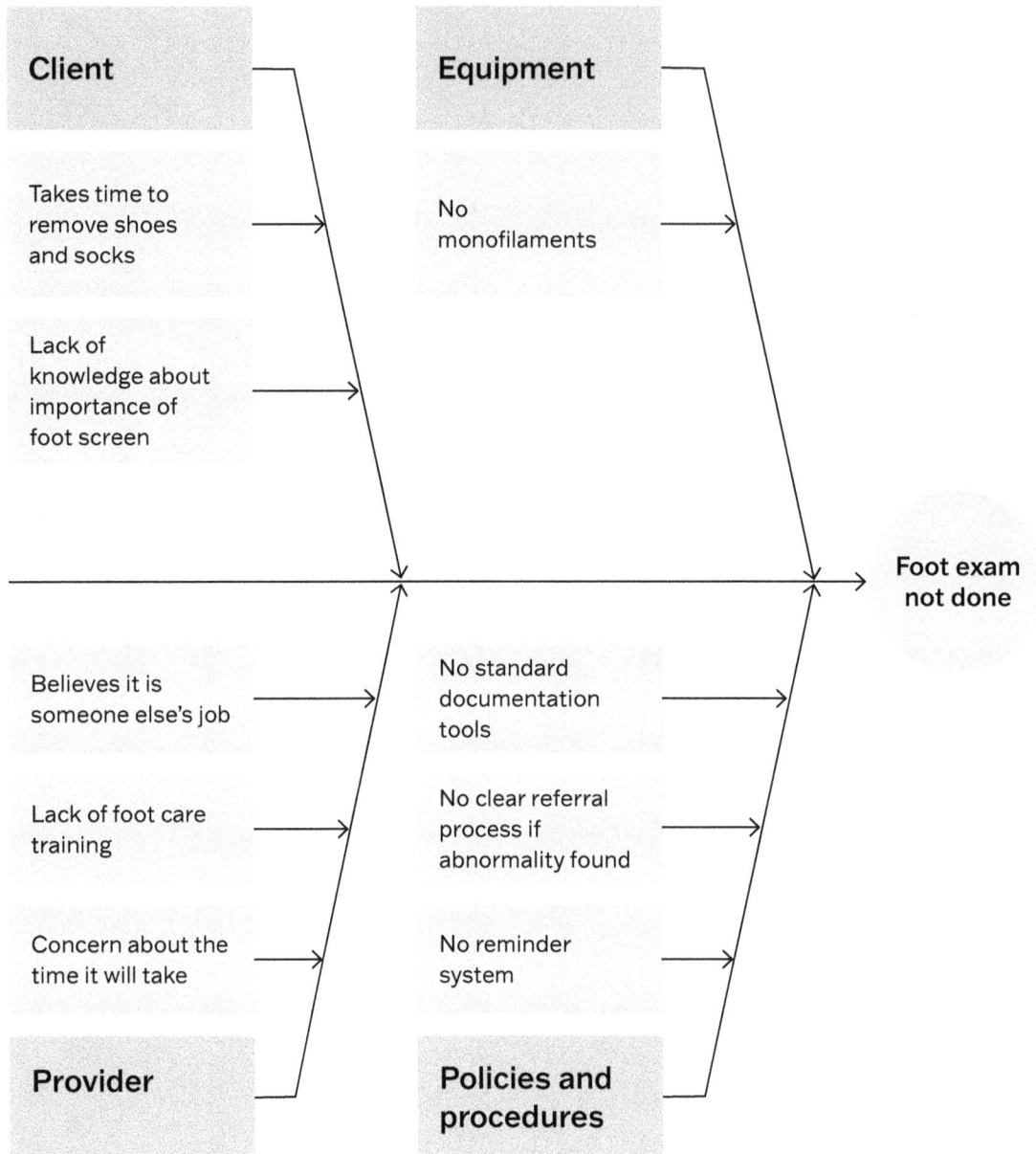

Figure 5.2 Example of a cause-and-effect diagram showing why clients with diabetes may not be receiving important items of care, namely foot examinations. Source: Halperin, Gilmour et al. 2019.

Driver diagrams

A driver diagram, or "action effect diagram",[40] is a visual tool for identifying opportunities to improve care systems and processes. It "visually represents a shared theory of how things might be better, building upon knowledge gleaned from research, observation and experience".[41] By setting out causal pathways between an improvement aim and the primary and secondary "drivers" for achieving the aim, a driver diagram can be used for these two purposes:

---

40   Reed, McNicholas et al. 2014.
41   Bennett and Provost 2015, 36.

- identify causes that underly variation in care
- systematically plan and test an improvement initiative to address the causes through tailored interventions.

A driver diagram is intended to be a living document that is updated as the PHC team builds and tests theories of improvement using, for example, plan-do-study-act cycles.[42]

> A driver diagram is intended to be a living document that is updated as the PHC team builds and tests theories of improvement.

A driver diagram usually includes the following columns:

- *aim* – the agreed improvement aim, or what you are trying to achieve. The aim should be high-level but specific enough to guide and evaluate an improvement initiative. For example, "Improve delivery of care to address identified gaps in chronic illness care".
- *primary drivers* – the main contributing causes of variation in care. These are the system components that you need to influence, to achieve the aim. For example, if your aim is "Improve delivery of care to address identified gaps in chronic illness care", one main cause of variation (a primary driver) may be the "availability and use of clinical information systems and decision support tools".
- *secondary drivers* – the factors or causes that contribute to the primary drivers. Several secondary drivers are likely to contribute to each primary driver (drawn using "relationship arrows"). For example, if a primary driver is "availability and use of clinical information systems and decision support tools", secondary drivers may include "training of staff in effective use of clinical information systems" and "functionality and user-friendliness of clinical information systems".
- *change ideas/interventions* – evidence-based change concepts or interventions to address the secondary drivers: that is, what you are going to do and how you are going to do it. For example, to improve "functionality and user-friendliness of clinical information systems", a PHC service would implement a range of strategies, such as: "ensure the information system is up-to-date, and client recall and reminder lists are maintained" and "encourage and support visiting specialists to enter information about clients' care into the local clinical information system".[43]

Each change idea should contribute to at least one secondary driver. Teams may develop SMART goals and action plans (see Chapter 6) to implement interventions, which are often tested and tailored using plan-do-study-act cycles. Some driver diagrams prioritise change ideas. This is done by determining whether the change is likely to have a high or low impact on the aim, and whether it will be easy or difficult to implement.[44] Addressing all of the identified secondary drivers should be sufficient to achieve the improvement aim.

---

42   Bennett and Provost 2015.
43   Bailie, Laycock et al. 2016.
44   Clinical Excellence Commission n.d.

Reading a driver diagram from left to right answers the question "What changes can we make that will result in an improvement?" Reading the diagram from right to left answers the question, "What are we trying to accomplish through these interventions?"

Developing a driver diagram can be a way of encouraging people in different roles to agree on some common goals and priorities. It supports systems thinking by encouraging PHC teams to explore the many factors that affect quality of care and how they are connected. The process helps to identify key leverage points in the system, and how activities and changes link to system components. These insights are helpful for measuring and monitoring improvement. A driver diagram can also be extended to develop a detailed program theory that includes aims, contributing factors, interventions, implementation activities and how the effectiveness of planned interventions will be measured.[45]

Figure 5.3 shows part of a driver diagram we developed following a wide-scale stakeholder survey about ways to improve the delivery of chronic illness care. Our study sought to identify drivers and change ideas at different levels of the health system. One of five primary drivers identified by survey respondents was "community capacity, engagement and mobilisation for health".[46]

A simple driver diagram template can be downloaded from the Institute for Healthcare Improvement website. See the Quality Improvement Essentials Toolkit.[47]

Pareto diagrams

Pareto diagrams are a data-analysis tool for identifying what matters most for improving the quality of care. It is useful for understanding variation (which is explained in Chapter 6). Named after a 17th-century Italian economist, Pareto analysis is based on the principle that 80 per cent of consequences (for example, gaps in best-practice care) come from just 20 per cent of causes. Identifying these "vital few" causes enables PHC teams to focus improvement efforts for maximum impact.

> A Pareto diagram is used for identifying what matters most for improving the quality of care.

A Pareto diagram is a frequency chart with the columns arranged from the longest (most frequently observed or recorded items) on the left of the horizontal (x) axis to the shortest (least frequent items) on the right. For example, the items might be errors or gaps in care identified in a clinical audit, causes of system problems identified by staff, or results of a client survey. The vertical (y) axis shows the number of times the item or event occurred. A cumulative percentage line is then drawn showing the added contribution of each item (with the cumulative percentage scale usually recorded on the right-hand side of the diagram). A horizontal line is drawn at the 80-per-cent mark to intersect the cumulative percentage line. The items to the left of where these lines intersect are the "vital few" factors that warrant

---

45   Reed, McNicholas et al. 2014.

46   Bailie, Laycock et al. 2016.

47   Institute for Healthcare Improvement 2017. Download from http://www.ihi.org/resources/tools/quality-improvement-essentials-toolkit.

the most attention. In principle, addressing these items will create the most improvement in quality of care.

Figure 5.4 charts the results of a survey to find out why clients did not attend their appointments. In our example, the reason given most frequently was lack of transport to get to the PHC service, followed by forgetting the appointment. The least reported reasons were being unable to get time off work or being away. For the Pareto analysis, a cumulative percentage line was drawn by adding on the number of clients who gave each reason, starting with the largest group. A horizontal line was then drawn to intersect the line at the 80-percent mark. Four "vital few" reasons were identified. The analysis suggested that focusing on transport needs, and systems for appointment scheduling and reminders would significantly improve attendance. A change in clinic opening hours may also warrant attention.

Pareto analysis can be useful for building team consensus to prioritise improvement action. Pareto analysis can also be applied to data at scale to inform policy directions and strategic planning to improve care. We used Pareto analysis to identify the "vital few" barriers to wide-scale system improvement in PHC, following investigation of stakeholders' views on system barriers to improving PHC. Our example of applied Pareto analysis is described in Chapter 20.

Run charts

A run chart is a simple tool for observing and understanding variation in quality of care over time. Data about process performance are gathered and displayed over time, enabling teams to observe patterns in the data. This may help to relate variation to changes in systems, care processes or the health service environment. Run charts can also be used to monitor changes in quality of care resulting from an improvement program, and whether improvements are sustained.

While conventionally used in healthcare settings with high client and staff numbers, such as hospitals, run charts can be useful for providing information about care processes in PHC settings. Examples might include the charting of how long clients wait to see a clinician or charting the percentage of clients who receive an examination recommended as part of best-practice care. When a planned change results in improvement (for example, a higher percentage of clients received the recommended examination), we would expect the median line of the run chart to shift.

Notes and arrows can be added to a run chart to show where change strategies have been tested (for example, using plan-do-study-act cycles), or to explain shifts or trends. Adding this information can help the team to understand patterns in the data and to plan change strategies. If an upward or downward "run" on a chart (a trend of 5 or more points) occurs without a deliberate change being made (for example, if average client waiting time continued to increase each week, or more examinations were missed), this would indicate a need to investigate and attend to the possible causes. By graphically displaying how well (or poorly) a process is working, a run chart may help the team to develop improvement aims, see the effect of changes, see whether changes are truly improvements and inform the refinement of ongoing improvement work.

A run chart may help the team see the effect of changes and whether changes are truly improvements.

Aim	Primary drivers	Secondary drivers
		Levels of health literacy and health-related behaviour in the community
Improve delivery of care to address priority evidence practice gaps in chronic illness care	Community capacity, engagement and mobilisation for health	Strength of links between the local health service and the community
		Level of cultural awareness among staff

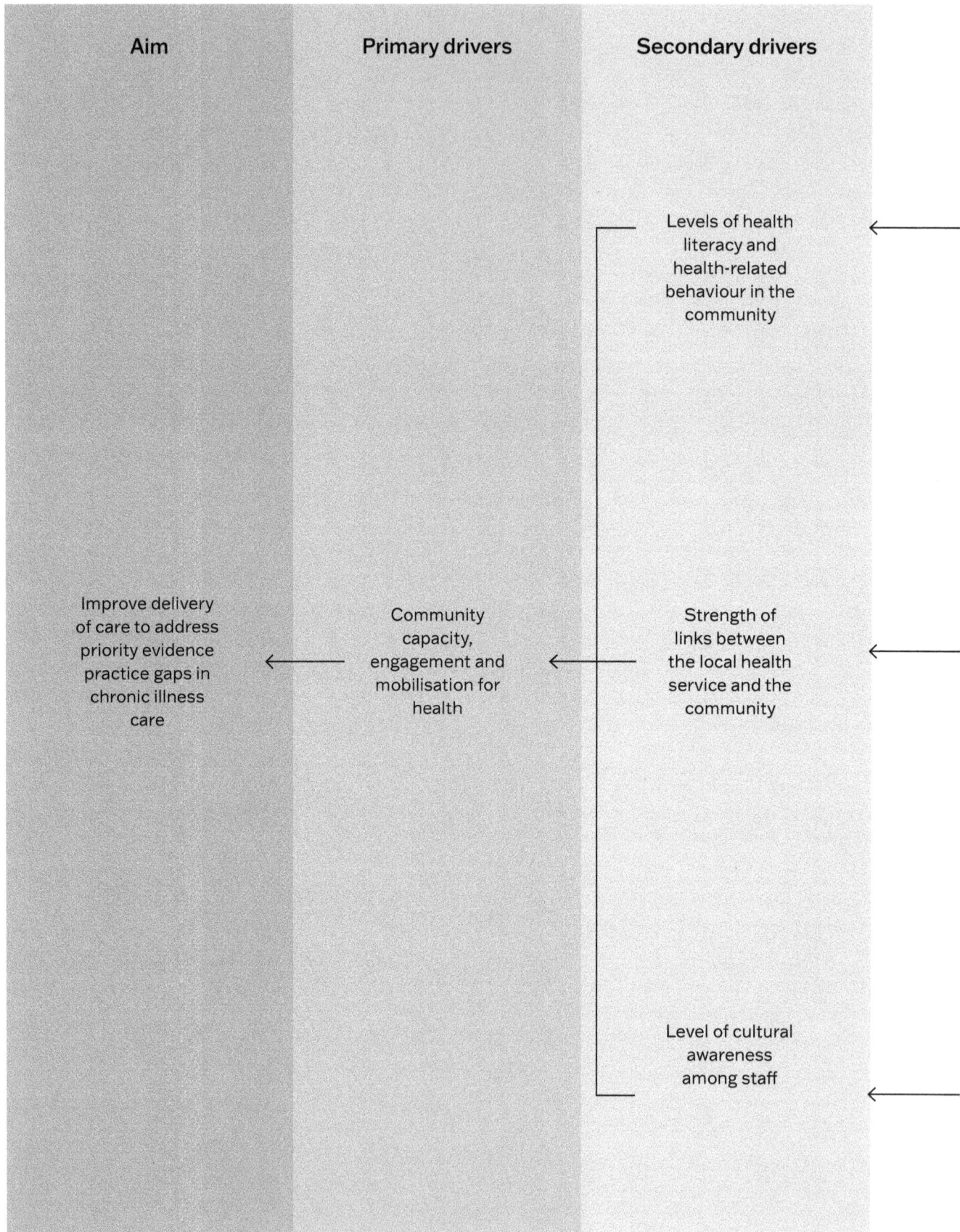

Figure 5.3 Example elements from a driver diagram. Source: Adapted with permission from Bailie, Laycock et al. 2016.

Change ideas/strategies

Literacy support for community members to complete necessary forms

Community awareness raising on when to seek care and self-management

Provide training for allied health teams to educate and inform families about health-related issues such as self-management, brief intervention and when to seek care

Identify and encourage initiatives that have improved community engagement

Develop and encourage use of metrics of success to improve community engagement

A community collaborative to share success on building links with communities

Cultural awareness program to assist health teams to value and respect contributions of Indigenous team members

Employment of more Indigenous staff

Consider how to provide services to visiting clients, including effective follow-up where required

Support community outreach initiatives from the health service

Strengthen cultural awareness training, including attention to issues affecting use of health services, client-centred care, clinical inertia

Ensure all staff attend cultural awareness training

Staff induction on what life is like in remote communities

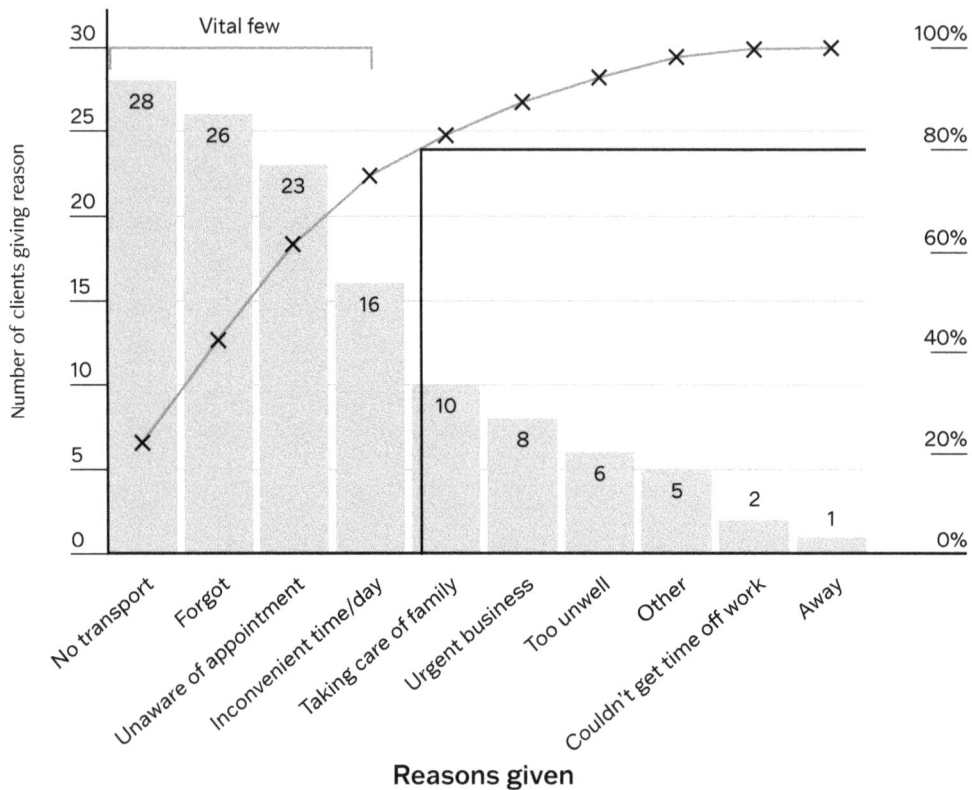

Figure 5.4 Pareto diagram example: reasons clients gave for not attending appointments.

Figure 5.5 charts the average time clients spent in the waiting room of a PHC practice. Long wait times can be a barrier to clients accessing PHC. In this hypothetical example, wait times were recorded and averaged each week for 10 weeks by the health centre receptionists. A run chart was developed, displaying a median wait time of 70 minutes. In response, a new appointment system was trialled. Recording and charting wait times for a further 10 weeks showed that the new appointment system led to greatly reduced wait times (median 25 minutes) and should be continued and refined.

A guide on using run charts in PHC has been developed by the United Kingdom Royal College of General Practitioners.[48] More advanced charting methods are available for teams seeking statistical rigour or reassurances that improvement is being sustained or the process is still in flux; your team could consider using a statistical process control chart for this purpose. The Institute for Healthcare Improvement's "Quality Improvement Essentials Toolkit" has guidance on using run charts and control charts.[49]

---

48   See https://gmpcb.org.uk/general-practice/gp-excellence/resources/rcgp-quick-guide-run-charts/.
49   Institute for Healthcare Improvement n.d.b.

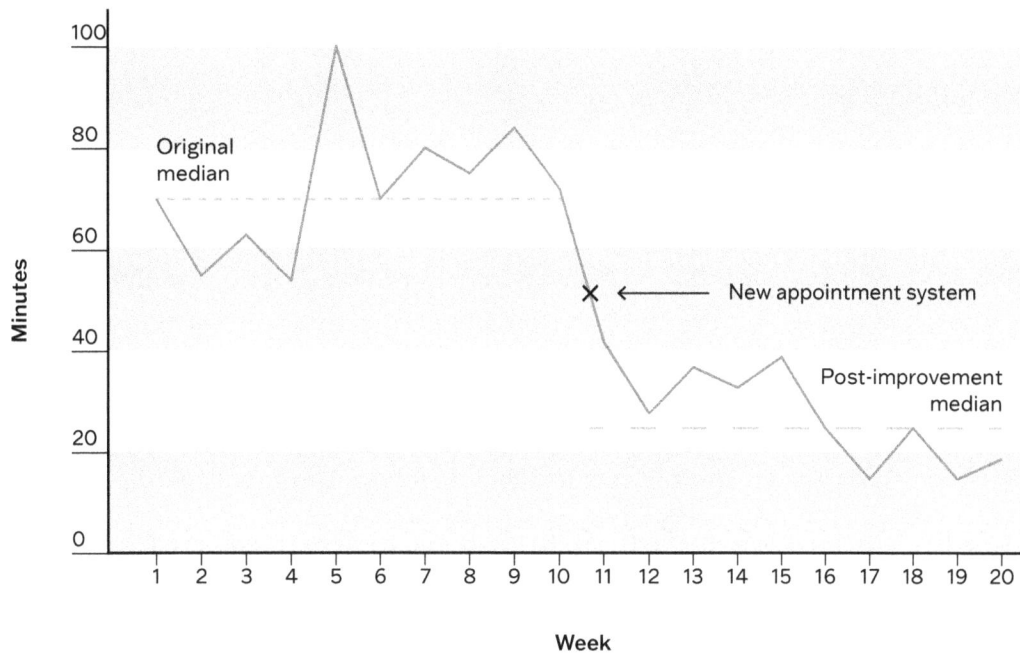

Figure 5.5 Run chart example: average client time in waiting room.

Use of continuous quality improvement tools

CQI tools should not be used in isolation; their use is only part of the CQI process or cycle. Different tools are used during different phases of the CQI cycle, as shown in Figure II.1 in the Part II Summary.

A CQI tool is typically used in these situations:

- in conjunction with other CQI tools – for example, a systems assessment tool may be used in conjunction with a clinical audit tool to assess the quality of diabetes care, with interpretation aided by information collected through a health centre and community survey
- as part of a CQI technique – for example, an audit tool is often used as part of "audit and feedback", a flowchart may be used as part of systems thinking
- to support a methodological approach, such as Lean or Six Sigma (see below).

In some cases, a PHC network or large health service may require the use of standardised tools as part of a system-wide approach to CQI and data management. This approach is useful for comparing the performance of your service or practice with others. It can be rewarding to know that your systems are working at a particularly high standard for your clients, and reassuring to know that other teams are experiencing a similar quality challenge. Importantly, such insights can start conversations between teams about what has worked well or not so well to improve care and can lead to the establishment of CQI collaboratives and other quality forums.

A continuous quality improvement tool is used as part of a continuous quality improvement process or cycle

Methodological approaches

Lean and Six Sigma methods

CQI tools may be used as part of a methodological approach to CQI. Lean and Six Sigma CQI methods originated in manufacturing industries in the 1980s and have become popular improvement approaches in health care. Lean focuses on eliminating waste in care processes through an ongoing system of improvement that adds value for clients (for example, by reducing wait times to see clinicians). It tends to be used to improve processes and workflows in large healthcare settings rather than for small changes to a care process or system.[50] Six Sigma is a data-driven system combining statistical analysis with quality management methods. It focuses on variation and is used to reduce client safety incidents (for example, incorrect diagnosis or treatment) and to remove defects from the processes involved in delivering care (for example, failing to follow up abnormal screening results).

Lean and Six Sigma are often used together in healthcare settings in a "Lean Six Sigma" approach. This approach uses five steps to improve care processes, as follows:

- *define* – clients, client needs and values, the process being measured, team objectives
- *measure* – identify data and metrics to measure improvement efforts
- *analyse* – collect and analyse data using proven techniques and tools (for example, clinical auditing, client surveys, systems assessment tools and other tools described in this chapter such as flowcharts, Pareto diagrams, cause-and-effect diagrams)
- *improve* – implement modifications to improve the process
- *control* – monitor performance to maintain improvement.

Lean Six Sigma has been found to be effective for improving care processes[51] but, to date, there is little reported use in PHC settings. Most publications in English describe studies conducted in the United States, mainly in hospital and specialist settings with the CQI objective of reducing demands on time (for example, through better client flow or shorter hospital stays), cost (for example, avoiding unnecessary procedures) or errors (for example, reducing medication errors, risk of infection).[52] There is need to investigate the use and effect of Lean and Six Sigma in PHC settings and in low- and middle-income countries, and to study the sustainability in implementing improvements based on these methods.[53]

Lean Six Sigma adopts widely used CQI tools and techniques (for example, clinical auditing, Pareto analysis). Use of these tools and techniques in your CQI program does not mean that you are using the Lean Six Sigma method. But your team may decide to use elements of Lean and Six Sigma approaches, such as removing a step that is perceived as wasteful in a client consultation process, to provide more time for other steps.

---

50   National Learning Consortium 2014.
51   Sollecito and Johnson 2019.
52   Niñerola, Sánchez-Rebull 2020.
53   Peimbert-García 2019.

Box 5.2 Questions to ask when considering the use of a CQI method

- Is there evidence that the CQI method is effective for improving PHC?

- Does use of the method require specialised training and additional resources? If so, are these available?

- Is the method suited to our PHC context?

- Will the method involve the whole team in learning and improvement?

- Does the method offer a systematic approach for implementing and sustaining improvement?

Summary

This chapter has presented some practical tools for improving the quality of PHC. They include tools for assessing care structures, conducting clinical audits, assessing systems, measuring client experiences of PHC, and for assessing health promotion. While developed for use in Australian PHC, they can be adapted for other settings or updated to reflect new evidence, treatments or technologies. We have also described some CQI tools for visualising PHC systems and processes. These tools can be used when engaging teams in collecting and analysing data, understanding variation in quality and planning improvement. CQI tools need to be selected based on the improvement purpose, the PHC setting and team, and available data.

There is much potential for the development of further CQI tools for use in PHC, and of new ways to visualise and assess PHC systems and processes. Examples are tools that integrate different knowledge systems (for example, Western and Indigenous knowledges), tools and processes that reflect the way specific groups conceptualise health and quality of care, and CQI tools that respond to the health and wellbeing challenges related to climate change. CQI tools, like PHC, should be responsive to the needs and values of populations and settings and should aim to advance healthcare equity.

In the next chapter, we describe CQI cycles and discuss the presentation and analysis of CQI data. Useful websites for downloading CQI tools and templates are listed at the end of Part II.

References

Bailie, J., A. Laycock, V. Matthews and R. Bailie (2016). System-level action required for wide-scale improvement in quality of primary health care: synthesis of feedback from an interactive process to promote dissemination and use of aggregated quality of care data. *Frontiers in Public Health* 4: 86. DOI: 10.3389/fpubh.2016.00086.

Bennett, B. and L. Provost (2015). What's your theory? Driver diagram serves as tool for building and testing theories for improvement. *Quality Progress* July: 36–43.

Bonomi, A.E., E.H. Wagner, R.E. Glasgow and M. VonKorff (2002). Assessment of chronic illness care (ACIC): a practical tool to measure quality improvement. *Health Services Research* 37(3): 791–820. DOI:10.1111/1475-6773.00049.

Brimblecombe, J. (2014). Good food planning tool. Menzies School of Health Research. Darwin: Menzies School of Health Research. https://www.menzies.edu.au/page/Resources/Good_food_planning_tool/.

Brimblecombe, J., R. Bailie, C. van den Boogaard, B. Wood, S. Liberato, M. Ferguson et al. (2017). Feasibility of a novel participatory multi-sector continuous improvement approach to enhance food security in remote Indigenous Australian communities. *SSM – Population Health* 3(C): 566–76. DOI: 10.1016/j.ssmph.2017.06.002.

Brimblecombe, J., C. van den Boogaard, B. Wood, S.C. Liberato, J. Brown, A. Barnes et al. (2015). Development of the good food planning tool: a food system approach to food security in indigenous Australian remote communities. *Health Place* 34: 54–62. DOI: 10.1016/j.healthplace.2015.03.006.

Chakraborty, A. E. Walke, R. Bainbridge, R. Bailie, V. Matthews, S. Larkins et al. (2023). VOICE – validating outcomes by including consumer experience: a study protocol to develop a patient reported experience measure for Aboriginal and Torres Strait Islander peoples accessing primary health care. *International Journal of Environmental Research and Public Health* 20(357). DOI: 10.3390/ijerph20010357.

Clinical Excellence Commission (n.d.). Quality Improvement Tools: driver diagrams. https://www.cec.health.nsw.gov.au/Quality-Improvement-Academy/quality-improvement-tools.

CRE-STRIDE (n.d.). http://cre-stride.org.

Cunningham, F., S. Ferguson-Hill, V. Matthews and R. Bailie (2016). Leveraging quality improvement through use of the systems assessment tool in Indigenous primary health care services: a mixed methods study. *BMC Health Services Research* 16(1): 583. DOI: 10.1186/s12913-016-1810-y.

Doyle, C., L. Lennox and D. Bell (2013). A systematic review of evidence on the links between patient experience and clinical safety and effectiveness. *BMJ Open* 3(1): e001570. DOI: 10.1136/bmjopen-2012-001570.

Grazia, A., L. Laura, B. James, E. Liz and R. Julie (2021). Process mapping in healthcare: a systematic review. *BMC Health Services Research*. DOI: 10.21203/rs.3.rs-80631/v1.

Halperin, I., J. Gilmour, P. Segal, L. Sutton, R. Wong, L. Caplan et al. (2019). Determining root causes and designing change ideas in a quality improvement project. *Canadian Journal of Diabetes* 43(4): 241–8. DOI: 10.1016/j.jcjd.2019.03.001.

Institute for Healthcare Improvement (2017). Quality improvement essentials toolkit. http://www.ihi.org/resources/tools/quality-improvement-essentials-toolkit.

Institute of Medicine (2001). *Crossing the quality chasm: a new health system for the 21st century.* Washington, DC: National Academies Press. DOI: 10.17226/10027.

Larson, E., J. Sharma, M. Bohren and Ö. Tunçalp (2019). When the patient is the expert: measuring patient experience and satisfaction with care. *Bulletin of the World Health Organization* 97(8): 563–9. DOI: 10.2471/BLT.18.225201.

Menzies School of Health Research and One21seventy (2015). Consumer's perspective of the quality of care tool. https://www.menzies.edu.au/page/Resources/Consumer_s_Perspective_of_Quality_of_Care_Tool/.

Menzies School of Health Research & One21seventy (2014). *Health centre and community survey.* Darwin: Menzies School of Health Research.

Menzies School of Health Research and One21seventy (2013). Vascular and metabolic syndrome management clinical audit tool. https://www.menzies.edu.au/page/Resources/Vascular_and_Metabolic_Syndrome_Management/.

Menzies School of Health Research and One21seventy (2012). *Systems assessment tool – all client groups.* Darwin: Menzies School of Health Research.

Naqshbandi Hayward, M., J. Paquette-Warren, S. Harris and on behalf of the Forge Ahead Program Team (2016). Developing community-driven quality improvement initiatives to enhance chronic disease care in Indigenous communities in Canada: the FORGE AHEAD program protocol. *Health Research Policy and Systems* 14(1): 55. DOI: 10.1186/s12961-016-0127-y.

National Learning Consortium (2014). *Continuous quality improvement (CQI) strategies to optimize your practice: primer.* Washington, DC: Health Information Technology Research Center.

Niñerola, A., M. Sánchez-Rebull and A. Hernández-Lara (2020). Quality improvement in healthcare: Six Sigma systematic review. *Health Policy* 124(4): 438–45. DOI: 10.1016/j.healthpol.2020.01.002.

Northern Territory Aboriginal Health Forum (2021). *Tobacco control guide.* Darwin: Northern Territory Government & Aboriginal Medical Services Alliance NT (AMSANT).

O'Donoghue, L., N. Percival, A. Laycock, J. McCalman, K. Tsey, C. Armit et al. (2014). Evaluating Aboriginal and Torres Strait Islander health promotion activities using audit and feedback. *Australian Journal of Primary Health* 20(4): 339–44. DOI: http://dx.doi.org/10.1071/PY14048.

One21seventy and Heart Foundation (2016). *Tobacco control audit tool.* Menzies School of Health Research. Darwin: Menzies School of Health Research.

One21seventy and Menzies School of Health Research (2012). *Health promotion systems assessment tool.* Darwin: Menzies School of Health Research.

Peimbert-García, R. (2019). Analysis and evaluation of reviews on Lean and Six Sigma in health care. *Quality Management in Health Care* 28(4): 229–36. DOI: 10.1097/qmh.0000000000000226.

Peiris, D., A. Brown, M. Howard, B.A. Rickards, A. Tonkin, I. Ring et al. (2012). Building better systems of care for Aboriginal and Torres Strait Islander people: findings from the Kanyini health systems assessment. *BMC Health Services Research* 12(1): 369. DOI: 10.1186/1472-6963-12-369.

Percival, N., L. O'Donoghue, V. Lin, K. Tsey and R.S. Bailie (2016). Improving health promotion using quality improvement techniques in Australian Indigenous primary health care. *Frontiers in Public Health* 4: 53. DOI: 10.3389/fpubh.2016.00053.

Point of Care Foundation (n.d.). Patient and family-centred care toolkit. https://www.pointofcarefoundation.org.uk/resource/patient-family-centred-care-toolkit/.

Puszka, S., T. Nagel, V. Matthews, D. Mosca, R. Piovesan, A. Nori et al. (2015). Monitoring and assessing the quality of care for youth: developing an audit tool using an expert consensus approach. *International Journal of Mental Health Systems* 9(28): 1–12. DOI: 10.1186/s13033-015-0019-5.

Reed, J., C. McNicholas, T. Woodcock, L. Issen and D. Bell (2014). Designing quality improvement initiatives: the action effect method, a structured approach to identifying and articulating programme theory. *BMJ Quality and Safety* 23(12): 1040–8. DOI: 10.1136/bmjqs-2014-003103.

Sollecito, W. and J. Johnson (2019). *McLaughlin and Kaluzny's continuous quality improvement in health care.* Burlington, MA: Jones & Bartlett Learning.

Thomas, D. (2020). Tobacco control research evidence to monitor and support a comprehensive approach to tobacco control in NT health services. Darwin: Northern Territory Aboriginal Health Forum. http://www.amsant.org.au/tobacco-control/.

Ward, J., S. McGregor, R. Guy, A. Rumbold, L. Garton, B. Silver et al. (2013). STI in remote communities: improved and enhanced primary health care (STRIVE) study protocol: a cluster randomised controlled trial comparing "usual practice" STI care to enhanced care in remote primary health care services in Australia. *BMC Infectious Diseases* 13(1): 425. DOI: 10.1186/1471-2334-13-425.

World Health Organization (2002). *Innovative care for chronic conditions: building blocks for action: global report.* Geneva: World Health Organization.

Using CQI cycles, and understanding and presenting data

Continuous quality improvement (CQI) cycles are data-driven ongoing cycles of learning and improvement. The cycles enable participants to use data to identify quality improvement priorities, set improvement goals, identify causes of poor system quality, plan and implement change, and find out whether a change led to improvement. Our approach starts with the assumption that there is always scope for improvement in some aspect of care. But how should local teams identify priority areas for improvement? Knowledge of developments in best practice among clinical leaders, of concerns about delivery of certain aspects of care, of predominant health issues or "burden of disease" in the health service population, of priority health concerns for local communities, and of the findings of previous clinical audits should all contribute to identifying important areas for improvement (for example, in chronic illness care or in some specific aspect of care). Sometimes the focus of CQI cycles is determined at a higher system level – for example, based on key performance indicators across a group of PHC services or practices. In all cases it is imperative that the local health service teams understand the basis or rationale for selection of the priority area for improvement, as their work and engagement will be integral to achieving the desired goals.

The next step is to identify the most appropriate resources on best-practice care relevant to the identified priority area for improvement (for example, care as recommended in the best-practice guidelines for diabetes care for the service setting). From this starting point, PHC teams select an appropriate audit tool (or adapt an existing tool or develop a new tool if necessary) and conduct an audit to determine which elements of care are being delivered relatively well or not so well. Those that are being delivered less well then become the priorities for improvement efforts. The CQI cycle described in this chapter in based on this approach.

It is essential that the data used for CQI are fit for purpose and presented in ways that help PHC teams and other healthcare stakeholders to identify and understand variation in quality of care. This chapter introduces a CQI cycle developed for PHC settings. Each phase of the cycle is explained, using examples to illustrate key concepts and processes.

The CQI cycle

As discussed in Part I, PHC is holistic care that is complex in its scope and the way it is delivered. PHC providers are diverse, widely dispersed and, while relatively independent in their practice, work closely with other providers. In a PHC setting, a CQI initiative is likely to involve diverse health professionals, clients, community groups and people who work in sectors that influence the social, cultural and environmental determinants of health. It may involve an entire PHC centre or practice team, and other service providers, in using CQI cycles to implement system change and improve the quality of care.

Plan-do-study-act (or PDSA) cycles are commonly used in CQI to achieve a specific goal. Through applied CQI research (described in Part III), our research group adapted the conventional PDSA cycle for use at the PHC centre or program level.[1] The resulting CQI cycle can be implemented over an extended timeframe (for example, over an annual audit and systems assessment cycle) compared with rapid PDSA cycles (which are discussed later in this chapter in the context of implementing improvement strategies).

As mentioned in the chapter introduction, the adapted CQI cycle is used by PHC teams to identify what is working well and not so well to deliver care or PHC programs, to collectively identify priorities for improvement and to plan and implement targeted improvement strategies. Four phases are continuously repeated to achieve, sustain and build on quality improvement (Figure 6.1):

- data collection
- data analysis
- participatory interpretation, goal setting and action planning
- implementation.

Data collection

Measuring quality and improvement

The purpose of measuring quality and improvement is to support the team to identify improvement priorities and to set and achieve their quality improvement goals. Planned systematic measurement, through data collection, provides the information needed to answer the question, "How will we know that a change is an improvement?" (see Chapters 2 and 4), and to know whether an improvement goal is met. Measurement should be continuous, reflecting the nature of CQI cycles. There are various purposes and opportunities for data collection:

- An improvement initiative is often based on data collected as part of the routine operations of the PHC practice or service (for example, to meet reporting requirements). Even when this is the case, the team is likely to need detailed baseline data at the start of an improvement initiative (for example, clinical audit data), to determine where system changes are needed and to serve as a baseline or benchmark for measuring improvement.
- As improvement strategies are implemented, data are collected to measure changes (planned and unintended), and to show whether the team is on track to achieve the goal (for example, by using short plan-do-study-act cycles). Various types of data are

---

1   Bailie, Si et al. 2007.

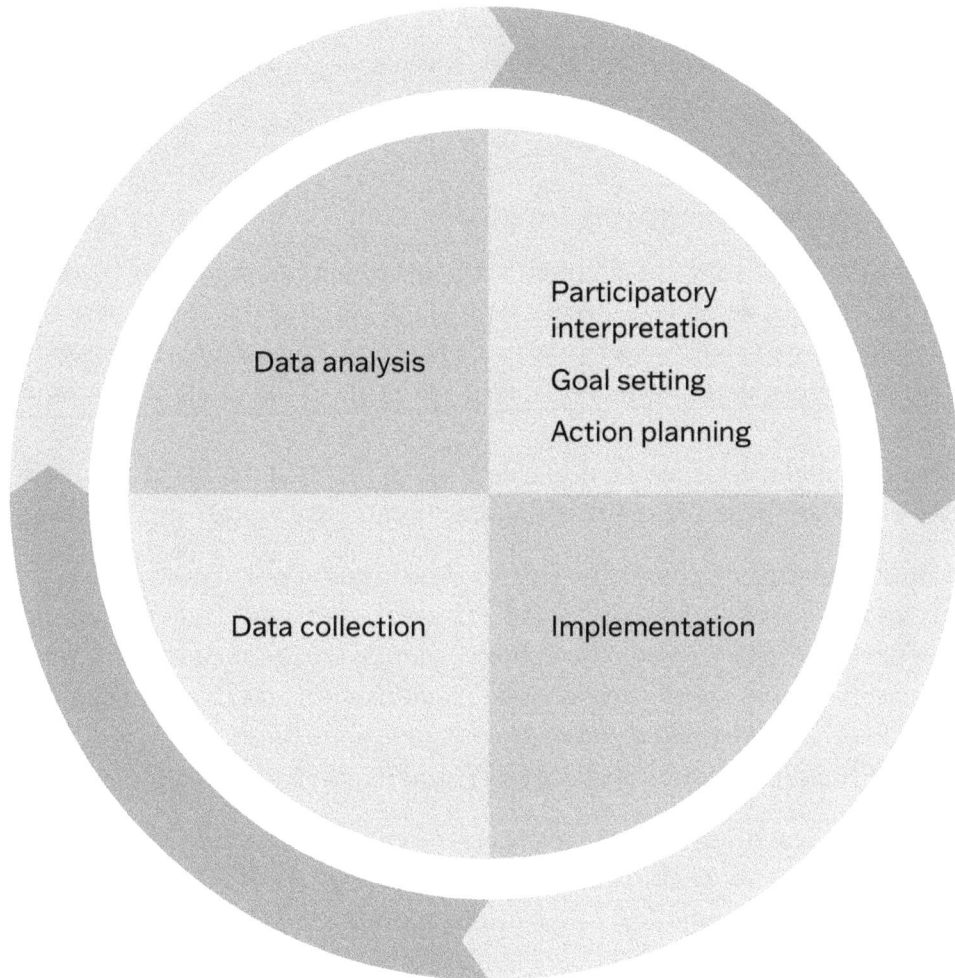

Figure 6.1 The CQI cycle in PHC. Source: Brands, Griffin et al. 2010; used with permission of Menzies School of Health Research.

collected and analysed to build a picture of what is changing and whether the changes are improvements. The learning gained is used to refine improvement strategies, or adjust goals and action plans, or both.

- Repeating the collection of data after a specific interval, using the same methods (for example, an annual clinical audit) shows what has been accomplished during the CQI cycle and identifies persistent gaps in care quality. This information is used for maintaining changes and for setting further goals and strategies for improvement.

What should be included in a plan for measuring improvement?

A plan for measuring improvement should specify:

- what data will be collected
- what methods will be used
- when and how often data will be collected
- who will be responsible for each element.

Measuring improvement answers the question, "How will we know that a change is an improvement?"

Aligning measures with improvement goals

Measures of improvement should align with the improvement goal your team has set (what will be achieved and by when: see "Goal setting" in this chapter) and relate directly to the factors you are aiming to change. Because goals focus on PHC system improvement, you are likely to need indicators that relate to PHC structures, processes and outcomes (rather than outcomes alone).

For example, a goal might be "Within 12 months, increase child immunisation rates by 50 per cent". These are possible measures of improvement (indicators) for this goal:

- child immunisation rates assessed by baseline and follow up audits
- family "knowledge about immunisation" surveys before and after an education campaign
- level of parent or carer engagement in the immunisation program tracked monthly
- staff satisfaction and experiences with the immunisation program continuously monitored
- proportion of clinical staff trained to provide immunisations at start and after 12 months
- number of completed immunisations at 6 and 9 months into the program.

Monitoring staff satisfaction and experiences is important for noting how changes made are affecting team interactions, workloads and other aspects of day-to-day care delivery. It aligns with the core value of including CQI as a routine agenda item in team or staff meetings.

Ensure that resources are available for measuring improvement, and that the measures, the scale of data collection and timeline are manageable for the team. The tools described in Chapter 5 can be used for measuring improvement over time.

Example: measuring improvement in child immunisation

Optimal immunisation program service delivery and childhood vaccine coverage remains an ongoing challenge in South Africa. Interventions aiming to improve immunisation service delivery in children under 24 months were co-designed with stakeholders in three clinics in Khayelitsha, Western Cape Province, South Africa. The prioritised interventions were implemented over a timeframe of 4–6 months and included weekly community radio sessions about immunisation; daily nurse-led education sessions at each clinic; service provider checklists to prompt delivery of all components of immunisation sessions; parent checklists to gather feedback and raise expectations about service quality; and health promotion materials (posters/postcards).

These indicators were used to measure improvement:

- service delivery outcomes for each clinic, including the number of vaccine doses delivered to children under 9 months per month

---

- parental engagement and knowledge, including changes in parents' and guardians' attitudes towards immunisation and interaction between parents or guardians and service providers
- parental satisfaction with immunisation services provided
- accessibility of services as reported by parents
- parents' and service providers' reported experience and outcomes, as a result of the changes.

Data collection methods included clinical audit, pre–post surveys, interviews and focus groups.[2]

Data analysis

Presenting data

In this section, we summarise graphs that are useful for presenting and analysing CQI data and provide examples of their use.

Bar graphs

A bar (or column) graph is used to visually compare categories of data or data values, or to track changes in values over time, or both. By visually quantifying data, bar charts can help teams to recognise and analyse anomalies, patterns or trends. The bars may be plotted horizontally or vertically. One axis of the graph shows the specific categories being compared, and the other axis represents a measured value, as a number or percentage.

Bar graphs are useful in CQI because they are simple to construct, easy to understand and versatile. For example, bar graphs can be used to visually quantify survey responses, clinical indicator and service delivery data, to compare data collected over consecutive audit cycles and to display demographic data. They can compare multiple indicators (Figure 6.2) or focus on a single item of care (Figure 6.3). Bars can be divided into parts that represent portions of a data category (Figure 6.3).

Figure 6.2 is a bar graph displaying data about delivery of a service. It shows the proportion of clients diagnosed with coronary heart disease who received specific items of care recommended in best practice care guidelines. By presenting audit data in a way that shows which items of care have been done well and less well (in this case by using two colours), the graph can help a team to identify priorities for improvement.

Figure 6.3 is a "stacked" bar graph, in which the bars are divided to represent portions of a data category. Each bar represents all (100 per cent) of the audited client records for that client group and audit year. In this example, the bars represent percentages of clients by record of tobacco smoking status in the last 12 months. By presenting data in this way, staff can see a change in practice over time (that is, continuing improvement in inquiry and recording of smoking status) and its possible impact on data about the number and percentage of clients who smoke tobacco.

---

2   Timothy, Coetzee et al. 2021.

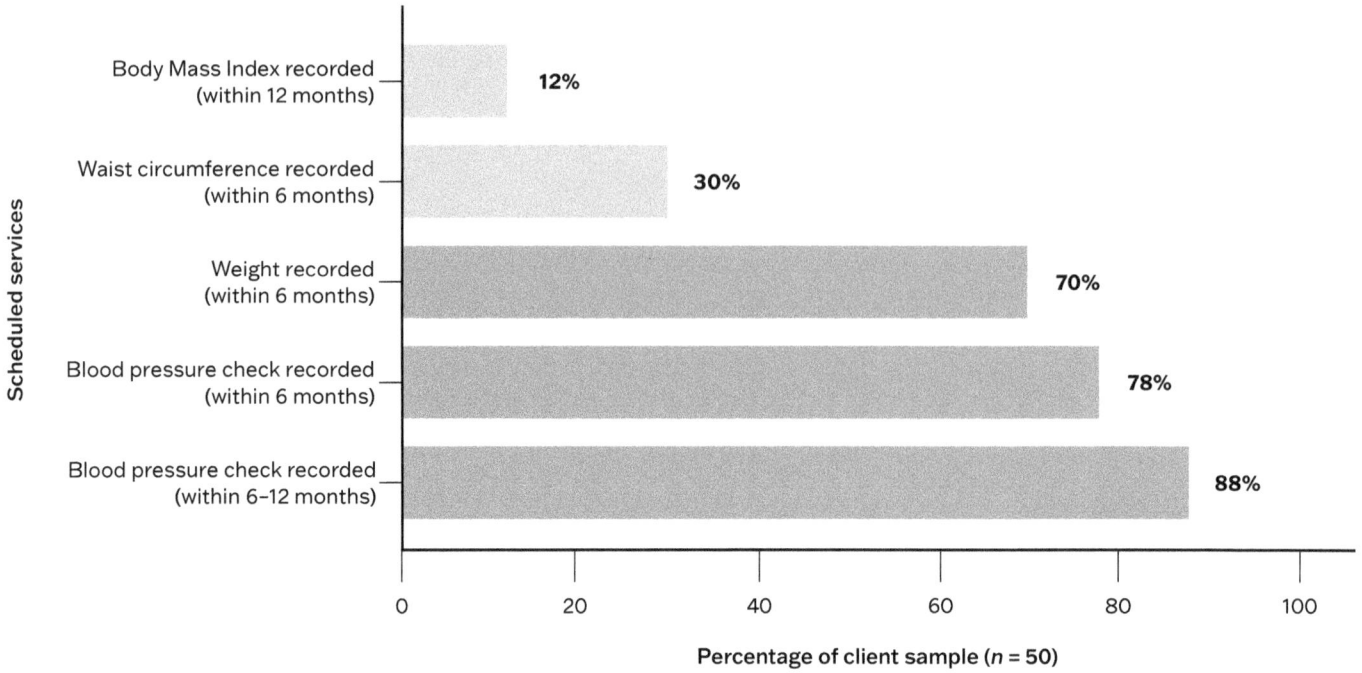

Figure 6.2 Bar graph example: proportion of clients with coronary heart disease by record of scheduled services.

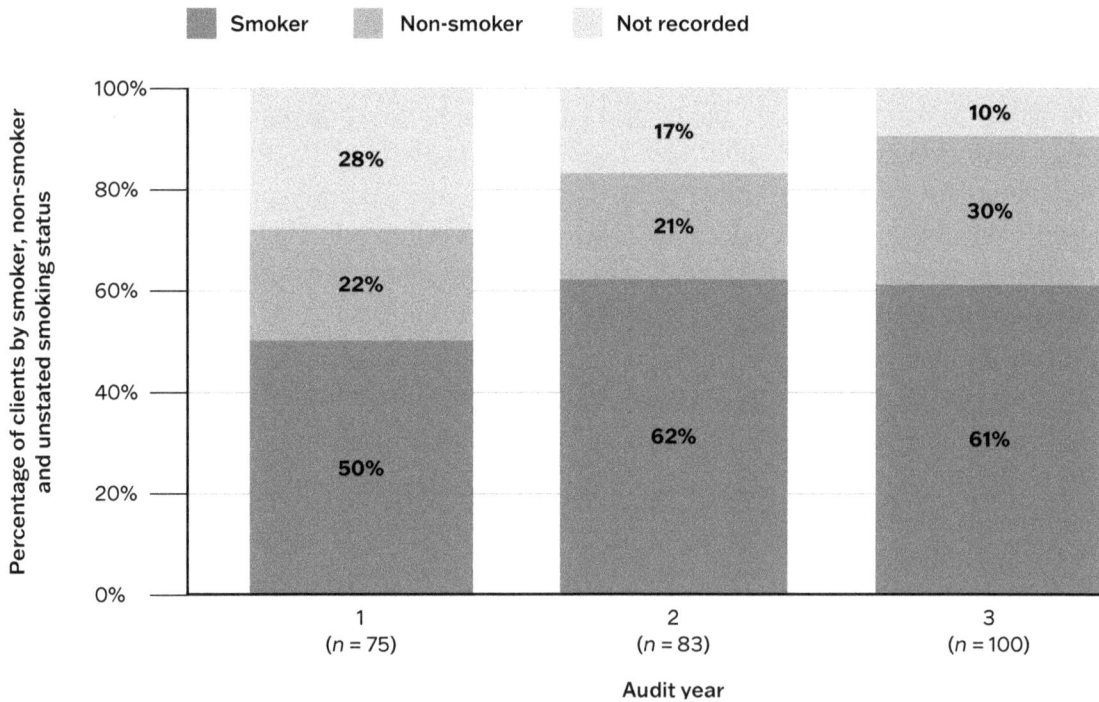

Figure 6.3 Stacked bar graph example: proportion of adult clients by recorded tobacco smoking status in the last 12 months and by audit cycle.

In Audit year 1, smoking status was not recorded in the health records of 28 per cent of adults in the client group. This dropped to 17 per cent in Audit year 2. By Audit year 3, only 10 per cent of clients, health records had no record of smoking status. This shows an improvement in practice over the three audit cycles. The percentage of smokers is consistent between Audit years 2 and 3 (61 per cent and 62 per cent respectively), suggesting that more than a third of clients for whom smoking status was not recorded in Audit year 2 were non-smokers.

Box 6.1 Best-practice design for bar graphs

- Use a zero-value baseline for meaningful comparison of data values.

- Use horizontal data labels to improve readability.

- Standard convention is to sort the bars from longest to shortest, unless there is a reason for ordering the category labels (for example, by audit years).

- Add value labels (numbers or percentages) where these are important.

See also "Pareto diagrams" in Chapter 5.

Box and whisker plots

A box and whisker plot displays variation in a set of data and is therefore useful for showing variation in PHC delivery.

Box and whisker plots show (Figure 6.4) these elements:

- the minimum and maximum values (ends of whiskers if no outliers)
- outliers that are values far away from most other values in the data set (or a distance that is greater than 1.5 times the length of the box)
- the range of service item delivery by dividing the dataset into quarters
- the box represents the middle 50 per cent of the dataset, and the line within the box represents the median (or middle value)
- the top whisker (and outliers if present) represents the top 25 per cent of the data
- the bottom whisker (and outliers if present) represents the bottom 25 per cent of the data
- the longer the box plot, the greater the range (or variation).

Figure 6.5 presents data from audits of PHC centre records about treatment and care for clients diagnosed with a mental illness. The box and whisker plots show mean health centre percentages for 269 clients attending at 17 Indigenous PHC centres in the three months prior to a clinical audit. The results show wide variation in service delivery. For example, psycho-health education of clients ranged from 0 to 100 per cent (the 25th to 75th centile is 15–80 per cent. Compare this with data for psycho-health education of family and/or carers: 75 per cent of data ranges between 0 and 38 per cent, suggesting a need for family and carer education programs in psycho-health.

Interpretation

Examples

Wide variation in service delivery (range 0–100%).	Majority of data values at lower end of range (between 0–20%) with a few values at higher levels – up to 93%.	Smaller variation in service delivery (range 70–100%).
Data values relatively equally dispersed across the range. 25th to 75th centile is 30–90%.		All data values at higher end with 75% of values in the 87–100% range.

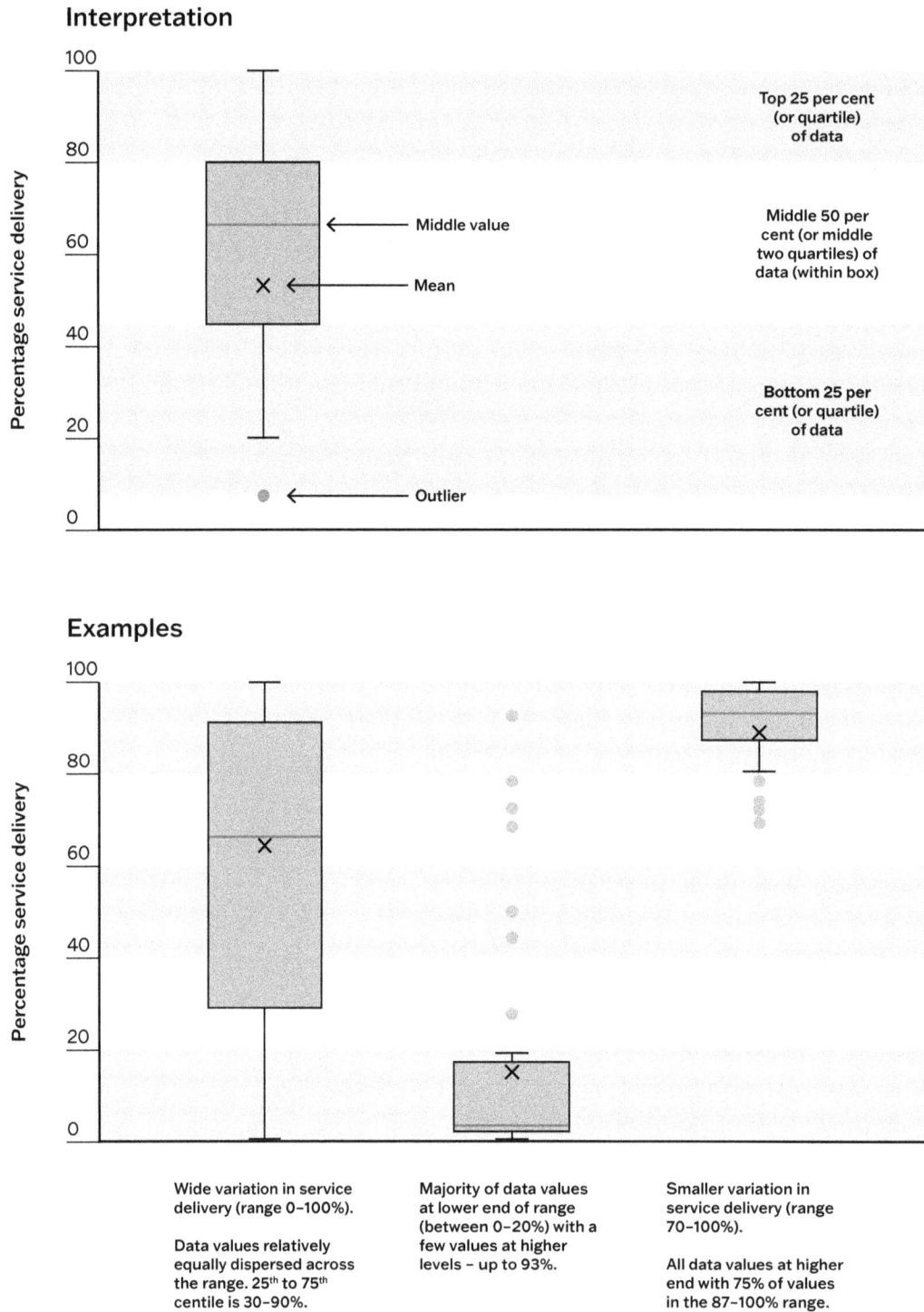

Figure 6.4 How to interpret box and whisker plots. Source: Matthews, Connors et al. 2015.

(*n* = number of health centres; number of audit records)

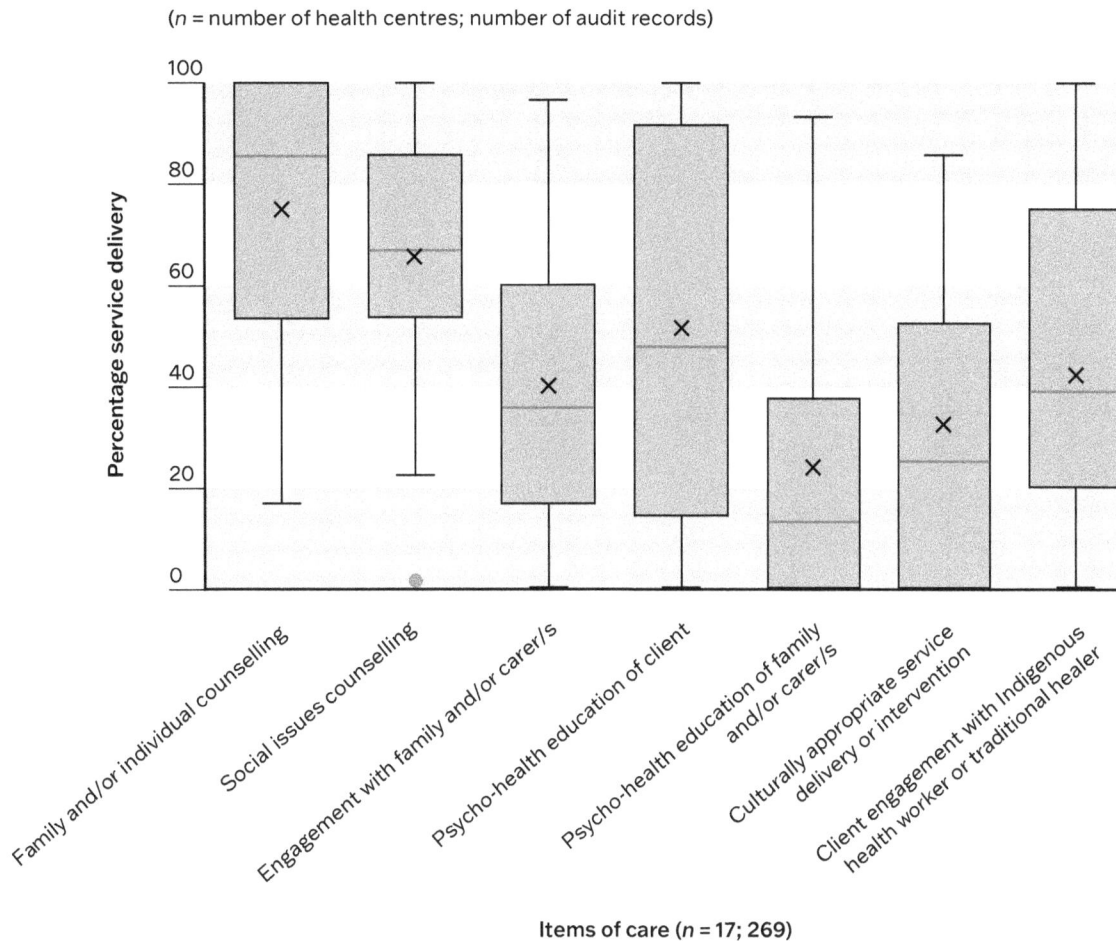

Figure 6.5 Box and whisker plot example: mean health centre percentage of mental health clients with a record of scheduled treatment and care in the last three months. Source: Matthews, Bailie et al. 2016.

Radar plots

A radar plot is designed to plot one or more series of quantitative values over multiple variables (three or more) on a two-dimensional plane. Sometimes called web, star or spider charts, radar plots are useful in CQI for these purposes:

- visually presenting a large amount of information in one graph
- comparing multiple variables (for example, of system performance) using a simple form
- integrating information about different quality concepts (for example, health outcomes, client satisfaction, cost)
- observing how the values change over time or between groups (for example, a group of health centres).

Radar plots have at least three axes, drawn from a central point. In most radar plots, the axes are equally distributed and drawn in the same way. Each axis represents a variable and is labelled. Values in a series are plotted on the axes and joined to form a shape. As each series is added (for example, the values for each year), variation in the size and in the shape of the plot shows changes or variation in care quality or systems.

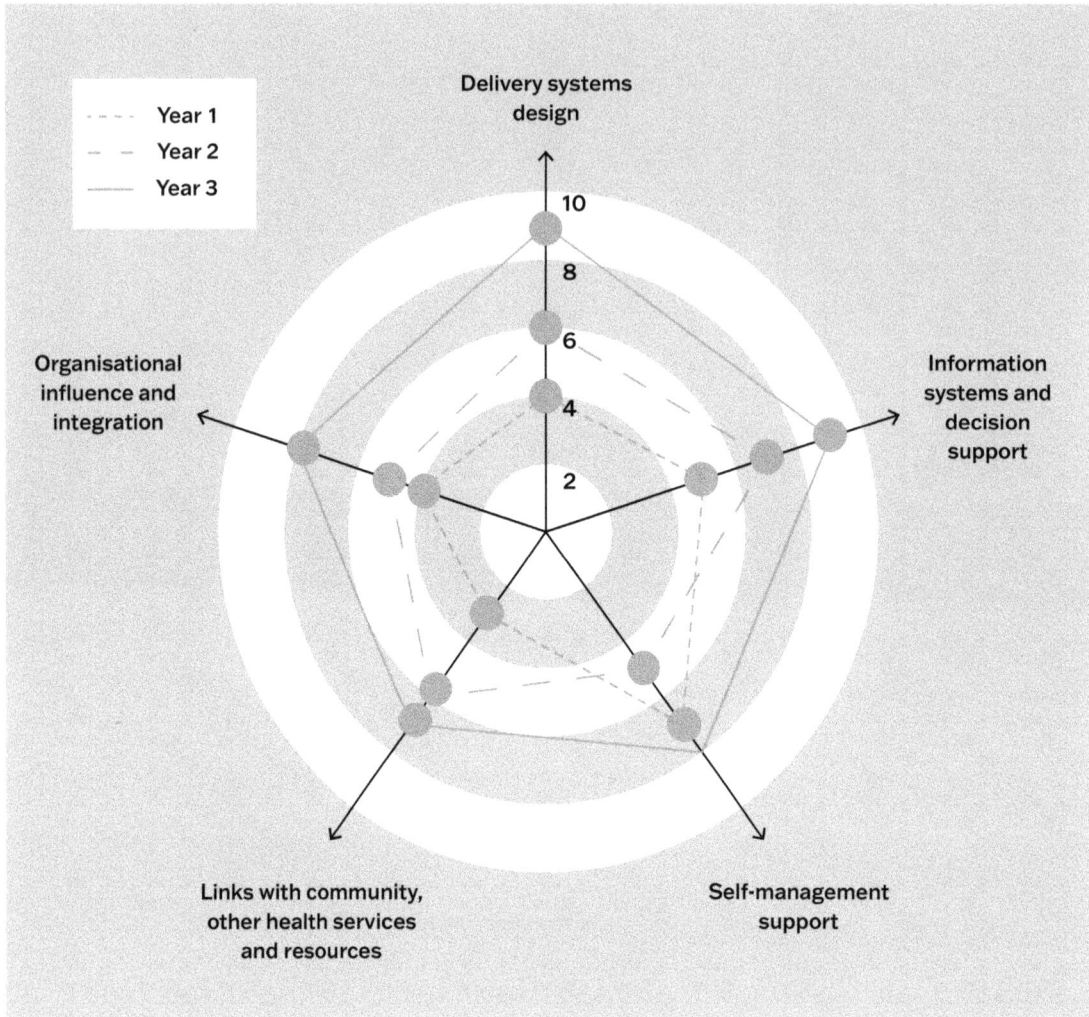

Figure 6.6 Radar plot example: a health centre's systems assessment scores over three annual audit cycles.

Figure 6.6 presents a health centre's systems assessment scores over three annual audit cycles. Five axes radiating from the centre show scores out of ten for the five main components of the system assessment (for example, information systems and decision support). Scores towards the middle indicate that parts of the system are less well developed and have greater potential for improvement. Scores towards the boundary indicate well-developed systems. In this example, increase in size of the "radar" shape shows overall improvement in the health centre's systems over time. For examples of radar plots used in this way, see Woods et al, 2017.[3]

_____

3   Woods, Carlisle et al. 2017.

Data tables and dashboards

While not classified as graphs, we include data tables and dashboards because they are commonly used to display data for CQI purposes.

Data tables are used to find values, compare values or communicate multiple units of measure in columns and rows format: for example, data about client numbers, attendance, demographics, clinical indicators or services delivered.

A data dashboard is a high-level summary of data, displayed on one page or computer screen, that helps the team or organisation to monitor performance and quickly identify opportunities for analysis and improvement. A data dashboard commonly includes graphs and data tables. For example, a diabetes dashboard might provide a snapshot of the number of clients with diabetes, numbers and percentages of clients who have received specific items of care within a specified timeframe, and data relating to important clinical indicators for diabetes management.

Box 6.2 General tips for presenting data

- Choose the appropriate type of graph, figure or table for presenting and understanding the data, and for your CQI purpose.

- Avoid detail that is not necessary for understanding the data (for example, repeated words/symbols, prominent grid lines and explanatory text on graphs).

- Avoid pie charts unless simple and representing only a few variables that add up to 100 per cent.

- Use colour with intention (for example, to highlight an important finding or changes over time).

- Avoid 3D effects and shading.

Online advice on data visualisation is readily available. We recommend the Evergreen Data website and textbooks for accessible advice on effective communication of data.[4]

This section has presented different ways to present data for analysis, but it is not necessary to have sophisticated data tools to produce useful reports for CQI. Your team's CQI reports should aim to give the team and managers an accurate picture of what is happening at that point in time, and from one cycle to the next.

> You do not need sophisticated data tools to produce useful reports for CQI.

---

4   To access Evergreen Data resources, see Evergreen 2024.

Understanding variation in quality

We have made many references to variation in quality of care. Understanding and addressing variation is the focus of much CQI work. It was the starting point for quality improvement pioneers such as Shewhart and Deming, who sought to understand and reduce variation in the quality of manufactured goods. Variations in health care include differences in:

- the proportion of diabetic clients with poor blood glucose control
- rates of screening for certain conditions over time
- waiting time to access a service
- rates of referral to smoking cessation programs
- the number and characteristics of clients seeking social support services
- the proportion of men and women attending for health checks
- performance between health services.

These are all examples of variation in outcomes. Outcomes are affected by care processes, which in turn are affected by care structures (remember Donabedian's theory?). To understand the underlying causes of variation in outcome, we look for variation in processes and structures that may explain them.

The quality improvement studies of our research network have consistently found wide variation in adherence to clinical best-practice guidelines between health services.[5] They also show variation among different aspects of care, with relatively good delivery of some aspects, such as physical checks for clients with chronic illness, and poor delivery of others, such as follow-up of abnormal clinical or laboratory findings.[6] These findings are evident in diabetes care,[7] eye care,[8] general preventive clinical care,[9] and in cardiovascular risk assessment.[10] They are consistent with CQI research findings in maternal care,[11] child health,[12] rheumatic heart disease[13] and sexual health.[14]

To respond effectively to variation – whether it be variation in performance between health services, or variation in care processes or service delivery at the health centre level – it is necessary to identify the sources of variation and understand what is causing it.

Sources of variation

Variation in care quality is often the result of the way systems are structured and how processes are managed, such as how services are accessed and delivered, the composition of PHC teams, how care is coordinated, how client referrals are organised and how information is recorded in clients' health records. Variation also has other, natural sources, such as differences in the

---

5   J. Bailie, Matthews et al. 2016; Burnett, Morse et al. 2016; Matthews, Burgess et al. 2017.
6   J. Bailie, Laycock et al. 2016; Schierhout, Matthews et al. 2016.
7   Matthews, Schierhout et al. 2014.
8   Burnett, Morse et al. 2016.
9   J. Bailie, Matthews et al. 2016; J. Bailie, Matthews et al. 2017.
10   Matthews, Burgess et al. 2017; Vasant, Matthews et al. 2016.
11   Gibson-Helm, Teede et al. 2015.
12   McAullay, McAuley et al. 2018.
13   Ralph, Fittock et al. 2013.
14   Nattabi, Matthews et al. 2017.

symptoms and health conditions that clients present with, differences relating to clients' age, gender and socio-economic circumstances, and differences in the skills and motivation of staff.

The variation found in the studies listed at the end of the previous section is largely explained by the way systems are structured and managed at the health service level[15] and at the policy level.[16] The variation is less likely to be caused by client characteristics. In addition, our CQI research has shown that PHC staff are highly motivated to improve the health of their clients,[17] indicating that system factors around PHC staffing, rather than the characteristics of staff, affect variation in care quality.

Causes of variation

It is important to understand the distinction between common and special causes of variation. This understanding enables teams to make decisions about the most appropriate action for improvement.

Common cause variation is the predictable, random variation that occurs naturally in stable processes.[18] It is the sum of many small variations from minor causes, which means that the variation cannot be traced back to a single root cause. Common cause variation can come from the way systems are structured and used, or from natural sources.

Example of common cause variation

A large PHC service used run charts to track wait times over 12 months for children referred to speech pathology services. Waiting times generally varied between 4 weeks and 5 months. Variation could be explained by a combination of factors. These included an ongoing nationwide shortage of speech pathologists, restricted places for new clients due to many children needing long-term therapy, the need to match the therapy needs of individual children to the specialised skills of individual speech pathologists, and parents' availability to attend appointments.

Special cause variation is unpredictable deviation that results from unexpected occurrences. It is not an inherent part of a process or system,[19] and can be traced back to a root cause. Like common cause variation, the source of special cause variation may be system based (for example, triggered by an unusual system error that resulted in a long delay in treatment for some clients) or naturally occurring (for example, the PHC practice records its first case of tuberculosis in 18 years for a client who is new to the practice).

Variation in quality of care can be caused by random error. It may be a result of the way records have been sampled and data analysed and displayed. Variation may be caused by different people recording information in different ways.

---

15   Burnett, Morse et al. 2016; Nattabi, Matthews et al. 2017; Schierhout, Matthews et al. 2016; Vasant, Matthews et al. 2016.
16   Bailie, Matthews et al. 2016; R. Bailie, Matthews et al. 2017; Matthews, Burgess et al. 2017.
17   J. Bailie, Schierhout et al. 2015; Larkins, Carlisle et al. 2019; Laycock, Harvey et al. 2018.
18   Bowen and Neuhauser 2013.
19   Bowen and Neuhauser 2013.

Example of special cause variation

A clinical audit of diabetes care indicated that care quality had reduced significantly since the previous audit. Staff examined client records to look for the reason for the variation and noted a pattern in data entry. Certain items of care had not been recorded on the same two days each week over an extended period, when a particular clinician was entering data. The variation reflected a change (omission) in the recording of care rather than a change in care delivery.

Responding to variation

When we understand variation, we can plan appropriate responses. In the last example, an appropriate response would be to train clinicians to enter data correctly in clinical information systems and to monitor the consistency of recording. Responding to variation in quality of care often involves prioritising and implementing a range of strategies.

Reducing variation "per se" is not the goal. We would not wish to lower the standard of care delivered by a high-performing PHC service to bring it in line with average performing services. The goal is to raise the standard of care that is not meeting expectations, so that high-quality care is consistent across services, and client outcomes are improved overall.

Responding to common cause variation

There is always some degree of random variation. If the current performance is acceptable, it is not necessary to make changes. If the variation is not within an acceptable range, action should be taken to improve care. Much CQI work focuses on refining systems to deal with common cause variation.

Responding to special cause variation

The external, non-routine factors that caused the variation should be identified and addressed. System change may not be needed, but a contingency plan may be necessary for managing risk and maintaining routine processes if it happens again.

> Much CQI work focuses on refining systems to manage and reduce common cause variation.

Variation can be caused by both common and special causes, particularly if a process is not stable and leads to unpredictable outcomes. When this is the case, special causes should be identified and prevented from happening again, followed by changes that target common causes of variation.

The examples offered above reinforce an important take-home message from earlier stories: that identifying the causes of variation and planning responses requires the participation of people with relevant knowledge and real-world experience.

Participatory interpretation

A participatory approach to data interpretation is a core concept in CQI. Bringing people together to interpret data collectively supports accurate and meaningful interpretation of the data. It is important to schedule time for this process as part of your CQI program.

Why is participatory interpretation of CQI data important?

The participatory interpretation of data is important for:

- telling the "story" of the data from multiple perspectives, enabling different worldviews and priorities to be taken into account
- helping to build a better understanding of health information for all in the team
- providing staff with a meaningful picture of their health centre's and practice's performance within the local setting and in the broader primary care context
- encouraging staff to reflect on the relevance and importance of using data to inform changes in PHC systems and processes
- helping to differentiate between what is clinically significant and what is statistically significant: for example, an increase in attendance rates may not be statistically significant, but to the health centre it may be clinically significant, because it shows a trend that is consistent with their efforts to improve attendance and with their experience "on the ground"
- enabling people to share insights and building collective knowledge. Participatory interpretation can be especially valuable for newer members of the team to hear from those with experience of previous CQI cycles, and for longer-term staff to hear new perspectives when making sense of data. Comparing and discussing results from previous audit or CQI cycles and from other PHC services also offers important information.[20]

Participatory interpretation captures experiential knowledge. As well as being important for meaningful data interpretation, this approach respects and affirms the experience that each person brings to the process. Depending on who is present, participatory interpretation can take account of the multiple priorities of PHC staff, other workers, management and clients.

When and how to facilitate data interpretation

The participatory interpretation of findings usually occurs after a preliminary analysis of data by a CQI facilitator, system administrator or leadership group. A preliminary analysis of data enables the facilitator to plan the session around the findings, so the group can use the time together to work out what the results mean, rather than what the results are.

The process should be designed to suit the needs of the service, practice or program and the team. Factors such as timing, staff availability and existing organisational planning methods might influence when and how the interpretation process is done. Participatory interpretation of CQI findings can be done in a staged approach (Figure 6.7) as different data are collected and become available, or it can be done when a CQI cycle has been completed: for example, combining results from a clinical audit, systems assessment and client experience or satisfaction data.

---

20   Brands, Griffin et al. 2010.

Preliminary analysis	The data are organised into a format that can be understood – e.g. graph, table, dashboard. The results and their significance for client care and population health may be summarised.
Summarised data	The preliminary analysis is presented to the team or group. The group includes as many of the staff, managers, governance team and client or community representatives as feasible.
Sense-making	Sense-making is facilitated in a way that draws on the expertise available and encourages the sharing of different perspectives to interpret the findings. What do outcomes say about the structures and processes of care? Are these findings consistent with findings from the use of other continuous quality improvement tools?
Systems thinking	Consider the bigger picture. What might the causes be? What are the effects? Do the continuous quality improvement findings align with other information available to the team? What else do we need to know to identify priorities for improvement?

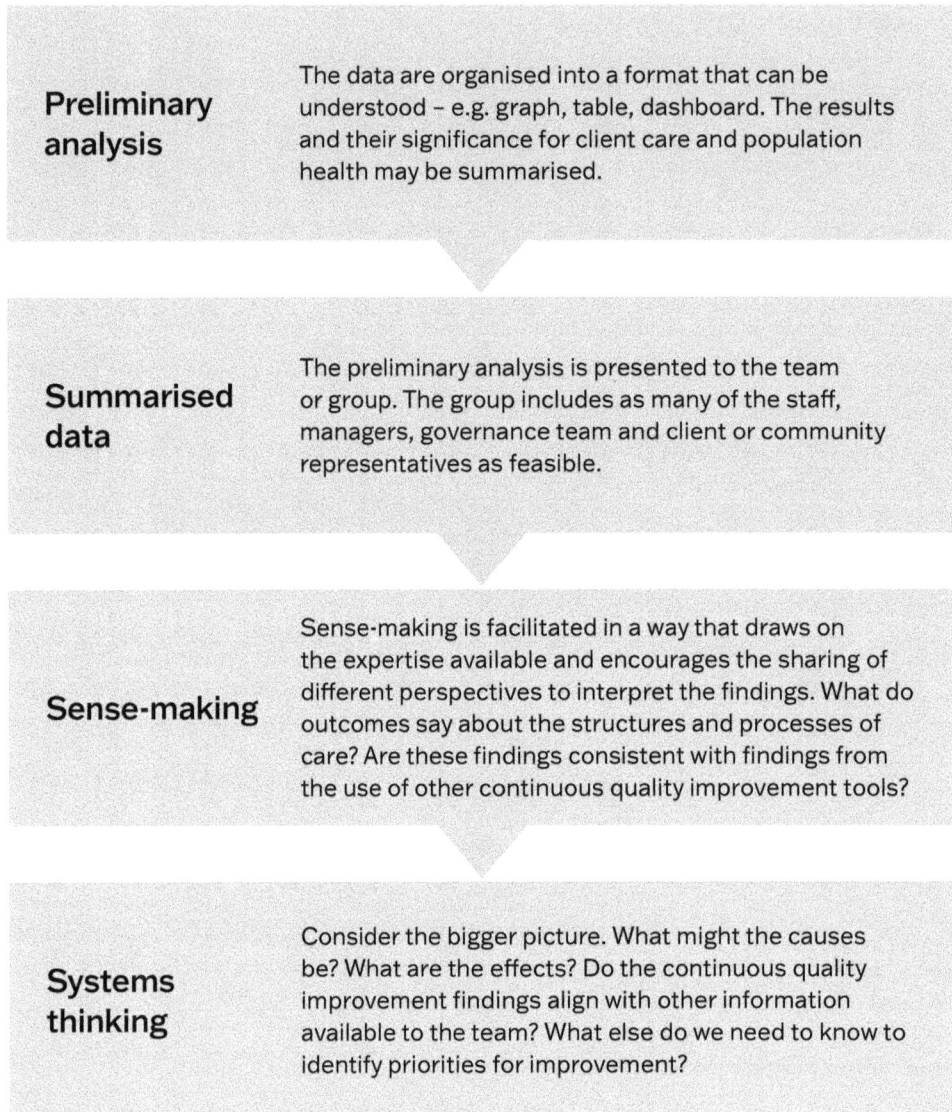

Figure 6.7 The participatory interpretation process.

The importance of local knowledge

It is vital that CQI data are interpreted in the context of the local PHC delivery model. There may be many influences within a PHC setting that are relevant to the interpretation of data. These might include, for example, cultural issues (such as around gender or understandings of health), the effect of health promotion activities on clinical data, the influence of individuals (positive or negative) on the team, and staff capacity. The following examples demonstrate the importance of a participatory approach to data interpretation.

The only staff member trained to use the point-of-care blood-testing machine was on leave for three months. This meant that regular blood glucose testing could not be done. Local knowledge about staff absences was necessary for understanding why delivery of this item of care was lower than expected.

The number of clients attending exercise classes for Elders and seniors had dropped significantly over several months, even though participant feedback continued to show a high level of satisfaction with the classes. The drop could not be explained by changes to class delivery or arrangements for transporting participants to the classes. It emerged through discussion that another agency was scheduling social outings for this age group on the same mornings each week.

It appeared from clinical audit data that 56 per cent of pregnant women had presented to the clinic before conception for folate supplements – a good news story. This finding didn't align with the experiences of clinicians. Through team discussion, it became apparent that the folate was included in the iron medication that women were already taking because they were anaemic, rather than folate being specifically prescribed.

The number of men presenting for health checks, and before their illnesses became serious, had increased each year for three years. The Aboriginal PHC service had been promoting men's health checks and had extended opening hours on two evenings each week. While these changes were viewed positively, community feedback confirmed that strategies for embedding culturally appropriate care across the service had most influence on men accessing care. These included employing more Aboriginal staff, training and mentoring in cultural safety for non-Indigenous staff and use of interpreters.

Using systems thinking

CQI tools are designed to collect data about the structure, processes and outcomes of care. Systems thinking is used to make sense of that data (often in conjunction with other techniques) and to plan improvement. Systems thinking is the ability to recognise, understand and synthesise the links, interactions and interdependencies between different parts of a system. It involves looking for these connections and understanding the context in which they occur.[21]

---

21   de Savigny and Adam 2009; Dolansky and Moore 2013.

> Systems thinking involves looking for connections between different parts of a system and understanding the context in which they occur.

The examples at the end of the previous section illustrate the use of systems thinking to interpret data. Take the first example. The team connected knowledge about how blood glucose testing was done (the process, equipment used and requirement for special training) with contextual knowledge about people and their roles (who was authorised to use the equipment) and organisational processes (timing of individual leave) to interpret audit data. Continued use of systems thinking will enable the team to plan sustainable system improvements, such as training more staff to use the blood glucose monitor, and coordinating staff leave dates to ensure blood glucose testing is always available to clients. The conversations can help staff to prioritise the next audit: for example, is there a need for data about the quality of preventive care the service or practice is delivering? In contrast, a team using linear thinking may incorrectly attribute the low rate of blood glucose testing to a drop in client attendance or to clinical inertia. Team members would risk focusing improvement efforts on a one-off campaign to educate (possibly already well-informed) clients and colleagues about the importance of diabetes screening and blood glucose monitoring.

Systems thinking includes these skills:

- dynamic thinking – viewing a problem as part of a pattern of system behaviour over time
- system-as-cause thinking – placing responsibility for what is happening on people inside the system who manage the policies and procedures, rather than on external forces
- forest thinking (also called helicopter view) – seeing the bigger picture and understanding the context in which system interactions occur, instead of focusing on details
- operational thinking – focusing on cause and effect, and understanding how system behaviour is generated
- thinking in feedback loops – seeing cause and effect as an ongoing process. A change may be modified when put into action, or it may lead to changes in other parts of the system. Feedback informs further action.[22]

When systems thinking is used, synergies between parts of the system can be anticipated. Unintended consequences, or negative effects of a change on another part of the system, can be mitigated. A systems thinking approach, which shifts the focus from individual PHC team roles and care processes to the systems in which they work, is essential for understanding and improving the quality of PHC.

---

22   de Savigny and Adam 2009.

Example: establishing a systems thinking approach to improving chronic illness care

The importance of a systems thinking approach for improving health outcomes was established in one of the earliest studies of the ABCD CQI research program. PHC teams in twelve Aboriginal and Torres Strait Islander communities identified resources and areas of strength and weakness in the systems relating to chronic illness care. The study found that all components of the "chronic care model"[23] were evident in, and influenced, every facet of PHC centre operations. The components delineated the connections between clients, PHC staff, families and communities. These specific findings were made:

- Organisational influence was strengthened by inclusion of chronic illness goals in business plans and appointment of chronic disease coordinators to conduct clinical audits, but weakened by lack of training in disease prevention and health promotion, and by the funding structure of the time.

- Community linkages were facilitated by PHC teams working with community organisations (for example, local stores) and running community-based programs (for example, Health Week), but weakened by a shortage of staff, especially Aboriginal and Torres Strait Islander health workers.

- Self-management was promoted through client education and goal setting with clients but hindered by limited focus on family and community-based activities due to understaffing.

- Information systems were facilitated by computerised information systems but weakened, at that time, by the systems' complexity and need for IT maintenance and upgrade support (information systems have greatly improved since the study, including the capacity of electronic information systems to support CQI).

- Decision support for clinicians was facilitated by access to clinical guidelines and their integration with daily care but limited by inadequate access to and support from specialists.

- Delivery system design was strengthened by provision of transport for clients to PHC centres, separate men's and women's clinic rooms, specific roles of PHC team members in chronic illness care, effective teamwork, and functional pathology and pharmacy systems, but weakened by staff shortage and high staff turnover.[24]

These findings demonstrated that a systems approach was needed to improve chronic illness care. The study influenced the development of the ABCD systems assessment tool[25] described in Chapter 5. Further versions of the tool have been developed to support the use of systems thinking and CQI cycles in other areas of comprehensive PHC.

---

23   Bonomi, Wagner et al. 2002.

24   Si, Bailie et al. 2008.

25   Menzies School of Health Research and One21seventy 2012.

In the following story, the PHC team in a remote community used systems thinking to understand a care delivery problem, and to make changes that would bring about sustained improvement.

Story: using systems thinking to make sense of data and plan improvement

"We have done many systems assessments with community health centre teams. We aim to involve all members of the team in the process, which uses the systems assessment tool[26] to capture subjective feedback from PHC teams 'on the ground' about how well their health centre systems are working.

When asked about patient follow-up and continuity of care, one team said they had a good system in place, and it was working well. But when we reviewed data from their review of clinical records, it actually showed that follow-up was quite poor: patients were falling through the cracks and missing out on care. This came as a shock to everyone: the GP, Aboriginal health practitioners, nurses and drivers who were part of the feedback session.

The team decided to focus on one group of patients to explore what was happening in their recall system: children and adults with acute rheumatic fever and rheumatic heart disease (ARF/RHD). With the local CQI facilitator they reviewed the current recall system, developing a flowchart to identify the weakness in the process. They discussed how those weaknesses affected processes such as providing monthly benzathine penicillin G injections, consultations with the visiting cardiologist and paediatrician, access to translators and education about ARF/RHD in their first language and linking patients with other services. They brainstormed why there were outstanding recalls; there was local knowledge in the room including community members on the PHC team.

They proceeded with a PDSA cycle that had the goal of decreasing the number of outstanding recalls for patients with ARF/RHD over the following two months. Team members reviewed the medical record of every patient in the community diagnosed with ARF/RHD, deleted out-of-date recalls and amended follow-up appointments. This decreased the number of outstanding recalls in the short term. The second PDSA cycle focused on system changes. A weekly recall list was printed for the team members who held the "portfolio" for that group of patients. The team reviewed the patient recall list at daily team meetings, where the knowledge of Aboriginal health practitioners and other local staff, who knew who and where families were, was key to contacting them and for keeping the data base up-to-date.

The team achieved their goal. They significantly decreased the number of outstanding ARF/RHD patient recalls that were printed off at the start of each week and have since put this system into place for other groups of patients. All staff who use the electronic patient information system are trained to enter data correctly as part of their orientation. The work the team did improved and

---

26   Menzies School of Health Research and One21seventy 2012.

streamlined the recall system, leading to better care and patient outcomes. How did they review this? They saw it in the next round of CQI data!"

– Kerry Copley and Louise Patel, CQI program coordinators, Aboriginal Medical Services Alliance Northern Territory.

For more information, see Aboriginal Medical Services Alliance Northern Territory n.d.

The process mapping and root cause analysis tools described in Chapter 5 are systems thinking tools.

Goal setting

Identifying strengths and priorities for improvement

The participatory interpretation of data shows the team what is being done well and not so well, and the influence of contextual factors on care. It is important to identify and acknowledge strengths, as well as areas where systems need to be improved. For example, consider what strengths and weakness a primary healthcare centre might have for diabetes care:

- strengths: diabetes audit and systems assessment data might indicate a good rate of follow-up for abnormal blood glucose results, that the measuring and recording of blood pressure is embedded as routine practice, that rates of self-management goal setting have improved and that links with the community are strong: that overall, the PHC centre is performing well in diabetes care. Focus on these achievements before discussing the identified gaps in quality of care.
- need for improvement: identified gaps might be low rates of diabetes screening and diagnosis for men, a significant client group with poor blood glucose control, lack of screening for emotional wellbeing, and poor follow-up or lack of records describing the action taken following abnormal blood pressure results.

Not all improvement needs can be tackled at the same time. The identified gaps should be discussed by the team to understand factors that may be contributing to the quality issues, factors that may have a positive influence, and which gaps in care should be prioritised. Remember, CQI is about continuous learning and improvement, not about assigning blame. Group discussion should focus on these points:

- the significance or urgency (or both) of clients' healthcare needs
- which system changes are more likely to improve the health of this group of clients
- what changes are practical and feasible in your PHC context
- small, incremental improvements that are likely to be sustainable.

S	**Specific**	Describing the system to be improved and the population of clients who will be affected
M	**Measureable**	The team needs to know if the goal has been achieved, or progress made towards the goal
A	**Achievable**	The goal should stretch the team, but should be realistic
R	**Results**	Results to be achieved should be clearly stated
T	**Time-bound**	A timeframe is needed for achieving the goal

Figure 6.8 SMART goals.

Developing SMART goals

After an improvement priority has been identified, an improvement goal is developed. We set improvement goals to answer the question:"what are we trying to accomplish?" (See Chapter 2.)

Agreeing about the goal is critical for a sense of direction and for team commitment, as is allocating the people and resources necessary to achieve the goal. Many organisations use SMART as a guide for developing goals (Figure 6.8).

A numerical goal should be set when possible. A numerical goal directs how achievement will be measured and helps the team to think about the level of support needed: for example, "increase child immunisation rates by 50 per cent within 12 months" rather than "increase child immunisation rates". Note that numerical goals are not always relevant. For example, goals might focus on improving community and health centre relationships, improving communication and confidence among staff members, or improving the physical environment of the health centre. Non-numerical goals still need to be measurable, for example, by conducting client and staff surveys or focus groups. An aspirational goal stretches the team to look for ways of overcoming barriers to improvement.[27]

---

27   Institute for Healthcare Improvement 2021.

Examples of SMART goals

- Within 3 months, establish a system to identify and follow-up all clients with type 2 diabetes who have abnormal blood pressure and blood glucose results.
- Within 12 months, increase child immunisation rates by 50 per cent.
- Within 18 months, increase screening and follow-up for social risk factors for women receiving antenatal and postnatal care by 60 per cent.

Improvement goals should be regularly reviewed during team meetings. You may need to revise a goal to take account of organisational change or unexpected events (for example, a disease outbreak, a severe weather event) or to refocus on a part of the system over which the team has more influence.

A note about terms: some people prefer the term "aims" to "goals". Others think of aims as general statements – "Our aim is to improve child immunisation rates" – and goals as more specific (for example, SMART goals). Some teams identify general aims or goals and set SMART "objectives". And concepts expressed in a language other than English may be most appropriate for your team. As a rule, use terms that feel right for your organisation and setting.

Action planning

Action planning is the process of identifying what actions need to be taken to achieve the improvement goal. We plan actions based on the question: "what changes can we make that will result in an improvement?" (See Chapter 2.)

> We plan actions based on the question: "what changes can we make that will result in an improvement?"

Action planning involves these activities:

- developing improvement strategies and measurable activities
- identifying the resources needed
- allocating tasks and responsibilities
- setting milestones and timelines for completing the various activities.

The action planning process may be done in the same session as goal setting, or as a follow-up activity, depending on the people available and the time allocated to the session. As with participatory interpretation of data and goal setting, action planning should be a collective activity. Input from people with different expertise and experiences is important because of the complex nature of improvement in PHC and the difficulty of predicting what will work. Involving as many team members as possible leads to shared understanding and ownership of the action plan. This is particularly important for people who will have a role in implementing the plan, or whose work will be affected by it. Without collective commitment to the action plan, implementation will lack direction and momentum.

Visualise your completed action plan in a way that can be shared and understood by all involved. Options could be a table, an extended driver (or "action effect") diagram,[28] or a chart developed with project management software. CQI action plans typically include the following components:

- goal/s
- strategies
- implementation activities or tasks
- responsibility – people responsible for each activity or task
- milestones or timeline
- resources – needed to complete the activities
- measures – for monitoring and evaluating progress.

Implementation

In our CQI cycle, implementation refers to implementing improvement strategies to achieve system changes in a PHC centre, practice or program. This should be distinguished from using the term specifically to refer to the translation of evidence into practice, and to embedding and sustaining system changes (as commonly used in the field of implementation science).

Implementing your team's action plan is essential for achieving your improvement goals. This is self-evident, but, consistent with other phases of the CQI cycle in PHC, teams need the right tools for the task. An essential tool in your team's implementation toolkit is the plan-do-study-act, or PDSA, cycle.

Plan-do-study-act (PDSA) cycles

PDSA cycles[29] are usually rapid, small-scale cycles used for developing and testing change strategies (Figure 6.9). PDSA cycles enable teams to gather ongoing feedback about how well their change strategies are working and to adapt those strategies to work more effectively. Multiple PDSA cycles may be needed to optimise a change strategy. The cycles are used to ensure that the strategy has its intended effect and is carried out in a sustainable way without creating unintended consequences.[30]

In Box 6.1, PDSA cycles are used to test a strategy to improve the delivery of follow-up care for adults who had a preventive health assessment with abnormal screening results. Many clients did not attend their follow-up appointments. A common reason given by clients was that they forgot about the appointment.

---

28   Reed, McNicholas et al. 2014.
29   Deming 2018.
30   Halperin, Gilmour et al. 2019.

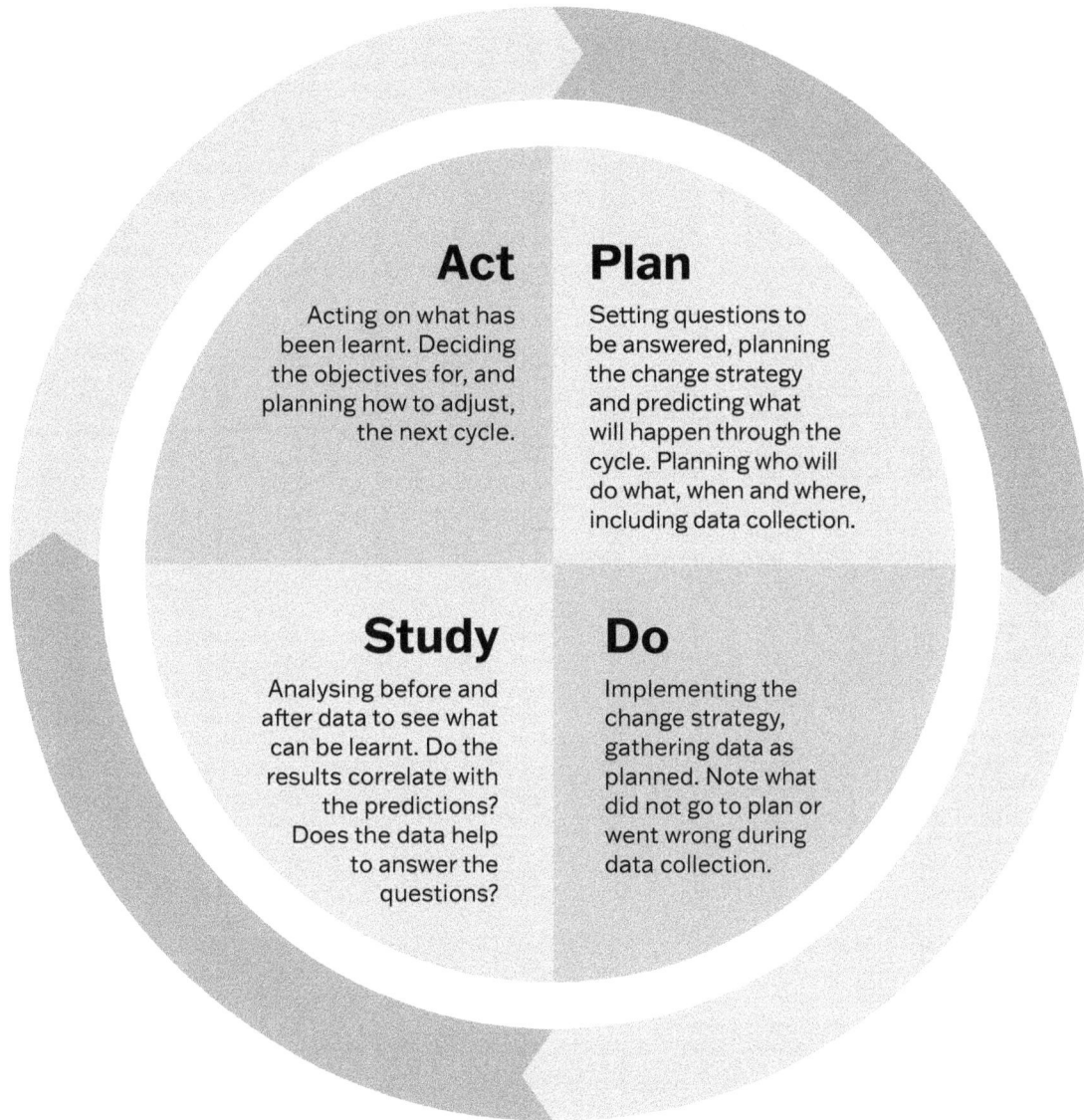

Act

Acting on what has been learnt. Deciding the objectives for, and planning how to adjust, the next cycle.

Plan

Setting questions to be answered, planning the change strategy and predicting what will happen through the cycle. Planning who will do what, when and where, including data collection.

Study

Analysing before and after data to see what can be learnt. Do the results correlate with the predictions? Does the data help to answer the questions?

Do

Implementing the change strategy, gathering data as planned. Note what did not go to plan or went wrong during data collection.

Figure 6.9 The Plan-do-study-act Cycle. Adapted from: Deming, W. Edwards. foreword by Kevin Edwards Cahill, *The New Economics for Industry, Government, Education, third edition*, The PDSA Cycle, page 91 © 2018 Massachusetts Institute of Technology, by permission of The MIT Press.

Box 6.1 Example PDSA cycles

Change strategy: remind clients of their follow-up appointments.

	PDSA cycle 1	PDSA cycle 2	PDSA cycle 3
Plan	Receptionist to set up system to send date and time reminder text to clients' mobile phones two weeks before, and one day before their appointments, with request to respond "yes" or "no", and a number to call to make another appointment if unable to attend.	Receptionist to call clients to remind them, or to reschedule the appointment.	Focus on non-attendees. When calling, reinforce the importance of following up on results. Assure clients that rescheduling is possible. Ask if they need support with transport to the health centre. Send reminder letter to clients who can't be reached by phone.
	Prediction: If clients have forgotten the appointment, this will prompt them to attend or to arrange a new appointment time.	Prediction: A personalised phone call will encourage clients to attend and help to promote a positive service–client relationship.	Prediction: A personalised caring approach and offer of transport (where possible) should encourage clients to attend or reschedule appointments.
	Measurement: Who – receptionist What – number of clients who are sent a text, number and type of responses (yes/no/none/callback), attendance How – data download from system, spreadsheet When – review after 4 weeks.	Measurement: Who – receptionist What – number of clients called, number and type of responses, attendance, time taken on calls How – spreadsheet When – review after 4 weeks.	Measurement: Who – receptionist and chronic care coordinator What – number of clients called and sent letters, responses, attendance How – spreadsheet When – review after 6 weeks.
Do	Receptionist sends reminder text to clients' mobile phones.	Receptionist calls clients with reminders, and records the response to her calls (for example: client confirms the appointment; client does not answer; when "hide caller ID" is used client does not answer).	Receptionist and chronic care coordinator contact clients as planned noting that this approach is generally well received by targeted clients, and many are grateful for the offer of transport.

	PDSA cycle 1	PDSA cycle 2	PDSA cycle 3
Study	Few clients responded, and those who respond "no" rarely make a new appointment time. Receptionist can't be sure the messages are being delivered. No improvement in attendance.	Many clients confirmed their appointments but still missed them. Several clients could not be reached by phone, even after changing to "show caller ID" (as clinic name). Trying to call every client with a follow-up appointment is overly demanding on receptionist's time. Little improvement in attendance.	Attendance of follow-up appointments increased from 60 per cent to 80 per cent.
Act	Team feels the approach is too impersonal or ineffective. See PSDA 2.	Team is aware that not many families in the community have motor vehicles. A more time-efficient approach is needed.	Maintain the focused personalised reminder system. Staff to check/update contact details at each client interaction.

Staying on track to implement improvement

Implementing CQI action plans and being part of improved quality of care is rewarding for everyone involved. Even so, day-to-day work and acute care demands, changes in staff or management, and unanticipated events may present obstacles to implementation, even for PHC teams who are experienced in CQI.

We recommended several strategies for staying on track to implement planned improvements.

- Communicate improvement plans to all who have a role in implementing CQI.
- Have CQI as a standing item on the agenda for staff meetings. This helps to keep track of the progress of each CQI cycle. It provides opportunities to discuss how strategies are going, and to plan any adjustments that are needed. It is important that information and action items for follow-up are shared among the team and others who are affected or involved.
- Share good news stories about improvements with colleagues and with the community (for example, on a website or in a community newsletter). Share positive feedback from the community among colleagues.
- Put up signs listing improvement goals and achievements. Signs can be displayed in areas used by staff and in client waiting areas.
- Prepare CQI progress reports for the management or governance group or board, or both.

It is important for CQI leaders, facilitators and managers to understand organisational and individual responses to change, and to respond effectively. People resist change for various reasons; they may even feel that their role or work is threatened by the planned changes to systems and care processes. Identifying or creating learning opportunities in CQI and innovation, and in managing change, will support implementation.

Example: implementing improvement strategies for better care coordination

Setting: An Australian health service experienced in using CQI. It has a main clinic with management and administrative staff located in a large regional town. Outreach clinics serve seven small rural communities.

Identified problems: Use of a triage process for clients visiting the main clinic and a lack of coordination meant that clients with diagnosed chronic diseases were required to visit multiple times for routine care. Many were missing important scheduled services. Chronic disease management plans were underused, reducing the potential for government funding of the service.

These strategies were implemented:

- With input from clinicians, managers and systems support staff, a "client-flow nurse" role was created to oversee clinic processes and liaise with clinicians, clients and other services to coordinate care. The role had flexibility to respond to changing local conditions.

- Client-flow processes were restructured. Clients due for chronic disease management appointments were identified and appointments were scheduled.

- Meetings of the clinic team each morning supported teamwork and communication for delivering care (for example, staff rosters, client appointments, hospital admissions and discharges).

- The plan included monitoring and evaluation to find out how well strategies were working and to adjust systems as needed.

Outcomes: Better team knowledge about the care needs of their clients and what was happening in the wider community, better care planning and coordination, increased government funds through chronic disease management plans, and improved community engagement.

> "I think the community started to really engage with us again . . . we'd seen some really positive things that were coming out of this service and the community started coming to us with their problems, rather than just trying to muddle through, or use the hospital as a GP service." – Nurse[31]

Finally, it is important to keep going with CQI cycles. If changes in the service environment interrupt CQI activities, picking up the process where the last CQI cycle paused and getting involved in practical tasks, for example analysing data, can help a team re-engage in CQI. Above all, don't abandon your CQI efforts when indicators of quality show minimal improvement. Remember, CQI aims for small changes that are realistic and achievable: changes that can be

---

31   Newham and Cunningham 2015, 27.

sustained. It takes time for small, incremental improvements in care quality to be reflected in data, as highlighted in the following reflection by a CQI facilitator.

Reflecting on the importance of ongoing engagement in CQI

"In the early days of the ABCD research program we discovered how important it was for PHC teams to look at data from one CQI cycle to the next. Each participating health service had its own 'community story' feedback reports for chronic illness care and preventive care that showed pie charts and bar graphs of clinical audit results and radar plots of the systems assessment results. These results were combined to show where the health team efforts were improving care. Some health services may not have achieved their systems improvement goals in the first CQI cycle, however the data showed positive changes over time. We could see the changes staff were making and they could see improvement in the care they were providing for their clients."

– Lynette O'Donoghue, CQI facilitator/researcher

Summary

This chapter has described how CQI cycles are used in PHC. We have worked through a CQI cycle that involves the four phases: data collection; data analysis (and understanding causes of variation); participatory interpretation, goal setting and action planning; and implementation. Examples have been used to illustrate concepts and processes within each phase. We presented different types of graphs that can be used in the data analysis phase; we also discussed variation in care quality. We have highlighted the importance of using local knowledge and systems thinking when interpreting data and planning system improvement, and the benefits of continued engagement in CQI cycles. In the next chapter, we describe CQI facilitation and techniques for engaging PHC teams and other PHC stakeholders in CQI cycles.

References

Aboriginal Medical Services Alliance Northern Territory (n.d.). Continuous quality improvement (CQI). http://www.amsant.org.au/cqi-new/.

Bailie, C., V. Matthews, J. Bailie, P. Burgess, K. Copley, C. Kennedy et al. (2016). Determinants and gaps in preventive care delivery for Indigenous Australians: a cross-sectional analysis. *Frontiers in Public Health* 4: 34. DOI: 10.3389/fpubh.2016.00034.

Bailie, J., A. Laycock, V. Matthews and R. Bailie (2016). System-level action required for wide-scale improvement in quality of primary health care: synthesis of feedback from an interactive process to promote dissemination and use of aggregated quality of care data. *Frontiers in Public Health* 4: 86. DOI: 10.3389/fpubh.2016.00086.

Bailie, J., V. Matthews, A. Laycock, R. Schultz, C. Burgess, D. Peiris et al. (2017). Improving preventive health care in Aboriginal and Torres Strait Islander primary care settings. *Globalization and Health* 13: 48. DOI: 10.1186/s12992-017-0267-z.

Bailie, J., G. Schierhout, F. Cunningham, J. Yule, A. Laycock and R. Bailie (2015). *Quality of primary health care for Aboriginal and Torres Strait Islander people in Australia. Key research findings and messages for action from the ABCD National Research Partnership Project*. Brisbane: Menzies School of Health Research.

Bailie, R., V. Matthews, S. Larkins, S. Thompson, P. Burgess, T. Weeramanthri et al. (2017). Impact of policy support on uptake of evidence-based continuous quality improvement activities and the quality of care for Indigenous Australians: a comparative case study. *BMJ Open* 7(10). DOI: 10.1136/bmjopen-2017-016626.

Bailie, R.S., D. Si, L. O'Donoghue and M. Dowden (2007). Indigenous health: effective and sustainable health services through continuous quality improvement. *Medical Journal of Australia* 186(10): 525–7. DOI: 10.5694/j.1326-5377.2007.tb01028.x.

Bonomi, A.E., E.H. Wagner, R.E. Glasgow and M. VonKorff (2002). Assessment of chronic illness care (ACIC): a practical tool to measure quality improvement. *Health Services Research* 37(3): 791–820. DOI: 10.1111/1475-6773.00049.

Bowen, M.E. and D. Neuhauser (2013). Understanding and managing variation: three different perspectives. *Implementation Science* 8(1): S1. DOI: 10.1186/1748-5908-8-S1-S1.

Brands, J., J. Griffin, R. Bailie, J. Hains, R. Cox, C. Kennedy et al. (2010). *Improving the quality of primary health care: a training manual for the One21seventy cycle.* Darwin: Menzies School of Health Research.

Burnett, A., A. Morse, T. Naduvilath, A. Boudville, H. Taylor and R. Bailie (2016). Delivery of eye and vision services in Aboriginal and Torres Strait Islander primary healthcare centers. *Frontiers in Public Health* 4: 276. DOI: 10.3389/fpubh.2016.00276.

de Savigny, D. and T. Adam, eds (2009). *Systems thinking for health systems strengthening.* Geneva: Alliance for Health Policy and Systems Research, World Health Organization.

Deming, W. Edwards (2018). *The New Economics for Industry, Government, Education. 3rd edn.* Cambridge, MA: MIT Press.

Dolansky, M. and S. Moore (2013). Quality and safety education for nurses (QSEN): the key is systems thinking. *Online Journal of Issues in Nursing* 18(3): 1. DOI: 10.3912/OJIN.Vol18No03Man01.

Evergreen, S. (2024). *Evergreen data: intentional reporting and data visualization.* https://stephanieevergreen.com/.

Gibson-Helm, M., H. Teede, A. Rumbold, S. Ranasinha, R. Bailie and J. Boyle (2015). Continuous quality improvement and metabolic screening during pregnancy at primary health centres attended by Aboriginal and Torres Strait Islander women. *Medical Journal of Australia* 203(9): e1–7. DOI: 10.5694/mja14.01660.

Halperin, I., J. Gilmour, P. Segal, L. Sutton, R. Wong, L. Caplan et al. (2019). Determining root causes and designing change ideas in a quality improvement project. *Canadian Journal of Diabetes* 43 (4): 241–8. DOI: 10.1016/j.jcjd.2019.03.001.

Institute for Healthcare Improvement (2021). Science of improvement: tips for setting aims. *How to improve.* https://www.ihi.org/how-improve-model-improvement-setting-aims

Larkins, S., K. Carlisle, N. Turner, J. Taylor, K. Copley, S. Cooney et al. (2019). "At the grass roots level it's about sitting down and talking": exploring quality improvement through case studies with high-improving Aboriginal and Torres Strait Islander primary healthcare services. *BMJ Open* 9 (5): e027568. DOI: 10.1136/bmjopen-2018-027568.

Laycock, A., G. Harvey, N. Percival, F. Cunningham, J. Bailie, V. Matthews et al. (2018). Application of the i-PARIHS framework for enhancing understanding of interactive dissemination to achieve wide-scale improvement in Indigenous primary healthcare. *Health Research Policy and Systems* 16: 117. DOI: 10.1186/s12961-018-0392-z.

Matthews, V., J. Bailie, A. Laycock, T. Nagel and R. Bailie (2016). *Aboriginal and Torres Strait Islander mental health and wellbeing care: final report, ESP Project.* Brisbane: Menzies School of Health Research.

Matthews, V., C. Burgess, C. Connors, E. Moore, D. Peiris, D. Scrimgeour et al. (2017). Integrated clinical decision support systems promote absolute cardiovascular risk assessment: an important primary prevention measure in Aboriginal and Torres Strait Islander primary health care. *Frontiers in Public Health* 5: 233. DOI: 10.3389/fpubh.2017.00233.

Matthews, V., C. Connors, A. Laycock, J. Bailie and R. Bailie (2015). *Chronic illness care for Aboriginal and Torres Strait Islander people: final report. ESP Project: priority evidence-practice gaps and stakeholder views on barriers and strategies for improvement.* Brisbane: Menzies School of Health Research.

Matthews, V., G. Schierhout, J. McBroom, C. Connors, C. Kennedy, R. Kwedza et al. (2014). Duration of participation in continuous quality improvement: a key factor explaining improved delivery of type 2 diabetes services. *BMC Health Services Research* 14(1): 578. DOI: 10.1186/s12913-014-0578-1.

McAullay, D., K. McAuley, R. Bailie, V. Mathews, P. Jacoby, K. Gardner et al. (2018). Sustained participation in annual continuous quality improvement activities improves quality of care for Aboriginal and Torres Strait Islander children. *Journal of Paediatrics and Child Health* 54(2): 132–40. DOI: 10.1111/jpc.13673.

Menzies School of Health Research and One21seventy (2012). *Systems assessment tool – all client groups*. Darwin: Menzies School of Health Research.

Nattabi, B., V. Matthews, J. Bailie, A. Rumbold, D. Scrimgeour, J. Ward et al. (2017). Wide variation in sexually transmitted infection testing and counselling at Aboriginal primary health care centres in Australia: analysis of longitudinal continuous quality improvement data. *BMC Infectious Diseases* 17: 148. DOI: 10.1186/s12879-017-2241-z.

Newham, J. and F. Cunningham (2015). *Continuous quality improvement success stories: identifying effective strategies for CQI in Aboriginal and Torres Strait Islander primary health care – study report*. ABCD National Research Partnership. Brisbane: ABCD National Research Partnership, Menzies School of Health Research.

Ralph, A., M. Fittock, R. Schultz, D. Thompson, M. Dowden, T. Clemens et al. (2013). Improvement in rheumatic fever and rheumatic heart disease management and prevention using a health centre-based continuous quality improvement approach. *BMC Health Services Research* 13: 525. DOI: 10.1186/1472-6963-13-525.

Reed, J., C. McNicholas, T. Woodcock, L. Issen and D. Bell (2014). Designing quality improvement initiatives: the action effect method, a structured approach to identifying and articulating programme theory. *BMJ Quality and Safety* 23(12): 1040–8. DOI: 10.1136/bmjqs-2014-003103.

Schierhout, G., V. Matthews, C. Connors, S. Thompson, R. Kwedza, C. Kennedy et al. (2016). Improvement in delivery of type 2 diabetes services differs by mode of care: a retrospective longitudinal analysis in the Aboriginal and Torres Strait Islander primary health care setting. *BMC Health Services Research* 16: 560. DOI: 10.1186/s12913-016-1812-9.

Si, D., R. Bailie, J. Cunningham, G. Robinson, M. Dowden, A. Stewart et al. (2008). Describing and analysing primary health care system support for chronic illness care in Indigenous communities in Australia's Northern Territory – use of the Chronic Care Model. *BMC Health Services Research* 8: 112. DOI: 10.1186/1472-6963-8-112.

Timothy, A., D. Coetzee, C. Morgan, M. Kelaher, R. Bailie and M. Danchin (2021). Using an adaptive, codesign approach to strengthen clinic-level immunisation services in Khayelitsha, Western Cape Province, South Africa. *BMJ Global Health* 6(3): e004004. DOI: 10.1136/bmjgh-2020-004004.

Vasant, B., V. Matthews, C. Burgess, C. Connors and R. Bailie (2016). Wide variation in absolute cardiovascular risk assessment in Aboriginal and Torres Strait Islander people with type 2 diabetes. *Frontiers in Public Health* 4: 37. DOI: 10.3389/fpubh.2016.00037.

Woods, C., K. Carlisle, S. Larkins, S. Thompson, K. Tsey, V. Matthews et al. (2017) Exploring systems that support good clinical care in Indigenous primary health-care services: a retrospective analysis of longitudinal systems assessment tool data from high-improving services. *Frontiers in Public Health* 5: 45 . DOI: 10.3389/fpubh.2017.00045.

While continuous quality improvement (CQI) tools and approaches differ, a common feature is that they harness the knowledge, skills, experience and views of a range of people involved in, or affected by, care. This is the essence of CQI. It is through participation, interaction, shared decision-making and ongoing engagement in CQI cycles that improvement needs are identified, and changes are implemented and sustained. People who are actively engaged in CQI processes are generally more invested in seeing their efforts succeed. The facilitation of these processes is crucial to improving care. This chapter shares knowledge and techniques for facilitating CQI in PHC settings.

What is facilitation?

Facilitation is a technique where an individual makes things easier for others, by providing support to help them develop their thinking and ways of working.[1] Put simply, it is a process of enabling groups or teams to work effectively together to achieve a common goal.[2] The humanistic principles of participation, engagement, shared decision-making and enabling that underpin facilitation[3] align well with the core principles of CQI.[4]

In health care, facilitation has been defined as the "active ingredient" that matches a proposed improvement to the individuals and teams involved and the context in which they work, thereby enabling successful implementation.[5] Facilitators are agents of change.

The focus of facilitation varies according to the underpinning theory being used (for examle, change management theory, community development theory) and the aim. Facilitation may focus on empowering participants, for example, by harnessing individual strengths to challenge existing practice and find new ways of thinking and doing to improve care. A common focus of CQI facilitation is on tasks and team processes for achieving defined goals.[6]

Some health services employ CQI facilitators, but often CQI facilitation is done by appointed CQI leaders within PHC services or practices, or in community-based programs. In some CQI models, external facilitators provide support across a network of PHC services and practices.[7] Facilitators may come from clinical or non-clinical backgrounds. Regardless of the model

---

1   Kitson, Harvey and McCormack 1998, adapted.
2   Schwarz 2002.
3   Hogan 2002.
4   Harvey and Lynch 2017.
5   Harvey and Kitson 2016.
6   Harvey, McCormack et al. 2018.
7   Best, Greenhalgh et al. 2012; Dogherty, Harrison and Graham 2010.

used, a key aim of a CQI facilitator is to drive and motivate a practice or system change and to act as a resource for making changes happen.[8]

Facilitation works to improve care

There is evidence that facilitation of team-based, goal-focused CQI that responds to local context can enhance the uptake of evidence-based care[9] and improve health outcomes.[10] International research found that PHC practices supported by facilitators are almost three times more likely to adopt evidence-based clinical guidelines.[11] This should not surprise, given the complexity of implementing best-practice guidelines across the scope of clinical PHC. Further evidence of the effectiveness of facilitation comes from a large trial in Vietnam engaging women with maternal and newborn care. Groups who received support from community workers trained as quality improvement facilitators demonstrated a significant reduction in neonatal mortality after three years.[12]

> International research found that PHC practices supported by facilitators are almost three times more likely to adopt evidence-based clinical guidelines.

Numerous factors at a local, organisational and health system level can influence the success of an improvement program. Effective facilitation is key to PHC staff making sense of data, identifying improvement goals and successfully tailoring evidence-based improvement interventions to context.[13] In Indigenous Australian settings, for example, facilitation is important for adapting CQI approaches to suit PHC settings,[14] and for adjusting CQI processes to respond to local needs.[15]

Example: embedding a CQI facilitator in a centralised support team

A study conducted across a network of eleven Aboriginal community controlled PHC services investigated barriers and enablers to implementing a CQI program. Participants in management and clinical roles identified dedicated facilitation support as a key enabler for initiating and sustaining CQI activity.

In this context, it was important for the CQI facilitation role to be embedded in a centralised team that offered integrated CQI delivery support to member services. The approach promoted a coherent and systems-based approach to planning and improvement across the organisation.[16]

---

8   Cranley, Cummings et al. 2017.
9   Baskerville, Liddy and Hogg 2012.
10   Persson, Nga et al. 2013.
11   Baskerville, Liddy and Hogg 2012.
12   Persson, Nga et al. 2013.
13   Harvey and Lynch 2017.
14   Brimblecombe, Bailie et al. 2017; Larkins, Carlisle et al. 2019; Percival, O'Donoghue et al. 2016.
15   Newham, Schierhout et al. 2016; Woods, Carlisle et al. 2017.
16   Newham, Schierhout et al. 2016.

Another study explored CQI implementation in six PHC services that had demonstrated significant improvement. Locally facilitated team meetings, community input to health service organisation, and shared decision-making contributed to CQI that responded to the sociocultural context of the service. The harnessing of collective intent and action were motivating for teams and supported the development of shared goals and improved health outcomes for service users.[17]

What does CQI facilitation look like?

As defined above, CQI facilitation is an enabling role, as opposed to persuading, directing or telling people what to do. A facilitator helps groups to work collaboratively to agree on areas for improvement and to create and sustain change in the way care is provided.[18] Working in this way stimulates learning. It helps to embed capacity for change within healthcare or program teams by influencing workplace culture, and by empowering and upskilling team or community members, or both, to facilitate change.[19] Sustainable change is more likely to result from CQI processes that actively involve a range of stakeholders in identifying improvement needs, and in planning and implementing changes.

> CQI facilitation is an enabling role.

Many CQI resources refer to "quality improvement teams". Bringing together a quality improvement team is best suited to large-scale organisations, such as hospitals, or to healthcare support organisations that serve a network of services or practices. It is not necessarily feasible to nominate a quality improvement team in a small health centre or practice, because the entire PHC team is likely to be involved in identifying improvement priorities and planning improvement strategies. When we refer to teams, we are referring to PHC or program teams.

Facilitating with PHC teams

Services with well-functioning CQI programs generally demonstrate good teamwork and collaboration, including supportive leadership for CQI. A striking feature of six high-improving PHC services studied by Larkins and colleagues was staff commitment to working together towards the same goal —improved health for their clients and their communities. Facilitators were likely to encourage teamwork through team meetings, shared decision-making and linking with CQI support networks.[20]

A range of strategies can be facilitated as part of a CQI process, such as these:

- educating participants in core concepts of CQI and how to use appropriate tools
- engaging staff, managers and other key stakeholders in CQI processes

---

17   Larkins, Carlisle et al. 2019.
18   Harvey and Lynch 2017.
19   Berta, Cranley et al. 2015.
20   Larkins, Carlisle et al. 2019.

- undertaking a baseline assessment that involves assessing readiness for CQI (motivation and capability); surveying the operating environment; and identifying who needs to be involved
- collecting data using CQI tools and methods (for example, undertaking an audit, surveying community perspectives)
- analysing and interpreting data, identifying improvement priorities and developing an action plan
- implementing improvement strategies, providing feedback on the activities in real time, and tracking progress
- repeating data collection to measure improvement and reflecting on CQI implementation (what worked well and less well)
- sharing results with a wider group as relevant, celebrating success, testing further changes as needed and sustaining improvement.[21]

The way in which the strategies are facilitated depends on the PHC context, the skills, knowledge and characteristics of the PHC team, management approaches, the focus of the improvement work and the evidence used for informing change.[22] Tailoring facilitation to needs and context leads to more effective CQI.[23]

> Tailoring facilitation to needs and context leads to more effective CQI.

Story: tailoring a CQI process to the needs of a PHC service

Experienced CQI facilitators were invited by a PHC team in a remote area to help develop an action plan to improve systems of care for clients with diabetes. It was a multidisciplinary team with resident nurses, Aboriginal health practitioners, a diabetes educator and health promotion staff, and two general practitioners who flew in and out on a weekly roster. Half the team were Aboriginal people from the community.

"We began by clarifying the quality problem. We looked at the data – how many clients had a diabetes diagnosis, HbA1c [blood glucose level] and blood pressure results and so on, and paid particular attention to trends over time. Did the data show things were improving or getting worse? We considered qualitative data. What was the feedback from the clients themselves and from the community? The large number of local Aboriginal staff made it a lot easier to understand the situation from a client perspective, as many had family members who had diabetes, or had a diagnosis themselves.

---

21 Harvey and Lynch 2017.
22 Harvey and Kitson 2015; Larkins, Carlisle et al. 2019; Laycock, Harvey et al. 2018; Øvretveit 2014.
23 Baskerville, Liddy and Hogg 2012.

Once we had a clear picture, we spent time mapping out those things that made effective diabetes management more difficult and what the health service could do to improve their systems of care, the patient experience and hopefully improve outcomes for their clients. We used a mind mapping tool to do this. This led to a prioritising process. We discussed what could they change straight away to improve care and what could be addressed down the track.

When the team had identified their priorities for improvement, we used the plan-do-study-act (PDSA) tool to set goals, plan measurement and outline the steps they would take to make changes. The team wrote out a plan. As we all know how easy it is to write a plan and not follow through on it, people were identified to take responsibility for ensuring each part of the plan was actioned. The manager of the team also put the CQI process for diabetes on their health centre meeting agenda to ensure it didn't get lost in the busyness of the health centre activities."

– Kerry Copley and Louise Patel, CQI program coordinators, Aboriginal Medical Services Alliance Northern Territory.

For more information, see Aboriginal Medical Services Alliance Northern Territory n.d.

Engaging clients, families, carers and communities in CQI

Engaging clients, their families or carers, and communities in CQI is consistent with concepts of client-centred and value-based care. It signals a shift in thinking from asking "What is the matter?" to asking "What matters to you or to us (or both)?".

Facilitation strategies for engaging clients, families/carers and communities are likely to focus on:

- working with organisational leadership to manage expectations and to clarify the expected contribution of clients and their families or carers, the resources required and potential risks and benefits
- developing mechanisms for community members and staff to share ideas, information and make joint decisions about quality improvement
- training and supporting community members to take on a community facilitator role
- engaging in genuine learning and sharing of perspectives through relationships as well as through structured learning opportunities (in some contexts, this involves building relationships with client participants through an appointed staff "partner")
- engaging clients and carers in quality improvement sessions and encouraging them to share their lived experience and local knowledge
- reaching out to clients through focus groups, interviews, surveys or gathering stories about clients' experiences, or a combination of these
- supporting staff to take on client input
- consulting client and community representatives on advisory committees and governing boards
- getting leadership commitment to implement suggestions or plans that come from client engagement in CQI. This may require advocacy with policy makers and funders.

Example: seeking community input about service quality

A health service providing PHC for an Indigenous community in a remote region of northern Australia held annual whole-of-community meetings to discuss the quality of care delivered. At the meetings, community members and service staff came together to share information and ideas, and to make joint decisions about quality improvement.

> "We go out yearly and hold open community meetings . . . Management staff will go out, put ourselves in front of the community . . . give an update on what we've done for the last twelve months . . . open that up to the community and our performance review begins at that point. You tell us from a grass roots perspective . . . and if we've got challenges then [they] will certainly let us know." – Indigenous service manager[24]

Community participation in health care is expected to build a better understanding of community needs and priorities,[25] build client expectations for quality care and strengthen community leadership for health.[26]

In many settings, knowledge about the ways in which social and cultural determinants (including historical and political events) affect health and access to care is important for improving service delivery.[27] Facilitation can bring care providers and community members together to support two-way learning for improving care.

Turner and colleagues studied the link between community participation and CQI in Aboriginal and Torres Strait Islander PHC services. Different mechanisms were used to encourage community engagement in quality improvement.

Example: engaging clients in identifying improvement priorities

The health service in an Aboriginal and Torres Strait Islander community was keen to introduce a culturally based model for care that supported clinicians to work with Indigenous families in a holistic and empowering way. There were regular discussions between groups of community people and health service staff for identifying improvement priorities in different areas of care.

> "There was a whole morning talking with the women [about maternal care]. It's a two-way conversation around what we already provide and what women really feel they need, and the issues around birthing in a different place when they have to leave town." – clinician[28]

---

24   Larkins, Carlisle et al. 2019.
25   McCalman, Bailie et al. 2018.
26   Wise, Angus et al. 2013.
27   Turner, Taylor et al. 2019.
28   Turner, Taylor et al. 2019, 1908.

Example: a facilitated partnership to improve health

In an Aboriginal and Torres Strait Islander community in northern Australia, there was strong participation in the health service and a whole-of-community approach to quality improvement. "Driving the health of the community" was a facilitated partnership between healthcare providers, service users and community members, which empowered the community for quality improvement. The health committee had representation from the local council, Elders and different health units and government agencies who came together for sharing, joint planning, and action, including group advocacy.

> "People are taking control of their own health and we've got a Health Committee here. That's been set up to look after the health in general of the community – things that work hand-in-hand with the clinical side." – community member[29]

In each of the examples in the boxes, the PHC service set out to create an environment where the health service was actively engaged with the community to build trust and improve the health and wellbeing of the community.

What characterises a good facilitator?

In this section, we summarise the skills, knowledge and attributes that are used to describe expert facilitators in the quality improvement literature.

- An experienced CQI facilitator is able to clarify the improvement task (for example, its purpose, complexity, and what is involved), and decide who needs to be closely involved in the work: the roles and expertise needed, groups to be included and collaborating organisations.
- In PHC settings, facilitators need a credible knowledge base in PHC (for example, core concepts, scope of clinical care and how it is provided), how data can be used for improvement, CQI tools and methods, and the local and organisational environment.
- Facilitators need skills to engage effectively with the people involved and in the proposed change. This requires the ability to develop positive and effective working relationships with managers, staff, other service providers and client representatives.
- Good CQI facilitators have skills to communicate clearly and consistently, to appraise evidence and prepare resource materials.
- Facilitators are able to set ground rules for group work, and work with participants to dismiss fears and manage expectations. They are respectful and can listen actively, build trust, and encourage participation and different points of view to arrive at team decisions and actions.
- Facilitators may need skills in negotiation and conflict management.
- Good facilitators are also reflective on their own practice.

---

29   Turner, Taylor et al. 2019, 1908.

- Facilitators have personal attributes that contribute to effective facilitation. Expert facilitators are described as empathetic, sensitive, flexible and pragmatic. They come across as credible and passionate about their work.[30]

It is not suggested that effective CQI facilitation depends on the facilitator having expertise in all aspects. Skills, knowledge and confidence are developed over time through informal and formal learning opportunities and on-the-ground experience. Furthermore, it takes experience to be able to act effectively in the moment: to decide if, when and how to intervene into discussions as a group works towards its goals. Over the course of a single meeting, multiple decisions may need to be made about when and how to act, particularly if the facilitator does not know the group well.[31]

> Facilitation skills, knowledge and confidence are developed over time through informal and formal learning opportunities and on-the-ground experience.

CQI facilitation may be shared across a PHC team, with members taking on roles according to their areas of expertise. This approach can help to sustain CQI in the event of a skilled facilitator leaving the service or program and has implications for where and how facilitator training is delivered.

Example: spreading facilitation skills across teams

For participants in Newham and colleagues' study of barriers and enablers to implementing a quality improvement program, developing CQI capability within PHC teams was seen as key to the uptake of CQI.

> "You need . . . one or two key people that have got the understanding and can drive it." – manager and clinician, service A

Staff talked about the importance of training local staff to facilitate learning and improvement.

> "I think it's very important that [the external CQI facilitator] come and teach the staff . . . and those people who are trained by [the facilitator] can act as champions and as trainers to other health workers." – manager and clinician, service B[32]

> Sharing CQI facilitation across a team can help sustain CQI in the event of a skilled facilitator leaving the service or program.

---

30   Dogherty, Harrison et al. 2013; Harvey and Kitson 2015; Harvey and Lynch 2017.
31   Shaw, Looney et al. 2010.
32   Newham, Schierhout et al. 2016, 250.

Supporting continuous learning and improvement

Continuous learning is a core concept of CQI. An understanding of adult learning principles and concepts supports effective CQI facilitation.

Facilitation and adult learners

People learn in different ways. In the 1960s, adult educator Malcolm Knowles identified principles of adult learning. These internationally accepted principles underpin current adult learning programs:

- our willingness to learn as adults is connected to what we want to learn more about
- we are independent and self-directed in our learning
- we bring life experiences and prior knowledge to learning
- our readiness to learn is often connected to a need to do something in real life (for example, work tasks)
- we are goal-oriented and problem-centred learners
- our motivation to learn comes from within.[33]

Other characteristics of adult learners should also be considered when planning and facilitating CQI learning activities. We tend to lead complex and busy lives, have set habits and preferences, and established attitudes (including attitudes about a learning situation). Some adults can be afraid of participation in group learning – we may fear embarrassment or a loss of dignity. Adults can resent being told what to do, particularly by a person in authority. We may also worry about keeping pace with the demands made on us in a learning environment (for example, to understand CQI data). These concerns can influence the way people engage with CQI processes.

Responding to learning and communication styles

Skilled facilitation takes account of individual learning styles and presents information in a range of ways to engage all group members. We all use a range of ways to learn, but we tend to respond to one method above others. These are some of the different learning preferences people have:

- taking in information visually (preferring charts, symbols, graphics)
- taking in information by reading and writing (preferring hand-outs, PowerPoint presentations and taking notes)
- hearing and discussing information (preferring group activities)
- doing a task and getting the feel for it (with hands-on, participatory learning in work settings).

Some adults are social and interpersonal learners; others prefer solitary learning activities. Personality styles influence learning, and the way individuals behave and respond in group sessions: introverted or extroverted; logical or emotional; task-oriented or process oriented. The ability of a facilitator to recognise and respond to these preferences and communication styles develops through learning and practice.

---

33 Knowles 1990.

Skilled facilitation takes account of individual learning styles and presents information in a range of ways to engage all group members.

Responding to diversity

Understanding who the participants are is important for successful facilitation outcomes and ultimately for effective improvement interventions. Diversity encompasses race, ethnic group, culture, gender, age, religion, ability/disability, sexual orientation, personality, cognitive style, knowledge bases (for example, Euro-Western and Indigenous knowledge systems) work roles, skill sets, education and more. These factors influence how people perceive themselves and how they perceive others. Those perceptions affect interactions within social settings, including the facilitation of CQI. It can be challenging to ensure that all group members feel safe to contribute to discussion when participants come from a range of backgrounds, or when the facilitator and participants come from different backgrounds.

Supporting cultural safety

Culture and language influence the way people learn, hold and share knowledge, and engage in group activities. In Indigenous health settings, culturally safe facilitation practice is crucial for engaging participants in CQI for client-centred care.

Cultural safety involves actions that recognise, respect and nurture the unique cultural identity of a person and safely meet their needs, expectations and rights. It is part of a rights-based approach to health care supported by the United Nations Declaration on the Rights of Indigenous Peoples. Cultural safety was first defined by a Māori nurse, Irihapeti Ramsden, in the cultural context of Aotearoa/New Zealand, in response to the harmful effects of colonisation and its ongoing legacy on the health and health care of Māori people.[34] It has been embraced in Australian health care involving Aboriginal and Torres Strait Islander peoples, and by some other nations with a history of colonisation, discrimination and disempowerment of First Nations peoples. Similar terms are used: for example, cultural awareness, cultural respect, cultural responsiveness and cultural competence.[35] Cultural safety is the term generally preferred by Aboriginal and Torres Strait Islander organisations, as being a more realistic aspiration.[36]

While being culturally aware involves sensitivity to the similarities and differences that exist between different cultures, working in a culturally safe way generally involves centring the cultural perspective of the other person, valuing and validating their experiences.[37] It involves being aware of culture, history and racism as determinants of health, being open to different cultural understandings of health and wellbeing, and being open to different models of health care (for example, Indigenous, Western and Eastern models). Services that provide care to First Nations communities, for example, can improve cultural safety by employing and investing in the career development of First Nations staff, supporting non-Indigenous staff to

---

34   Papps and Ramsden 1996.
35   Cross, Bazron et al. 1989.
36   Congress of Aboriginal and Torres Strait Islander Nurses and Midwives (CATSINaM) 2014.
37   Lowitja Institute 2022.

develop and uphold culturally safe and respectful practices, and having strong representation of First Nations peoples in management and governance positions.[38] Services can create an environment where their First Nations clients feel welcome and set up mechanisms for effective engagement with the community.

> Working in a culturally safe way generally involves focusing on the cultural perspective of the other person, valuing and validating their experiences.

CQI facilitators who strive to work in a culturally safe way appreciate and validate cultural differences. Those within the dominant culture engage in critical self-reflection to question how their beliefs, values and practices inform how they work. They recognise how the systems of power and privilege affect health worker teams, and work to prevent bias and racism.[39]

CQI facilitation that honours Indigenous ways of knowing, being and doing[40] is able to draw on participants' cultural strengths to interpret data and plan interventions that reflect community values and priorities. Establishing a culturally safe space at the outset is essential.

Example: creating a culturally safe space for CQI training

Louise Patel and Kerry Copley are non-Indigenous CQI leaders/program coordinators with experience in facilitating CQI training workshops with Aboriginal and Torres Strait Islander staff.

> "We start the day by acknowledging the traditional custodians of the land we are working on and by building a relationship with those in the room – connection before content. In a PowerPoint presentation, we confirm the importance of family (with photos) and where we come from (our homes and work history), our close working relationship with each other and the relationship we have with PHC staff and community. We've been in these roles for twelve years now, so we are familiar with cultural and health issues around PHC, and people know and trust us. We can tell stories to make CQI real.

> We share the history of the workshops; how senior Aboriginal health practitioners saw the need for CQI training specifically for the Aboriginal and Torres Strait Islander health workforce. We invite the participants to share their learnings – that we all have important knowledge to offer. English is not the first language for many, and we assure participants it's okay to ask for clarification, or to stop us if we don't use plain language. We reinforce that we want the environment to be a safe place to talk, discuss issues and tell stories – confidentiality and respect are high priorities. We only take photos with permission."

---

38 Australian Health Practitioner Regulation Agency and National Boards 2020.
39 Gollan and Stacey 2021.
40 Martin-Booran Mirraboopa 2003.

Establishing a safe environment for sharing experiences and working collaboratively can be challenging when the focus of improvement intersects with people's lived experience. The following example describes strategies used to achieve cultural and psychological safety in workshops to improve skills in mental health care.

Example: facilitating workshops to improve responses to mental health needs

Danielle Cameron is a Yuibera woman from the Birragubba nation in Queensland, Australia, a quality improvement researcher and facilitator specialising in mental health, trauma and workforce development.

"Walking into a room, I need to know who the traditional custodians are of the area I am working in, also if there has been any 'sorry business' and whatever else may be going on in the community. I ask what people need to enhance their learning experience. I talk about where my family is from and always honour the land I am on.

I normally start off with an icebreaker to create safety and help people relax – this is especially important when talking about social and emotional wellbeing. As a facilitator, it is a fine line between that storytelling process and ensuring that you are creating safety for others so they can feel they can be open, but they don't become traumatised. I generally walk around the room, keeping a warm and engaging tone and connecting with everyone so they know they are heard and seen. I think it is so important to know the material, so you can then focus on how you work the room.

I discuss suicidal ideation and other complex mental health concerns, so I always check in with people and use a thumbs-up and thumbs-down strategy for when they need to take a break. I use somatic grounding techniques. It's very important that people feel okay when they leave."

Resources and training for culturally safe PHC practice are offered through specialised consultants, community groups, health care, education and training providers. They include online resources and training relevant to specific First Nations settings.

Managing relationships and group dynamics

As highlighted in Part I, PHC is delivered through diverse organisational models, settings and staff. The facilitation of CQI needs to respond to each group and context. Individual engagement, behaviours and group dynamics can be influenced by multiple factors.

- Staff may feel they are being diverted from their primary role of providing care.
- Top-down power structures in health care, where traditionally doctors and medical specialists are in charge and nurses and other staff defer to their authority, may intimidate less senior team members.
- Other power relationships, such as the influence of governing boards, board members, practice owners or Indigenous Elders, may inhibit some individuals in the group.
- Managers and leaders may expect to, and be expected to, lead decision-making.

- Individual staff may feel a sense of ownership over a particular area of care and feel threatened by that area coming under scrutiny.
- Individuals may fear that changes to systems and processes will negatively affect their jobs, status or work environment.
- Individuals from diverse cultural and linguistic backgrounds need to feel culturally safe.
- Individuals may have differing perceptions of the role and value of other staff members: this can be a strength or a point of tension in the team.

These tensions need careful management by a CQI facilitator. People are more likely to participate actively in a CQI process if they feel heard and believe the improvement plan is relevant for them and the work they are doing.

The following tips (Box 7.1) were developed by highly experienced CQI facilitators who work with PHC teams.

Box 7.1 Tips for facilitating groups

Before a group session

If you are "external" to the services or practice, find out about the group you are working with and the context – team size, skill or role mix, how long people have been in the team, their experience in using CQI and issues such as workforce turnover and changes in management. Don't go in blind.

Have a plan for how you will facilitate the discussion but be prepared to change the plan in response to where the team is at and what happens on the day.

At the start

Discuss ways of working. Set group rules for interacting in a safe and respectful way. This process often follows an icebreaker activity.

Take time to connect with the group. Find out what matters to them in relation to the topic or topics you are discussing, and their expectations for the session. You will need to get buy-in to tease out their priorities for improvement and get input for planning change.

Acknowledge that change can be difficult, especially if people feel they have little influence on the direction of the change. Ensure everyone knows that their input matters.

Throughout the session

Always remember that as the facilitator you set the tone for the discussion.

Create and maintain a safe space where people feel valued, respected and comfortable to contribute.

- Model respect for different roles and cultures within the team and how that adds value and brings different perspectives to the discussion.

- Make sure everyone has opportunities to contribute to the discussion and planning. This may mean creating different ways for people to have a voice. Not everyone feels comfortable speaking up in a large group or in front of managers.

- Make clear the expectation that everyone will be professional and respectful and that the session isn't an opportunity to air grievances. When that happens (and it does), have a strategy for managing it. You might simply thank the person for their comment and put it into a "parking space" for later, while reminding everyone of the purpose of the discussion.

Be real! People connect with others who are genuine and congruent. A good facilitator makes connections with people and builds rapport by being open, honest and true to themselves.

– Kerry Copley and Louise Patel, CQI program coordinators, Aboriginal Medical Services Alliance Northern Territory.

For more information, see Aboriginal Medical Services Alliance Northern Territory n.d.

Facilitation is a complex task. Skills and confidence in facilitating CQI processes develop over time through formal and informal learning opportunities and through practice. Strategies for developing facilitation skills and knowledge may include:

- undertaking relevant training
- observing and learning from experienced facilitators
- identifying a mentor facilitator
- joining or building a network of people in similar roles to share learning
- taking opportunities to facilitate CQI processes and other group work
- building a tool kit of quality improvement tools and techniques for working with groups.

A wealth of resources is available about facilitating groups. Check online sources for resources that meet your needs. Encourage others who facilitate CQI in similar settings to share useful resources.

Features of effective facilitation

We have adapted the characteristics of facilitation from those identified by Harvey and Kitson in their guide to implementing evidence-based practice in health care:

- participation and involvement of key stakeholders
- development of a shared understanding of the improvement activity
- ownership and control of the CQI process by the people who are responsible for making change
- sensitivity to the local context and culture
- iterative processes integrated into routine systems and processes
- linkage of local initiatives to wider system changes
- provision of feedback on improvement activities through simple real-time mechanisms
- empowerment and enablement of others in decision-making and action
- management of group dynamics and supporting learning.[41]

---

41   Harvey and Kitson 2015.

Finally, facilitation should give PHC teams ownership of their CQI data and process and acknowledge their efforts in delivering quality care with the resources they have available. This is particularly important in settings where there is a high acute care load and a high burden of client illness. It helps to embed a culture of CQI. In the following examples, CQI facilitators reflect on key aspects of their role.

Supporting ownership of CQI

"In the early days of the CQI research, we were testing the CQI tools and the language we used, continually improving the protocols and noting what resources we needed to support PHC teams in their CQI processes. When we facilitated audits and systems assessments on the ground, we were making notes at every point about what was happening in the clinic on that day – visiting service providers, issues, how busy the clinic was – anything that would add to the data story when we fed back the results, that would help the team to understand and interpret their data. That's when I really started to see that how I facilitated CQI was important for helping to embed CQI in those health services."

– Lynette O'Donoghue, CQI facilitator, Menzies School of Health Research

Building trust and respect

"Reciprocal trust and respect grew as relationships developed between the CQI research facilitators and local participating health services and teams. That process fostered two-way learning. It was critically important for engagement in CQI that each health service's CQI story was their own and confidentiality was paramount – it was up to services how they wanted to share their feedback reports."

– Lynette O'Donoghue, CQI facilitator, Menzies School of Health Research

Acknowledging and supporting the work of PHC teams

"I have worked in remote health centres for eighteen years now. My role for the last eleven years has been as a CQI facilitator. I assist the local staff to develop, implement and evaluate quality activities that address their local needs . . . I love being able to show people how to manage what they do and see the improvement in their [key performance indicators] and just generally in the way they work, because they work very hard and – like we say in CQI – it's about working smarter not harder."

– Eva Williams, CQI facilitator, Northern Territory Department of Health [42]

CQI facilitation should give PHC teams ownership of their CQI data and process and acknowledge their efforts in delivering quality care.

---

42   Northern Territory Remote Locum Program and Aboriginal Medical Services Alliance of the Northern Territory (AMSANT), n.d.

Useful group techniques

Brainstorming

Brainstorming can help a team to quickly generate ideas. Designed to encourage spontaneous ideas, lateral thinking and creative problem solving, brainstorming enables people to participate without feeling bound to represent their role, to present alternative views, to offer critique or find group consensus. In CQI, brainstorming is used in conjunction with CQI tools, for purposes such as these:

- to identify the possible causes of a quality problem identified through a clinical audit and systems assessment
- to develop a cause-and-effect diagram
- to develop a driver diagram (see Chapter 5)
- to generate change ideas (possible solutions to identified problems) for strategy development and testing through plan-do-study-act cycles.

Brainstorming requires a facilitator and clear rules. Criticism, rejection or discussion of ideas is avoided (unless for clarification). Ideas are generated rapidly and are recorded for later discussion. They should be specific enough for the group to make meaning of them (for example, "staff don't have cultural competency training" rather than "training").

Brainstorming aloud has potential to trigger ideas amongst the team. Silent brainstorming limits the potential for dominance by individuals; it may be more productive with reserved team members, or when participation is influenced by hierarchical work relationships. Writing each idea on a new note also makes it easier to sort ideas into categories afterwards, and to prioritise ideas based on how many people had similar thoughts.

Five Whys brainstorming

Five Whys (also known as the Toyoda technique after Sakichi Toyoda, who developed it) is a specific brainstorming technique used to identify the underlying cause of a quality problem that has been identified through a CQI process (Box 7.2). It is useful when doing root cause analysis. Use of Five Whys can help the team to understand what is really happening, rather than what appears to be happening – which may simply be another symptom of the problem. It can help the team to understand the system issues that underlie gaps in care processes or delivery of care. This understanding enables effective action to be taken to address a problem and to prevent it from happening in the future.

- The team starts with a clear problem statement and asks the question: "Why is this happening?"
- The answer is recorded. The question "Why is that?" is asked.
- This process is repeated three more times (at least) until the team reaches the root cause of the problem.
- By then asking, "What can we do to change this?", you can develop and test a solution.

Box 7.2 Example of the Five Whys technique

Problem statement: A number of our elderly clients missed out on their vaccination.

1. **Why** did the elderly clients miss out on their vaccinations?

   The clients were not flagged as eligible for the vaccination by the electronic client information system.

2. **Why** weren't the clients flagged as eligible for the vaccination in the information system?

   Dates of birth for these clients were incorrectly formatted or were missing from their client records.

3. **Why** were the dates of birth incorrectly formatted or missing from their client records?

   Staff were unclear about the required format. Some elderly clients could not specify their date of birth, so that data field was not filled in.

4. **Why** were staff members unclear about the required format, or what to do when birthdates are unknown?

   Staff haven't received training in how to enter data and there is no advice on the electronic template for entering this information or for estimating date of birth.

5. **Why** haven't staff received training or advice on how to enter data in the electronic template?

   The information technology support team is under-resourced. Team members don't have capacity to train staff in data entry and updating the system to include this advice hasn't been a priority. They don't appreciate the importance of these data in the delivery of care.

Yarning

Yarning is an Indigenous way of communicating: a conversational process for sharing stories and for developing and passing on knowledge. Yarning is used by many Indigenous peoples as a way of learning collectively, sustaining relationships and preserving and passing on cultural knowledge.[43]

When used appropriately as a research method by and with Indigenous peoples, yarning can help to promote cultural safety, empower participants to tell their stories in their own way and create meaningful data. Yarning has potential for engaging Indigenous participants in CQI. It can be an informal process of "having a yarn" about a topic, with the facilitator taking on the information provided throughout the conversation. Collaborative yarning can be used to identify priorities, to analyse and interpret data, and to generate improvement projects in community settings.[44]

---

43   Atkinson, Baird and Adams 2021.

44   Bessarab and Ng'Andu 2010; Geia, Hayes and Usher 2013; Walker, Fredericks et al. 2014.

Six Thinking Hats®

Six Thinking Hats® is a technique created by Edward De Bono based on a principle of parallel thinking: group members thinking in the same direction at the same time to create a broad discussion about a topic.[45] In CQI, use of the Six Thinking Hats® technique can stimulate analytical thinking and evaluate potential improvement strategies from several perspectives. It can encourage individuals with entrenched views to consider other viewpoints and, as a facilitated CQI process, can prevent conflict between people with opposing perspectives.

Six different coloured hats symbolise different thinking roles. The facilitator wears a blue hat, which represents management of the thinking process. The group is given a short time to think about the improvement issue or strategy from each role perspective and to share thoughts with the group, before mentally and sometimes actually switching hats. The hats can be used in different orders and combinations to suit the purpose of the CQI session, and particular hats can be revisited if more exploration is needed.

The most promising improvement strategies can be tested using PDSA cycles, or further developed in collaboration with other PHC stakeholders. Table 7.1 presents the coloured hats and the thinking they represent with example questions. Parallel thinking can, of course, be facilitated without using the concept of hats.

Table 7.1 Using the Six Thinking Hats® technique.

Hat	Think about . . .	Example questions
White	Data Facts Information	What data do we have about this issue? What other data do we need to decide next steps?
Yellow	A positive view Optimism Identifying benefits	What would be the benefits of using this strategy?
Black	Risks Negatives Cautions	What could go wrong? What negative outcomes or obstacles might there be?
Green	New ideas Possibilities Creative thinking	What improvement strategy could we use? Is there another way of looking at this? How can the strategy or idea be developed?
Red	Emotion Gut feeling Intuitions	What do you feel about this?

---

45   de Bono 2000.

Hat	Think about . . .	Example questions
Blue	Managing the process Summarising information Moving forward	What are our findings so far? What should we do next?

Questions adapted from Advancing Quality Alliance (Aqua) 2024.

Many resources are available about the Six Thinking Hats®. Training is available.[46]

Using Six Thinking Hats®

"One of the benefits of using Six Thinking Hats® with a team is that it puts everyone in the position of having to consider the topic from each viewpoint, rather than just the ones that they are personally more comfortable with.

The Thinking Hats is a great tool to use with Aboriginal Health Boards and Community members as well as primary healthcare teams. It can be used to really get to the root of a problem and then to use that information to formulate a plan to drive the improvement process.

It gives everyone a voice and can be a fun and energising way to conduct a discussion that can lead to a much clearer picture of what the important next steps should be."

– Kerry Copley, CQI program coordinator, Aboriginal Medical Services Alliance Northern Territory

---

Stakeholder mapping

The complex and comprehensive nature of PHC and the systems focus of CQI mean that most improvement initiatives involve multiple stakeholders. Stakeholder mapping is a useful technique. It is relevant to understanding the causes of variation in care quality and identifying who needs to be engaged in developing improvement plans and progressing improvement strategies. This will include individuals, groups and organisations who are affected by, and influence, the quality of care and the effectiveness and sustainability of the CQI initiative.

After the quality issue or improvement goal has been identified, stakeholder mapping involves three steps:

- listing stakeholders and organising them into groups (for example, clients, carers and families; other PHC teams, other health professionals, other service providers; managers; community groups, councils; support organisations, researchers)
- conducting a stakeholder analysis by "mapping" their relationships to the quality problem and to each other (for example, using sticky notes)

---

46 de Bono n.d.

- identifying potential roles for stakeholders in developing and implementing improvement programs and interventions.

Many online resources are available to support stakeholder mapping and analysis. The usefulness of these resources will vary, based on the variables that are most relevant to your CQI project.

Resources for stakeholder mapping

"I think that good old-fashioned sticky notes are probably most helpful for stakeholder mapping – then you can organise and reorganise and fiddle with placements until you get the categories and relationships right. There are digital tools available that work pretty well to visualise and communicate relationships, as well as diagrams and matrices to help think through concepts, but sticky notes are the most flexible, simple and easy way to get started."

– Katie Conte, public health and systems thinking researcher

Developing a power–interest grid

As part of stakeholder mapping, a power–interest grid technique may be helpful for prioritising whom to engage in your improvement initiative and how to manage their involvement. This technique puts stakeholders into categories according to their influence and interest.

When putting stakeholders into categories, consider the positions of individuals within their organisation and their abilities to exercise change, and their interest in the quality problem.[47] The example at Figure 7.1 offers a general guide for engaging stakeholders according to their power and interest.

The improvement goal will influence the strategies you use to engage different stakeholders. For example, while important to actively engage stakeholders with high power and high interest, building relationships and gaining support from influential stakeholders with less interest in your project may be necessary for achieving your goal. Stakeholders with low power and low interest in the quality issue may require less regular and detailed communication, but if you aim to empower an interested group through the CQI process, you will be wanting to engage them actively in the project.

Continuous quality improvement collaboratives

CQI collaboratives are "groups of professionals coming together, either from within an organisation or across multiple organisations, to learn from and motivate each other in order to improve the quality of health services".[48] These collaboratives are widely adopted as an approach to shared learning and improvement in health care. There is some evidence that collaboratives can improve care processes, client outcomes, service use or cost (or both).[49]

---

47   Mukerji, Halperin et al. 2019.
48   de Silva 2014.
49   de Silva 2014; Lindenauer 2008; Schouten, Hulscher et al. 2008; Wells, Tamir et al. 2018.

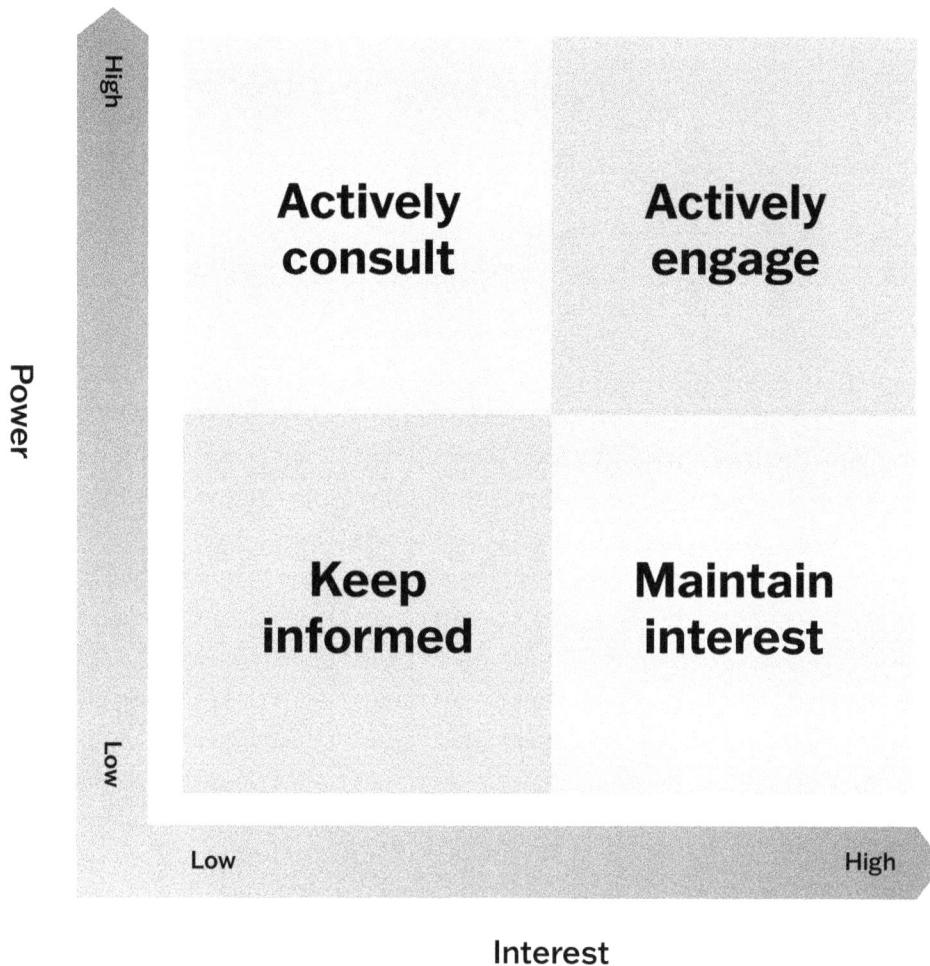

Figure 7.1 Example elements of a power-interest grid.

Many CQI collaboratives are based on the Institute for Healthcare Improvement's "Breakthrough Series" approach,[50] which uses a series of learning workshops, action periods, local support and continuous measurement. Some collaboratives use aspects of the chronic care model (see Chapter 1) and communities of practice approach.[51] The underpinning theory of change is that teams learn faster and are more effective in implementing improvement ideas and assessing their own progress when collaborating and benchmarking with other teams. Effective teams are, in turn, able to improve the quality of care they deliver.[52]

CQI collaboratives have been successfully applied in PHC.

CQI collaboratives have been successfully applied in PHC. In Australia, for example, a Primary Care Collaboratives project aimed to improve CQI capacity in general practices, Aboriginal and Torres Strait Islander health services and pharmacies by building capacity in the regional organisations that support them. Fifty teams engaged 341 frontline services in collaboratives,

---

50   Institute for Healthcare Improvement 2003.
51   de Silva 2014.
52   Wells, Tamir et al. 2018

nominating diverse topics including diabetes, cardiovascular disease, data quality, e-health and men's health. After initial challenges, repeated CQI cycles recorded greater than 30 per cent improvement in the measured competence of participants in quality improvement activities.[53]

Facilitating CQI collaboratives

Quality improvement collaboratives may be large or small scale. Regardless of scale, a CQI collaborative has five essential features:

- identifying a specified topic based on a shared quality problem (for example, large variations in care or gaps between best and current practice)
- engaging clinical and CQI experts in sharing evidence, change concepts and CQI methods, consolidating ideas and providing support for improvement
- bringing together multi-professional teams from multiple sites to share findings, innovations and lessons learnt from their improvement efforts
- working with participants to set clear and measurable goals, and to plan and undertake data collection to test changes on a small scale, using CQI tools and processes
- facilitating planned activities that promote collaboration to learn and share ideas, innovations and experiences (for example, meetings, site visits, web-based activities, coaching and feedback) over a limited time.[54]

The facilitation of a CQI collaborative is structured around these features.

Box 7.3 offers tips for facilitating a CQI collaborative.

Box 7.3 Facilitation tips – CQI collaboratives

At the outset

- Get buy-in from senior leaders (clinical and administrative) in the participating organisations ahead of the start date. Time, resources, work, and supportive conditions will be needed to make and sustain improvements.

- Ensure there is solid IT infrastructure for collecting data and sharing practice.

- Establish participants' reasons for taking part and the main objectives of the collaborative.

- Clarify expectations and adjust the collaborative to meet participants' needs. Be realistic and open about what is possible.

- Develop a "theory of change" that links activities and planned outcomes.

- Team building may be needed to encourage collaboration and develop the trust needed to share data and less successful lessons amongst participants.

---

53   Knight, Dhillon et al. 2019.
54   Schouten, Hulscher et al. 2008; Wells, Tamir et al. 2018.

During the learning activities

- Emphasise mutual learning and open sharing of outcome data and details of practice.

- Ensure participants set SMART goals (see Chapter 6).

- Use simple measurement tools.

- Equip and support teams to deal with data and change challenges, and to adapt ideas.

- Pay attention to motivating and empowering participants and teams.

- Use multiple methods of communication to build a close participant network.

Towards the end of the collaborative

- Plan for sustaining the improvements, involving organisation leaders.

- Plan for continued use of CQI by participants in their PHC services.

- Promote the benefits of maintaining an informal CQI learning network after the collaborative ends.[55]

Example: the Childhood Anaemia Collaborative, Northern Territory, Australia

The Childhood Anaemia Collaborative brought interested Aboriginal community controlled health services together over two years (from mid-2019 to 2021) to focus on improving the prevention and rates of testing and treatment of anaemia in Aboriginal children.

Services who participated shared their data for anaemia care and met online once a month. Online activities enabled small teams in widely dispersed services to participate, and to continue working together during the Covid-19 pandemic. Dashboards were used to display monthly data and trends over time, enabling teams to benchmark data, track progress and identify areas for improvement.

Based on the improvement priorities identified through analysis of their health service's data, each of the participating teams undertook monthly plan-do-study-act cycles to implement and test strategies for improving the quality of anaemia care. The collaborative enabled teams to discuss their experiences and exchange improvement ideas, strategies and resources.[56]

---

55   de Silva 2014; Øvretveit, Bate et al. 2002.
56   Copley and Patel 2021.

Summary

CQI facilitation is an individual role as well as a process involving individuals and groups. Facilitation enables staff and others involved in CQI processes to put evidence into practice to improve care. CQI facilitators need skills in improvement methods, interpersonal communication, group processes, negotiation and empowering others. Leadership and management are important components of facilitation: management of people, meetings, projects and change. The ability to tailor facilitation to the local context and to participants is crucial.

A range of facilitation techniques is available to support the implementation of CQI cycles. The techniques we have described in this chapter reflect core concepts of CQI. All of the techniques focus on improving systems and processes rather than individual performance, recognition that those who work in the system have the knowledge and insight to improve the system, the use of data and systematic planning at the local level, and continuous learning and improvement.

References

Aboriginal Medical Services Alliance Northern Territory (n.d.). Continuous quality improvement (CQI). http://www.amsant.org.au/cqi-new/.

Advancing Quality Alliance (Aqua) (2024). *Six Thinking Hats*. Quality, Service Improvement and Redesign (QSIR) Tools. https://aqua.nhs.uk/qsir-tools/.

Atkinson, P., M. Baird and K. Adams (2021). Are you really using yarning research? Mapping social and family yarning to strengthen yarning research quality. *AlterNative: An International Journal of Indigenous Peoples* 17(2): 191–201. DOI: 10.1177/11771801211015442.

Australian Health Practitioner Regulation Agency and National Boards (2020). *The National Scheme's Aboriginal and Torres Strait Islander Health and Cultural Safety Strategy 2020–2025*. https://www.ahpra.gov.au/About-Ahpra/Aboriginal-and-Torres-Strait-Islander-Health-Strategy/health-and-cultural-safety-strategy.aspx.

Baskerville, B., C. Liddy and S. Hogg (2012). Systematic review and meta-analysis of practice facilitation within primary care settings. *Annals of Family Medicine* 10(1): 63–74. DOI: 10.1370/afm.1312.

Berta, W., L. Cranley, J. Dearing, E. Dogherty, J. Squires and C. Estabrooks (2015). Why (we think) facilitation works: insights from organizational learning theory. *Implementation Science* 10(1): 141. DOI: 10.1186/s13012-015-0323-0.

Bessarab, D. and B. Ng'Andu (2010). Yarning about yarning as a legitimate method in Indigenous research. *International Journal of Critical Indigenous Studies* 3(1): 37–50. DOI: 10.5204/ijcis.v3i1.57.

Best, A., T. Greenhalgh, S. Lewis, J. Saul, S. Carroll and J. Bitz (2012). Large-system transformation in health care: a realist review. *Milbank Quarterly* 90(3): 421–56. DOI: 10.1111/j.1468-0009.2012.00670.x.

Brimblecombe, J., R. Bailie, C. van Den Boogaard, B. Wood, S. Liberato, M. Ferguson et al. (2017). Feasibility of a novel participatory multi-sector continuous improvement approach to enhance food security in remote Indigenous Australian communities. *SSM – Population Health* 3(C): 566–76. DOI: 10.1016/j.ssmph.2017.06.002

Congress of Aboriginal and Torres Strait Islander Nurses and Midwives (CATSINaM) (2014). *Towards a shared understanding of terms and concepts: strengthening nursing and midwifery care of Aboriginal and Torres Strait Islander peoples*. Canberra: CATSINaM.

Copley, K. and L. Patel (2021). *The Northern Territory Continuous Quality Improvement Strategy*. Darwin: Aboriginal Medical Service Alliance Northern Territory.

Cranley, L., G. Cummings, J. Profetto-McGrath, F. Toth and C. Estabrooks (2017). Facilitation roles and characteristics associated with research use by healthcare professionals: a scoping review. *BMJ Open* 7: e014384. DOI: 10.1136/bmjopen-2016-014384.

Cross, T., B. Bazron, K. Dennis and M. Isaacs (1989). *Towards a culturally competent system of care: a monograph on effective services for minority children who are severely emotionally disturbed.* Washington, DC: Georgetown University Child Development Center.

de Bono (n.d.). *de Bono.* www.debono.com.

de Bono, E. (2000). *Six Thinking Hats.* London: Penguin.

de Silva, D. (2014). *Improvement collaboratives in health care. Evidence scan no. 21.* London: Health Foundation.

Dogherty, E., M. Harrison and I. Graham (2010). Facilitation as a role and process in achieving evidence-based practice in nursing: a focused review of concept and meaning. *Worldviews on Evidence-Based Nursing* 7(2): 76–89. DOI: 10.1111/j.1741-6787.2010.00186.x.

Dogherty, E., M. Harrison, I. Graham, A. Vandyk and L. Keeping-Burke (2013). Turning knowledge into action at the point-of-care: the collective experience of nurses facilitating the implementation of evidence-based practice. *Worldviews on Evidence-Based Nursing* 10(3): 129–39. DOI: 10.1111/wvn.12009.

Geia, L., B. Hayes and K. Usher (2013). Yarning/Aboriginal storytelling: towards an understanding of an Indigenous perspective and its implications for research practice. *Contemporary Nurse: A Journal for the Australian Nursing Profession* 46(1): 13–17. DOI: 10.5172/conu.2013.46.1.13.

Gollan, S. and K. Stacey (2021). *Australian Evaluation Society First Nations Cultural Safety Framework.* Melbourne: Australian Evaluation Society.

Harvey, G. and A. Kitson (2016). PARIHS revisited: from heuristic to integrated framework for the successful implementation of knowledge into practice. *Implementation Science* 11: 33. DOI: 10.1186/s13012-016-0398-2.

Harvey, G. and A. Kitson (2015). *Implementing evidence-based practice in healthcare: a facilitation guide.* London: Taylor & Francis Ltd.

Harvey, G. and E. Lynch (2017). Enabling continuous quality improvement in practice: the role and contribution of facilitation. *Frontiers in Public Health* 5: 27. DOI: 10.3389/fpubh.2017.00027.

Harvey, G., B. McCormack, A. Kitson, E. Lynch and A. Titchen (2018). Designing and implementing two facilitation interventions within the "Facilitating Implementation of Research Evidence (FIRE)" study: a qualitative analysis from an external facilitators' perspective. *Implementation Science* 13: 141. DOI: 10.1186/s13012-018-0812-z.

Hogan, C. (2002). *Understanding facilitation: theory and principles.* London: Kogan Page.

Institute for Healthcare Improvement (2003). *The Breakthrough Series: IHI's collaborative model for achieving breakthrough improvement.* Innovation series 2003. Cambridge, MA: Institute for Healthcare Improvement.

Kitson, A., G. Harvey and B. McCormack (1998). Enabling the implementation of evidence based practice: a conceptual framework. *Quality in Health Care* 7(3): 149–58. DOI: 10.1136/qshc.7.3.149.

Knight, A., M. Dhillon, C. Smith and J. Johnson (2019). A quality improvement collaborative to build improvement capacity in regional primary care support organisations. *BMJ Open Quality* 8(3): p.e000684–e84. DOI: 10.1136/ bmjoq-2019-000684.

Knowles, M. (1990). *The adult learner: a neglected species.* Houston, TX: Gulf Publishing.

Larkins, S., K. Carlisle, N. Turner, J. Taylor, K. Copley, S. Cooney et al. (2019). "At the grass roots level it's about sitting down and talking": exploring quality improvement through case studies with high-improving Aboriginal and Torres Strait Islander primary healthcare services. *BMJ Open* 9(5): e027568. DOI: 10.1136/bmjopen-2018-027568.

Laycock, A., G. Harvey, N. Percival, F. Cunningham, J. Bailie, V. Matthews et al. (2018). Application of the i-PARIHS framework for enhancing understanding of interactive dissemination to achieve wide-scale improvement in Indigenous primary healthcare. *Health Research Policy and Systems* 16: 117. DOI: 10.1186/s12961-018-0392-z.

Lindenauer, P.K. (2008). Effects of quality improvement collaboratives. *BMJ* 336(7659): 1448–9. DOI: 10.1136/bmj.a216.

Lowitja Institute (2022). *Tools for supporting culturally safe evaluation.* Melbourne: Lowitja Institute.

Martin-Booran Mirraboopa, K. (2003). Ways of knowing, being and doing: a theoretical framework and methods for Indigenous and indigenist re-search. *Journal of Australian Studies: Voicing Dissent* 27(76): 203–14. DOI: 10.1080/14443050309387838.

McCalman, J., R. Bailie, R. Bainbridge, K. McPhail-Bell, N. Percival, D. Askew et al. (2018). Continuous quality improvement and comprehensive primary health care: a systems framework to improve service quality and health outcomes. *Frontiers in Public Health* 6: 76. DOI: 10.3389/fpubh.2018.00076.

Mukerji, G., I. Halperin, P. Segal, L. Sutton, R. Wong, L. Caplan et al. (2019). Beginning a diabetes quality improvement project. *Canadian Journal of Diabetes* 43(4): 234–40. DOI: 10.1016/j.jcjd.2019.02.003.

Newham, J., G. Schierhout, R. Bailie and P.R. Ward (2016). "There's only one enabler; come up, help us": staff perspectives of barriers and enablers to continuous quality improvement in Aboriginal primary health-care settings in South Australia. *Australian Journal of Primary Health* 22(3): 244–54. DOI: 10.1071/PY14098.

Northern Territory Remote Locum Program and Aboriginal Medical Services Alliance of the Northern Territory (AMSANT) (n.d.). *Continuous Quality Improvement in the NT.* eLearning module. https://www.rahc.com.au/elearning-resources/elearning

Øvretveit, J. (2014). *Perspectives on context: how does context affect quality improvement?* London: Health Foundation.

Øvretveit, J., P. Bate, P. Cleary, S. Cretin, D. Gustafson, K. McInnes et al. (2002). Quality collaboratives: lessons from research. *Quality and Safety in Health Care* 11: 345–51. DOI: 10.1136/qhc.11.4.345.

Papps, E. and I. Ramsden (1996). Cultural safety in nursing: the New Zealand experience. *International Journal for Quality in Health Care* 8(5): 491–7. DOI: 10.1093/intqhc/8.5.491.

Percival, N., L. O'Donoghue, V. Lin, K. Tsey and R. Bailie (2016). Improving health promotion using quality improvement techniques in Australian Indigenous primary health care. *Front Public Health* 4: 53 DOI: 10.3389/fpubh.2016.00053.

Persson, L., N. Nga, M. Målqvist, D. Thi Phuong Hoa, L. Eriksson, L. Wallin et al. (2013). Effect of facilitation of local maternal-and-newborn stakeholder groups on neonatal mortality: cluster-randomized controlled trial. *PLOS Medicine* 10(5): e1001445–e45. DOI: 10.1371/journal.pmed.1001445.

Schouten, L., M. Hulscher, J. van Everdingen, R. Huijsman and R. Grol (2008). Evidence for the impact of quality improvement collaboratives: systematic review. *BMJ* 336(7659): 1491–4. DOI: 10.1136/bmj.39570.749884.BE.

Schwarz, R. (2002). *The skilled facilitator: a comprehensive resource for consultants, facilitators, managers, trainers, and coaches.* New York: Jossey-Bass.

Shaw, E., A. Looney, S. Chase, R. Navalekar, B. Stello, O. Lontok et al. (2010). "In the moment": an analysis of facilitator impact during a quality improvement process. *Group Facilitation* 10: 4–16.

Turner, N., J. Taylor, S. Larkins, K. Carlisle, S. Thompson, M. Carter et al. (2019). Conceptualizing the association between community participation and CQI in Aboriginal and Torres Strait Islander PHC services. *Qualitative Health Research* 29(13): 1904–15. DOI: 10.1177/1049732319843107.

Walker, M., B. Fredericks, K. Mills and D. Anderson (2014). "Yarning" as a method for community-based health research with Indigenous women: the Indigenous women's wellness research program. *Health Care for Women International* 35(10): 1216–26. DOI: 10.1080/07399332.2013.815754.

Wells, S., O. Tamir, J. Gray, D. Naidoo, M. Bekhit and D. Goldmann (2018). Are quality improvement collaboratives effective? A systematic review. *BMJ Quality and Safety* 27(3): 226–40. DOI: 10.1136/bmjqs-2017-006926.

Wise, M., S. Angus, E. Harris and S. Parker (2013). *National appraisal of continuous quality improvement initiatives in Aboriginal and Torres Strait Islander primary health care: final report.* Melbourne: Lowitja Institute.

Woods, C., K. Carlisle, S. Larkins, S.C. Thompson, K. Tsey, V. Matthews et al. (2017) Exploring systems that support good clinical care in Indigenous primary health-care services: a retrospective analysis of longitudinal systems assessment tool data from high-improving services. *Frontiers in Public Health* 5: 45. DOI: 10.3389/fpubh.2017.00045.

Embedding a culture of CQI

The final chapter in Part II builds on the content of the previous chapters to discuss what is meant by a culture of CQI, and how to embed and sustain such a culture. We begin by considering the concept of organisational culture, and how it translates into a quality culture in PHC services. The chapter then discusses leadership for CQI and team building for change management. We draw attention to some tools that can be used to promote understanding of the current culture of your PHC service and organisation and what to think about when selecting an appropriate tool for this purpose.

What is organisational culture in health care?

"Organisational culture" is defined as the shared values, beliefs and norms of an organisation that shape members' attitudes, feelings and behaviours – or the way things are done.[1] In healthcare organisations, it represents the shared ways of thinking, feeling and behaving. Poor organisational culture is often blamed for failures in service delivery, and the need for culture change is frequently suggested as a remedy for improving performance.[2]

There are many theories relating to organisational culture and two distinct views. One view sees culture as something an organisation "has": a characteristic that can be assessed and then adjusted as required around an aspect of organisational culture, such as "client-centredness". The other view sees culture as something that cannot be separated from the organisation itself: something that just "is". This view prompts reflection, learning and action but is less optimistic about the potential to bring about cultural change within an organisation.[3]

In Edgar Schein's commonly used definition, organisational culture is discovered or developed as a group adapts to the external environment, and to the way its internal structures function.[4] Schein described three layers of organisational culture: artefacts and rituals (aspects of culture that are visible); adopted values (shared ways of thinking); and the shared assumptions that underpin them. Box 8.1 offers examples relevant to PHC. Together, the layers form the culture of an organisation.

---

1   Davies, Nutley and Mannion 2000; Shortell, O'Brien et al. 1995.
2   Malik, Buljac-Samardžić et al. 2020; Mannion and Davies 2018.
3   Mannion and Davies 2018.
4   Schein 2010.

Box 8.1 Three layers of organisational culture

Artefacts and rituals (what's visible) – such as how the health service is structured, how facilities are designed, role boundaries, care pathways, rules and procedures, reward systems and dress codes. Artefacts may include how CQI is implemented and how safety risks and complaints are managed.

Adopted values (shared ways of thinking) – such as the service's or practice's mission and strategic goals. These values provide the rationale for what is visible and may reflect prevailing views on client needs and autonomy, the type of evidence that influences decision-making, and expectations about quality and service performance.

Shared assumptions – are tacit beliefs that are "taken for granted" and which underpin values, decision-making and day-to-day practice. Examples might be assumptions about levels of health literacy among clients, or about which professional group holds most power in the health service. Understanding these "hidden" assumptions is crucial for understanding the culture of an organisation.[5]

Organisational culture matters, because it influences what matters to the organisation, how people work together, attitudes towards change, and how the organisation learns and uses new knowledge. It influences service outcomes. A recent review of international evidence found a consistent link between positive organisational culture and positive client outcomes across multiple studies, settings and countries.[6]

Team culture also matters, because teams can form subcultures within the organisation that influence the quality of care provided. In addition, teams need to work with other teams in a PHC service rather than as "siloed" work units to deliver high-quality client-centred care. A PHC team may be a driving force for quality improvement or may undermine continuous quality improvement activities. It is not surprising that ideas of organisational and team culture are central to quality improvement.

The look and feel of a continuous quality improvement culture

Organisations and teams with a strong improvement culture promote CQI as an everyday whole-of-organisation process and continually strive for learning and improvement. There is a "vision" of providing better care, shared thinking and an underlying assumption that investing time and effort in CQI pays off in better systems of care, in working smarter not harder, and in better outcomes for clients. An early United States study linked the implementation of CQI with a participative, flexible and risk-taking organisational culture.[7] Risk-taking in this context does not imply risking client safety, but means being prepared to innovate systems of care: to shift the status quo. The study, which involved 61 hospitals, found that more bureaucratic and hierarchical cultures were a barrier to implementing CQI, while cultures that fostered openness,

---

5   Mannion and Davies 2018 (adapted).
6   Braithwaite, Herkes et al. 2017.
7   Shortell, O'Brien et al. 1995.

collaboration, teamwork and learning led to more successful improvement initiatives with lasting effect.[8] These findings reflect current thinking about organisational culture and CQI.

While every PHC practice, service or health organisation is different, some common features have been identified in organisations with a strong CQI culture:

- leadership for continuous quality improvement at all levels
- boards, senior and middle managers share the same vision and goals for continuous quality improvement
- continuous quality improvement links with the strategic plan, policies, other reporting and performance frameworks
- devolved decision-making
- open communication across the organisation
- teamwork and diversity are valued
- safe to make mistakes
- focus on outcomes not just processes
- strong external links – working with other organisations
- strong community engagement
- staff and management open to change and new ideas
- improvement strategies are in place
- continuous quality improvement is routine
- active management of continuous quality improvement (for example, a continuous quality improvement facilitator role)
- continuous quality improvement training available for all managers and staff.

These features work together to create a culture of CQI.

In Chapter 7, we referred to work undertaken by Larkins, Turner and colleagues to identify features of Aboriginal and Torres Strait Islander PHC services that had demonstrated significant improvement in the quality of care. The researchers found that health services with a strong CQI culture had many features identified in international studies (such as those listed above). But these services also had some novel features specific to Aboriginal and Torres Strait Islander PHC:

- The services took account of the historical and cultural context of the community in the way they worked. Trusting and respectful relationships were developed between staff and clients.
- There was "two-way" learning, integrating cultural knowledge and knowledge of clinical care.
- Staff were caring. They were seen to go the extra mile for their clients.
- Communities were actively driving health improvement.[9]

As shown in Figure 8.1, the common and novel features operated at different levels:

- *micro-system level* – interactions between individual clients and staff (caring staff, clients and community members engaged with PHC service)
- *meso-system level* – within the health service (health service CQI supports, teamwork and collaboration, prepared workforce, two-way learning)

---

8   Shortell, O'Brien et al. 1995.
9   Larkins, Carlisle et al. 2019; Redman-MacLaren, Turner et al. 2021; Turner, Taylor et al. 2019.

- *macro-system level* – in the broader context (linkages and partnerships with external organisations, understanding and responding to historical and cultural contexts, health service external policies, communities driving health improvement).

Continued research by the group has highlighted the significance of PHC teams and communities having a shared purpose around improving the health of the community.[10] We see these features as evidence of a strong CQI culture in Aboriginal and Torres Strait Islander PHC contexts. A culture of CQI may have unique features in other PHC contexts. It is important to be open to difference and avoid taking a one-size-fits-all approach when evaluating the CQI culture in your PHC setting.

Embedding and sustaining the culture

A literature review by Willis and colleagues identified six guiding principles for sustaining cultural change in health systems: align vision and action; make incremental changes; foster distributed leadership across the organisation; promote staff engagement; create collaborative relationships; and continuously assess and learn from change.[11] The principles are strikingly similar to principles for guiding CQI, supporting the evidence that continuously implementing CQI helps to embed and sustain a CQI culture. The skills and knowledge needed to put these shared principles into practice include:

- skills in quality improvement and change management
- skills in leadership, team building and collaboration
- an understanding of the current organisational culture and context of the organisation
- the ability to engage clients and families or communities in CQI, so that improvement interventions can be tailored to local needs.[12]

We presented tools and strategies for developing CQI skills, and for engaging clients and communities in CQI in the previous chapters. We focus here on leadership for CQI, team building for change management, and understanding the current culture of an organisation.

Leadership

Leadership for CQI is essentially about leading change. Capable and passionate leaders can inspire others by setting out a vision for change, engaging others in improvement activities, leading implementation and demonstrating outcomes that align with staff or community priorities for improving care. Leadership for CQI can come from people in different roles and at different levels of a service or PHC support organisation. It can be formal or informal, strategic, operational or clinical.[13] A "distributed leadership" approach, built on a foundation of good relationships, has been linked to improvements in service outcomes.[14]

> Leadership for CQI is about leading change.

---

10   Carlisle, Matthews et al. 2021.
11   Willis, Saul et al. 2016.
12   Hart, Dykes et al. 2015.
13   Øvretveit 2009.
14   Fitzgerald, Ferlie et al. 2013.

Macro
- Linkages/partnerships with external organisations
- Understanding and responding to historical/cultural context
- Health service external policies
- Communities driving health improvement

Meso
- Health service CQI supports
- Teamwork and collaboration
- Prepared workforce
- Two-way learning

Micro
- Users/community engaged with the service
- Caring staff

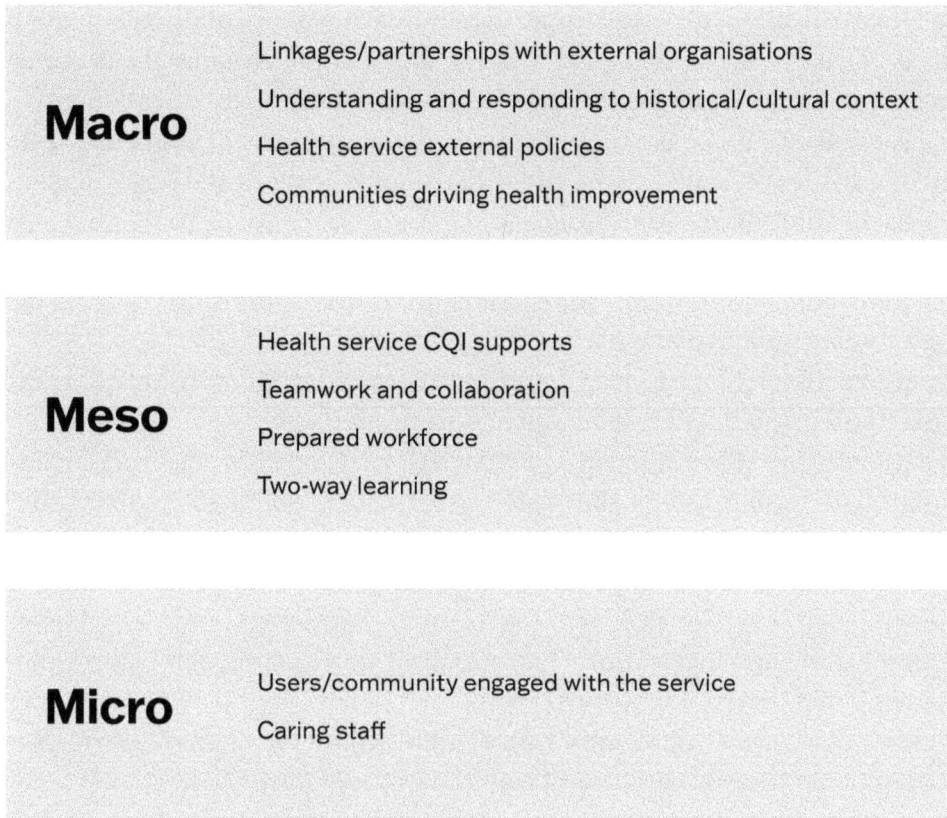

Figure 8.1 Factors influencing quality improvement at high-improving Aboriginal and Torres Strait Islander PHC services (Carlisle, Matthews et al. 2021).

When people are engaged in CQI, they are more likely to understand and trust data, to work as a team and to see their CQI efforts result in better care outcomes for clients and communities. This in turn creates positive attitudes towards change and willingness to participate in CQI activities.[15] And when more people adopt a CQI way of thinking, it more quickly becomes the way things are done.

A CQI approach can, in turn, be applied in leadership development programs. A case study with health service managers from geographically remote settings found that workplace-based action learning projects for continuous quality improvement provided managers with opportunities to apply their learning. The context-specific application of skills helped in understanding real-world competence. CQI based learning projects can also potentially produce the type of data needed for evaluating program impact and lead to better client outcomes.[16]

Tips for CQI leadership in PHC

We offer tips for PHC leaders about how to embed and sustain an organisational culture of CQI. Key messages from our experience are reinforced by international literature.

- Develop your skills and capabilities for CQI.

---

15   Gardner, Dowden et al. 2010; Riley, Parsons et al. 2010; Schierhout, Hains et al. 2013; Wise, Angus et al. 2013.

16   Onnis, Hakendorf et al. 2019.

- Share responsibility for quality improvement with leaders at different levels and work together. Work to your individual strengths (for example, in communication, negotiation, finance, or community engagement) to collaboratively lead improvement.
- Take responsibility for strengthening poor systems that result in poor-quality processes or outcomes. Advocate and collaborate with senior managers and policymakers to develop solutions and embed system changes.
- Be prepared to invest time and resources into implementing CQI. Work to maintain staff engagement. Enable staff training in CQI and provide support for leadership development. Create time for teams to engage in CQI processes.[17]
- Use data effectively. Make a clear distinction between collecting data for accountability purposes and using data for learning and improvement.[18]
- Work to create a "no blame, no shame" culture that fosters respect, measurement and learning. It is natural for people to fear that their performance will be judged negatively, possibly with personal consequences, when gaps are identified in care quality. Have strategies for overcoming resistance to change and getting staff involved in change processes.[19]
- Actively engage teams in CQI. Aim for input and engagement in all phases of the CQI cycle and encourage innovation. Tap into staff motivation; celebrate small and large successes; build on what is working well.
- Involve clients, carers and communities in co-producing change. Be open to different, context-specific ways of thinking about and implementing CQI.[20]
- Have a systematic, coherent approach to CQI and commit for the long term. Remember: improvement is usually made in small increments over continuous CQI cycles. There are no quick fixes.[21]
- Identify and work with champions of change, both in the PHC service and the community.

Team building for change management

Competent leadership is essential, but successful and sustainable CQI also requires capable teams.[22] Building a capable, well-prepared PHC team is a key leadership function. It begins with identifying the skills and knowledge needed across the team, recruiting the right people and properly orienting new staff (for example, to the organisation, job, team, population, context). Those who join a PHC team need these supports:

- a shared sense of purpose
- clear roles and responsibilities
- understanding of each other's roles
- a safe workplace with open lines of communication.

Successful and sustainable CQI requires capable teams.

---

17   King's Fund 2017.
18   Shojania and Grimshaw 2005; Sollecito and Johnson 2019; Wensing, Wollersheim and Grol 2006.
19   Willis, Saul et al. 2016.
20   Larkins, Carlisle et al. 2019.
21   King's Fund 2017.
22   Hart, Dykes et al. 2015.

Workplace systems need to be designed to support teamwork and coordinated care, and team members need to feel confident in using the systems. Opportunities to do training and professional development as a team, or to share new learning with other team members, also build a sense of teamwork. Training needs to be matched to the team, the nature of the PHC work and the context. Examples might include cross-cultural competency training for cross-cultural teams and for teams working with people from cultural backgrounds other than their own, and training in mental health first aid or trauma-informed care.

As stated above, staff who are actively engaged in CQI are more likely to work as a team. The use of participatory CQI processes – including some of the group techniques described in Chapter 7 – can act as an effective team-building strategy.

> "Probably the most powerful aspect of continuous quality improvement is that opportunity to reflect, and particularly if you can reflect with your team. It helps to strengthen the understanding between the team members, strengthen the knowledge and skill set between the team members, and strengthen the cohesiveness of the team."
> – Dr Christine Connors, executive director, Population and Primary Health Care, Top End Health Services Northern Territory[23]

Online resources and expert services are available for team building. They should be selected based on organisational and team needs, and available resources.

Understanding the current organisational culture

Some understanding of the current organisational culture is important for facilitating and evaluating cultural change. Specific tools have been developed for measuring organisational culture in health care.[24] Some of these tools are categorised as CQI tools. A systems assessment tool, for example, measures aspects of organisational culture and can measure a shift when use is repeated over time (for example, improvement in teamwork or links with the community). Quantitative tools for assessing organisational culture tend to cover the visible dimensions of culture (Schein's "artefacts and rituals"), such as leadership, teamwork, training, organisational structures and processes. Qualitative and mixed-methods tools cover both visible dimensions and those that are less tangible, such as trust, commitment, power, blame and support for each other.[25]

These tools can provide a general picture of organisational culture, but they may have limitations for understanding the underlying causes and dimensions of organisational culture and for identifying the nuanced strategies needed to bring about or sustain change.[26] Questions have also been raised about whether tools developed for assessing organisational culture in, for example, Western settings, are transferable to non-Western settings.

Other tools worth considering are critical reflection tools that encourage staff to reflect on shared values and beliefs. Evaluation approaches, such as principles-focused evaluation, can be used to explore members' and clients' views on how well an organisation adheres to

---

23   Northern Territory Remote Locum Program and Aboriginal Medical Services Alliance of the Northern Territory (AMSANT) n.d.
24   Scott, Mannion et al. 2003; Simpson, Hamilton et al. 2019.
25   Malik, Buljac-Samardžić et al. 2020.
26   Malik, Buljac-Samardžić et al. 2020.

its espoused principles and values.[27] Evaluation tools designed to stimulate thinking about program or service success in specific settings (such as Indigenous health services) may help alleviate concerns about the transferability of tools. The selection of a suitable tool for assessing the organisational culture of an organisation will be based on the purpose of the assessment and how you intend to use the findings, the healthcare setting (for example, community controlled service, private practice) and the resources available. An understanding of the current organisational culture will often develop as CQI processes are implemented.

Example: embedding a CQI culture in a PHC service

A large, well-established metropolitan PHC service was experienced in using CQI, but management was concerned that the organisation's approach to quality improvement was stop-start, rather than continuous, and that this had prevented CQI from gaining real traction. Some staff had a low level of awareness of CQI and their potential role in improving systems of care. The management team identified the need for CQI to be considered within the context of the business of the whole organisation. They identified the need for a CQI framework that would guide quality improvement work across the service.

The Quality, Safety and Reporting team took the lead to develop the strategy. First, they reviewed literature on quality and quality improvement, focusing on literature relating to their client population (Aboriginal and Torres Strait Islander peoples). The team then held a series of face-to-face meetings with staff and managers (at senior and team levels), and the executive team, to develop a draft framework for their review. This process reinforced the role of managers in leading and supporting CQI initiatives within their teams.

Developing the framework enabled the health service to articulate the organisation's understanding, commitment and approach to CQI. The finalised framework aimed to:

- guide employees, and particularly managers, in a systematic approach to improving organisational and service-delivery level systems, processes and outcomes

- provide information to support orientation, induction and training activities that enable everyone to contribute towards continually improving the delivery of quality services.

"Defining QI [quality improvement] roles and responsibilities was one of the most important pieces of work we achieved. This was a gap identified early on, which prevented successful CQI from occurring more often . . . We have embedded [our health centre's] approach to CQI in the broader context of organisational performance management, quality management and clinical and practice governance" – executive manager[28]

---

27   Bailie, Laycock et al. 2021.
28   Newham and Cunningham 2015, 15, 16.

Lesson learnt

Strategies must include the whole of the organisation and connect activity to broad organisational aims and goals to be sustainable and successful.

The following example describes an approach to Covid-19 testing and management in a PHC service with an embedded culture of CQI.

Example: applying CQI in a Covid-19 response

The PHC service in the remote island community of Galiwin'ku in Australia's Northern Territory serves a population of approximately 3,000 mostly Aboriginal residents. Comprehensive PHC is delivered by Northern Territory Health and is provided by a multidisciplinary team including resident staff and fly-in, fly-out health professionals. Seriously ill residents are evacuated by air to hospital. Policy support and funding for CQI has been provided for more than a decade.

The PHC team drew on their CQI experience to develop a Covid-19 surge response plan. The plan was developed collaboratively with information systems and public health teams and was designed to scale up in the event of a surge in Covid-19 cases in the community. It includes a vaccination program, detailed Covid-19 screening, treatment and management protocols, and a standardised approach for recording and entering client data into a centralised client information system. All staff undertook training before using the client information system. Five community members were trained in rapid antigen testing (RAT), data entry and tasks considered essential for community engagement.

The PHC clinic offers walk-in and in-home RATs with culturally appropriate hand-outs about testing and managing Covid-19. Community residents are encouraged to do the testing at the clinic, where red and green zones are set up according to people's known exposure to Covid-19, and where client data (name, contact details, number of people living in the house, age, RAT results) can be recorded immediately in the client information system. A recall list is printed each day and is used to guide home assessments for reviewing medium- and high-risk Covid-19 positive clients. Review data are entered into the system for triage, treatment planning and recall. Acutely unwell people are transferred to a larger clinic in the regional town.

CQI processes were built into the plan, including these features:

- monitoring the procedures used for administering RATs with residents (red and green zones in the clinic, home testing) to ensure processes are effective, timely and acceptable

- trialling a system for recording the data from positive RATs and home assessments each day, with attention to data quality and confidentiality

- daily checking of data reports and recall lists to ensure data are accurately captured and clients are appropriately triaged

- getting feedback from clients about their experiences and care priorities (for example, the need for community-based treatment options)

- refining community information processes, Covid-19 testing and management, data entry and data reporting to improve health service systems for responding to Covid-19.

– Amanda Robinson, medical practitioner, Dani Jordan, CQI facilitator, Shawn Cartwright, occupational therapist, Mark Ramjan, nurse/midwife education and research consultant, Northern Territory Health, Northern Territory.

Summary

The final chapter in Part II has explored the concept of organisational culture, with a focus on embedding and sustaining a culture of CQI in PHC services. A positive culture of CQI enables evidence to be used effectively for improving care. It supports the use of CQI tools and techniques into routine care and the effective facilitation of CQI. To this end, we have briefly discussed leadership for CQI, team building for change management and offered tips for leaders. Tools for understanding the current culture of an organisation have been suggested and examples of an embedded CQI culture have been included. It is important to remember that implementing CQI cycles can help to gradually shift organisational or team culture in a positive direction as changes to systems and processes are collaboratively developed, tested, evaluated and adopted.

"CQI is everybody's business" is a widely used motto in Aboriginal and Torres Strait Islander PHC. It embraces the concept of a CQI culture, reinforcing the message that all people who work or access health services have a voice and a role in improving high-quality care.

References

Bailie, J., A. Laycock, K. Conte, V. Matthews, D. Peiris, R. Bailie et al. (2021). Principles guiding ethical research in a collaboration to strengthen Indigenous primary healthcare in Australia: learning from experience. *BMJ Global Health* 6(1): e003852. DOI: 10.1136/bmjgh-2020-003852.

Best, A., T. Greenhalgh, S. Lewis, J. Saul, S. Carroll and J. Bitz (2012). Large-system transformation in health care: a realist review. *Milbank Quarterly* 90(3): 421–56. DOI: 10.1111/j.1468-0009.2012.00670.x.

Braithwaite, J., J. Herkes, K. Ludlow, L. Testa and G. Lamprell (2017). Association between organisational and workplace cultures, and patient outcomes: systematic review. *BMJ Open* 7(11): e017708. DOI: 10.1136/bmjopen-2017-017708.

Carlisle, K., V. Matthews, M. Redman-MacLaren, K. Vine, N. Turner, C. Felton-Busch et al. (2021). A qualitative exploration of priorities for quality improvement amongst Aboriginal and Torres Strait Islander primary health care services. *BMC Health Services Research* 21(1): 431. DOI: 10.1186/s12913-021-06383-7.

Davies, H., S. Nutley and R. Mannion (2000). Organisational culture and quality of health care. *Quality in Health Care* 9: 111–19. DOI: 10.1136/qhc.9.2.111.

Davis, M., E. Mahanna, B. Joly, M. Zelek, W. Riley, P. Verma et al. (2014). Creating quality improvement culture in public health agencies. *American Journal of Public Health* 104(1): e98–e104. DOI: 10.2105/AJPH.2013.301413.

Fitzgerald, L., E. Ferlie, G. McGivern and D. Buchanan (2013). Distributed leadership patterns and service improvement: evidence and argument from English healthcare. *Leadership Quarterly* 24(1): 227–39. DOI: 10.1016/j.leaqua.2012.10.012.

Gardner, K., M. Dowden, S. Togni and R. Bailie (2010). Understanding uptake of continuous quality improvement in Indigenous primary health care: lessons from a multi-site case study of the Audit and Best Practice for Chronic Disease project. *Implementation Science* 5: 21. DOI: 10.1186/1748-5908-5-21.

Hart, C., C. Dykes, R. Thienprayoon and J. Schmit (2015). Change management in quality improvement: the softer skills. *Current Treatment Options in Pediatrics* 1(4): 372–9. DOI: 10.1007/s40746-015-0028-2.

King's Fund (2017). Making the case for quality improvement: lessons for NHS boards and leaders. https://www.kingsfund.org.uk/publications/making-case-quality-improvement#what-should-nhs-leaders-do-.

Larkins, S., K. Carlisle, N. Turner, J. Taylor, K. Copley, S. Cooney et al. (2019). "At the grass roots level it's about sitting down and talking": exploring quality improvement through case studies with high-improving Aboriginal and Torres Strait Islander primary healthcare services. *BMJ Open* 9(5): e027568. DOI: 10.1136/bmjopen-2018-027568.

Malik, R., M. Buljac-Samardžić, N. Akdemir, C. Hilders and F. Scheele (2020). What do we really assess with organisational culture tools in healthcare? An interpretive systematic umbrella review of tools in healthcare. *BMJ Open Quality* 9(1): e000826. DOI: 10.1136/bmjoq-2019-000826.

Mannion, R. and H. Davies (2018). Understanding organisational culture for healthcare quality improvement. *BMJ* 363: k4907. DOI: 10.1136/bmj.k4907.

Newham, J. and F. Cunningham (2015). *Continuous quality improvement success stories: identifying effective strategies for CQI in Aboriginal and Torres Strait Islander primary health care – study report.* ABCD National Research Partnership. Brisbane: ABCD National Research Partnership, Menzies School of Health Research.

Northern Territory Remote Locum Program and Aboriginal Medical Services Alliance of the Northern Territory (AMSANT) (n.d.). *Continuous Quality Improvement in the NT.* eLearning module. https://www.rahc.com.au/elearning-resources/elearning.

Onnis, L., M. Hakendorf, M. Diamond and K. Tsey (2019). CQI approaches for evaluating management development programs: a case study with health service managers from geographically remote settings. *Evaluation and Program Planning* 74: 91–101. DOI: 10.1016/j.evalprogplan.2019.03.003.

Øvretveit, J. (2009). *Evidence: leading improvement effectively.* London: Health Foundation.

Redman-MacLaren, M., N. Turner, J. Taylor, A. Laycock, K. Vine, Q. Thompson et al. (2021). Respect is central: a critical review of implementation frameworks for continuous quality improvement in Aboriginal and Torres Strait Islander primary health care services. *Frontiers in Public Health* 16: 9. DOI: 10.3389/fpubh.2021.630611.

Riley, W., H. Parsons, G. Duffy, J. Moran and B. Henry (2010). Realizing transformational change through quality improvement in public health. *Journal of Public Health Management Practice* 16(1): 72–8. DOI: 10.1097/PHH.0b013e3181c2c7e0.

Schein, E. (2010). *Organizational culture and leadership.* San Francisco, CA: Jossey-Bass.

Schierhout, G., J. Hains, D. Si, C. Kennedy, R. Cox, R. Kwedza et al. (2013). Evaluating the effectiveness of a multifaceted, multilevel continuous quality improvement program in primary health care: developing a realist theory of change. *Implementation Science* 8: 119. DOI: 10.1186/1748-5908-8-119.

Scott, T., R. Mannion, H. Davies and M. Marshall (2003). The quantitative measurement of organizational culture in health care: a review of the available instruments. *Health Services Research* 38(3): 923–45. DOI: 10.1111/1475-6773.00154.

Shojania, K. and J. Grimshaw (2005). Evidence-based quality improvement: the state of the science. *Health Affairs* 24(1): 138–50. DOI: 10.1377/hlthaff.24.1.138.

Shortell, S., J. O'Brien, J. Carman, R. Foster, E. Hughes, H. Boerstler et al. (1995). Assessing the impact of continuous quality improvement/total quality management: concept versus implementation. *Health Services Research* 30(2): 377–401. https://pubmed.ncbi.nlm.nih.gov/7782222.

Simpson, D., S. Hamilton, R. McSherry and R. McIntosh (2019). Measuring and assessing healthcare organisational culture in the England's National Health Service: a snapshot of current tools and tool use. *Healthcare* 7(4): 127. DOI: 10.3390/healthcare7040127.

Sollecito, W. and J. Johnson (2019). *McLaughlin and Kaluzny's continuous quality improvement in health care.* Burlington, MA: Jones & Bartlett Learning.

Turner, N., J. Taylor, S. Larkins, K. Carlisle, S. Thompson, M. Carter et al. (2019). Conceptualizing the association between community participation and CQI in Aboriginal and Torres Strait Islander PHC services. *Qualitative Health Research* 29(13): 1904–15. DOI: 10.1177/1049732319843107.

Wensing, M., H. Wollersheim and R. Grol (2006). Organizational interventions to implement improvements in patient care: a structured review of reviews. *Implementation Science* 1: 2. DOI: 10.1186/1748-5908-1-2.

Willis, C., J. Saul, H. Bevan, M. Scheirer, A. Best, T. Greenhalgh et al. (2016). Sustaining organizational culture change in health systems. *Journal of Health Organization and Management* 30(1): 2–30. DOI: 10.1108/JHOM-07-2014-0117.

Wise, M., S. Angus, E. Harris and S. Parker (2013). *National appraisal of continuous quality improvement initiatives in Aboriginal and Torres Strait Islander primary health care: final report*. Melbourne: Lowitja Institute.

Part II Summary

Using CQI in comprehensive PHC

Part II has described how CQI can be used in a comprehensive approach to PHC. We have discussed how evidence is used to guide clinical practice, sources of data for CQI, and the principles that guide decisions about generating information to measure care quality. Principles and features of CQI facilitation have been described, supported with examples from PHC settings. Tools and techniques for facilitating CQI cycles in PHC have been included, along with some useful types of graphs for presenting CQI data. We have discussed variation in quality and introduced a CQI cycle that acknowledges the complexity of improving comprehensive PHC. Finally, we have discussed the importance of organisational culture for embedding and sustaining CQI.

Figure II.1 brings this information together to align the tools, techniques and types of graphs with the phases of the CQI cycle. Note that several tools, techniques and graphs are suited to more than one stage.

Whatever CQI tools and techniques you use, participatory approaches, facilitation and ongoing commitment to improving the quality of care are keys to success. CQI efforts need to be sustained to make a positive difference for PHC clients and populations. Changes need to be grounded in an organisational culture that actively supports CQI.

● Tools　　● Techniques　　　Graphs

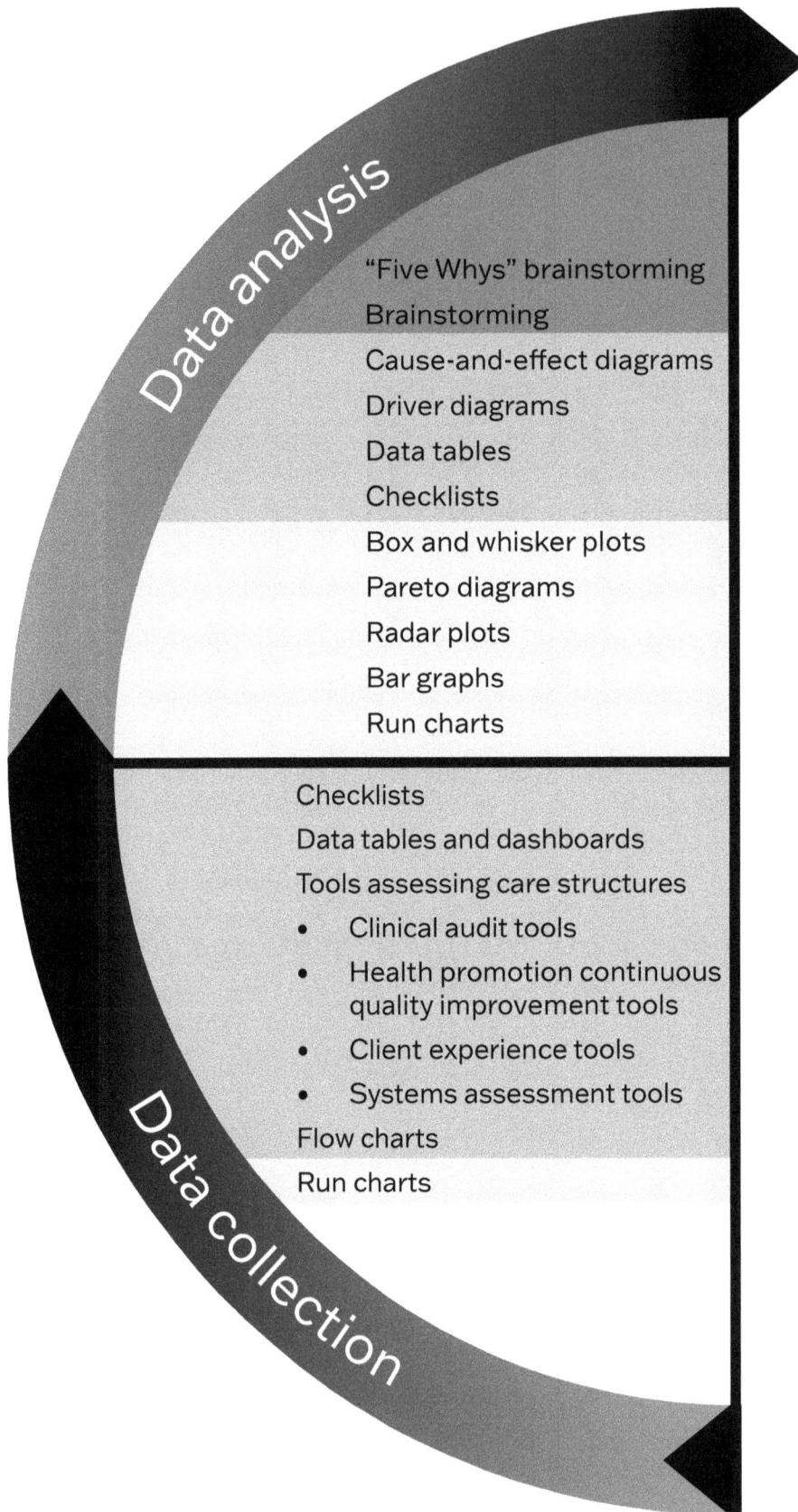

Data analysis

"Five Whys" brainstorming

Brainstorming

Cause-and-effect diagrams

Driver diagrams

Data tables

Checklists

Box and whisker plots

Pareto diagrams

Radar plots

Bar graphs

Run charts

Checklists

Data tables and dashboards

Tools assessing care structures

- Clinical audit tools
- Health promotion continuous quality improvement tools
- Client experience tools
- Systems assessment tools

Flow charts

Run charts

Data collection

Figure II.1 Use of CQI tools, techniques, and types of graphs in a CQI cycle.

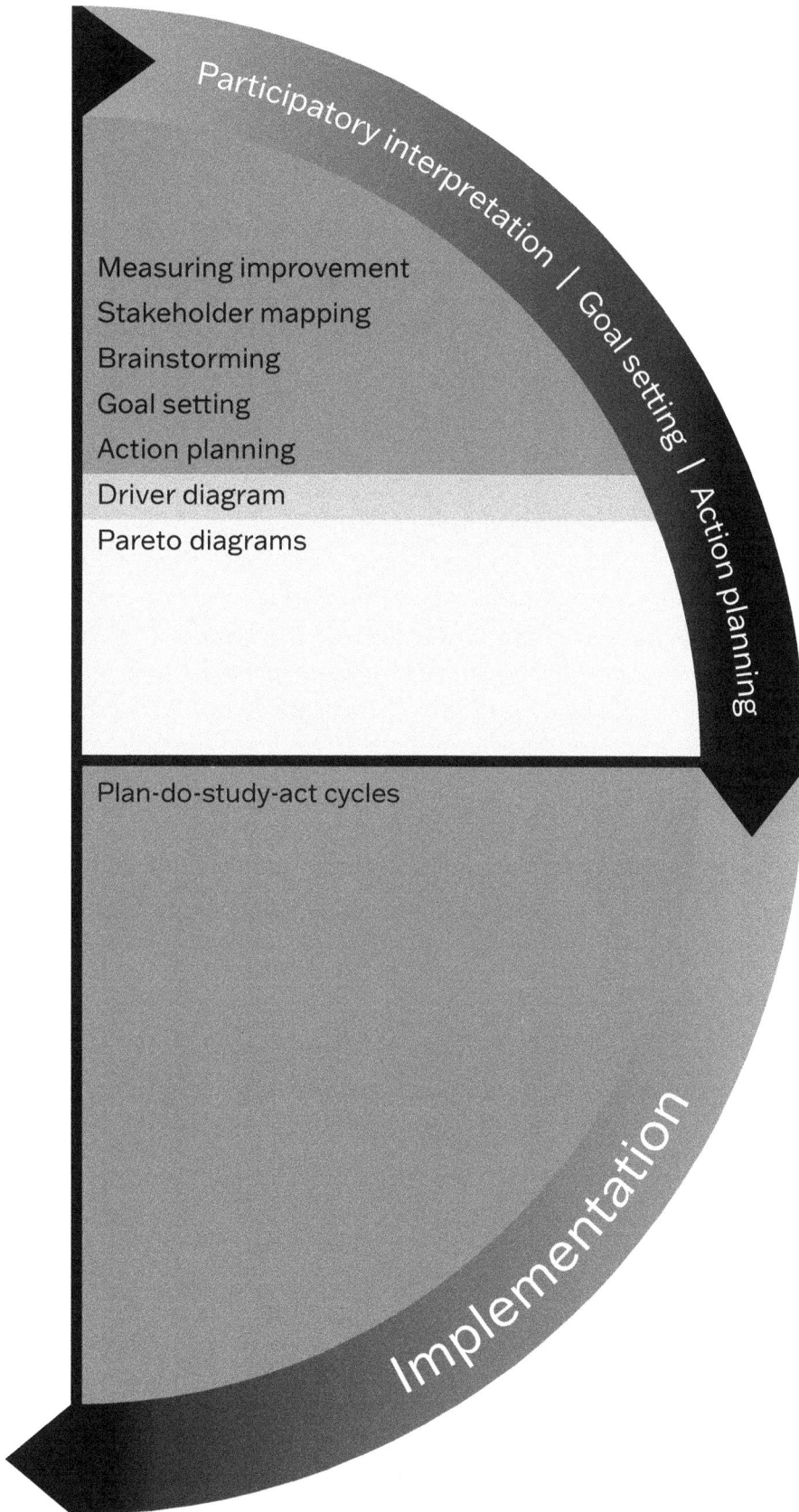

Participatory interpretation | Goal setting | Action planning

Measuring improvement
Stakeholder mapping
Brainstorming
Goal setting
Action planning
Driver diagram
Pareto diagrams

Plan-do-study-act cycles

Implementation

Further resources

Downloadable templates and instructions for the selected tools, and for other CQI tools, are available on the following websites.

Agency for Healthcare Research and Quality: https://www.ahrq.gov/ncepcr/tools/transform-qi/

Clinical Excellence Commission, Quality Improvement Academy: https://www.cec.health.nsw.gov.au/Quality-Improvement-Academy/quality-improvement-tools/

Institute for Healthcare Improvement's "Quality Improvement Essentials Toolkit": http://www.ihi.org/resources/tools/quality-improvement-essentials-toolkit

National Health Service Improvement Hub: https://www.england.nhs.uk/improvement-hub/

Menzies School of Health Research: https://www.menzies.edu.au/

The Point of Care Foundation: https://www.pointofcarefoundation.org.uk/resource/patient-family-centred-care-toolkit/

University Centre for Rural Health: https://ucrh.edu.au/

Quality improvement toolkits have been developed for specific countries and/or health issues. An example is the National HIV service quality improvement tool kit developed by the Federal Ministry of Health of Ethiopia and published by the World Health Organization (2018), available at https://www.afro.who.int/publications/national-hiv-service-quality-improvement-tool-kit.

The World Health Organization has collated tools to support the integration of stakeholder and community engagement in quality-of-care initiatives for maternal, newborn, child and adolescent health. A large number of online resources are available at https://www.who.int/groups/Quality-of-care-network/tools-to-support-the-integration-of-stakeholder-and-community-engagement-in-quality-of-care-initiatives-for-maternal-newborn-and-child-health.

We encourage you to search for resources and examples that are relevant to the continuous quality improvement needs of your primary healthcare team, practice or service – and to regularly update your search.

Using CQI to improve primary health care

Part III describes an approach to implementing continuous quality improvement (CQI) in primary healthcare (PHC) settings. We have tried and tested this approach over almost two decades and are able to show the data on clinical performance and change over time in a range of Australian Aboriginal and Torres Strait Islander PHC services. It is not the only approach, but it is one for which there is a strong evidence base – stronger than for any other approach to CQI in PHC as far as we are aware. Chapter 9 describes the approach.

Chapters 10 to 19 each focus on an area of PHC that has been identified as a priority in the Aboriginal and Torres Strait Islander PHC context: diabetes prevention and management; preventive health; child health; maternal health; youth health; mental health and wellbeing; cardiovascular disease; rheumatic fever and rheumatic heart disease; sexually transmissible infections; and eye health. Each chapter describes the background and rationale for focusing on the area of care and presents and discusses CQI findings, based on data collected using clinical audit tools. Chapter 14 differs from other chapters as it describes how a youth health audit tool was developed and applied; as a case study, it offers insights and guidance for teams undertaking these processes in areas of PHC with less developed guidelines.

The findings are largely based on CQI data collected between 2005 and 2014, which more than ten years later remain the most recent and comprehensive set of CQI data available in Australia, with ongoing relevance for improving the quality of PHC.

The Audit and Best Practice for Chronic Disease CQI research program

A brief history

The Audit and Best Practice for Chronic Disease (ABCD) National Research Partnership originated in 2002 in the Top End of Australia's Northern Territory. It built on substantial prior research and evaluation of CQI methods, using participatory action research to explore the feasibility and acceptability of CQI tools and processes in Aboriginal and Torres Strait Islander PHC. From 2010, with growth and support from service providers and researchers around Australia, the ABCD partnership explored variation in clinical performance, examined strategies for improving primary care, and worked with health service staff, management and policymakers to implement successful improvement strategies.[1] By the end of 2014, the ABCD partnership had generated the largest and most comprehensive dataset on quality of care in Aboriginal and Torres Strait Islander PHC settings.

The work was extended through the Centre for Research Excellence in Integrated Quality Improvement. The 2015–19 phase of research resulted in further evidence on the effectiveness of CQI, factors that support its use by PHC teams and services, priorities for achieving large-scale health improvement, and the importance of Aboriginal and Torres Strait Islander leadership and participation in PHC services and research in this sector. From 2020, an Indigenous-led collaboration, the Centre for Research Excellence: Strengthening Systems for Indigenous Health Care Equity (CRE-STRIDE), focused on embedding CQI into PHC practice and expanding its use to tackle the social, cultural and environmental determinants of health.[2] Ongoing research is based on growing evidence of the importance of community-driven, culture-strengthening interventions in Indigenous PHC settings.

Table 9.1 sets out the evolution of the ABCD CQI research program between 2002 and 2024, listing the key focus and aims of each phase of research.

---

1   R. Bailie, Si et al. 2010.
2   R. Bailie, J. Bailie et al. 2017; Laycock, Conte et al. 2020.

Table 9.1 ABCD CQI research program 2002–24 – focus and aims of each phase of research.

	2002–2004	2005–2009	2010–2014	2015–2019	2020–2024
	ABCD project	ABCD Extension	ABCD National Research Partnership	One21seventy (service support, 2010–2016)	CRE-STRIDE
				Centre for Research Excellence in Integrated Quality Improvement	
Focus	Exploring feasibility and acceptability of CQI tools and processes	Exploring scalability and expansion of CQI. Developing a CQI cycle for PHC	Supporting wide-scale implementation and developing a model for CQI	Embedding CQI approaches in systems	Strengthening leadership and engagement in system-wide CQI
Aim	Explore whether a CQI approach was feasible and effective in Indigenous PHC[3]	Identify support requirements for large-scale implementation of the ABCD model[4]	Understand variation in quality of care and strategies for improvement[5]	Provide PHC services with training, tools and support for CQI, including a web-based data analysis and reporting system[6]	Strengthen Aboriginal and Torres Strait Islander research leadership for CQI.
				Accelerate and strengthen large-scale CQI efforts[7]	Apply Indigenous knowledge and methodologies.
					Extend CQI processes and tools to enhance community linkages and tackle social and cultural determinants of health.[8]

Source: Adapted with permission from Bailie, Potts et al. 2021.

3 R. Bailie, Si et al. 2004.
4 R. Bailie, Si et al. 2008.
5 R. Bailie, Si et al. 2010.
6 Cunningham, Ferguson-Hill et al. 2016.
7 J. Bailie, Laycock et al. 2020.
8 See CRE-STRIDE n.d.

This CQI research in Aboriginal and Torres Strait Islander PHC has made a large contribution to original research on CQI in PHC internationally, with over 180 papers published in the peer-reviewed literature between 2002 and mid-2023.

The ABCD participatory action research program produced evidence-based CQI tools and resources for PHC teams. These included a clinical systems assessment tool and eight clinical audit tools. The findings presented in the following 10 chapters resulted from the use of these tools. An audit and systems assessment tool for health promotion, a tobacco control audit tool and a food systems assessment tool were also developed (see Chapter 5).

Clinical audit tools based on clinical practice guidelines

As explained in Part II, the ABCD clinical audit tools and associated protocols are based on evidence and the service items listed in the relevant Australian and international guidelines for recommended care. Like the clinical guidelines, the ABCD audit tools were developed in consultation with expert reference groups. These groups comprised clinical experts, PHC practitioners with experience working in Aboriginal and Torres Strait Islander PHC and others with understanding of quality improvement and experience in using audit tools. The ABCD audit tools and processes for each area of clinical care (for example, child health) are designed to help PHC teams to identify items of care (for example, growth monitoring) that are being delivered well and less well, and priorities for improvement.

Systems assessment tool based on primary healthcare systems research

The ABCD systems assessment tool is designed to be used in conjunction with each clinical audit tool. The tool was also developed collaboratively and is based on internationally accepted models that reflect the way health systems work and interact at organisational, practice, client and community levels: namely the Chronic Care Model and associated Assessment of Chronic Illness Care tool developed in the United States, and the Innovative Care for Chronic Conditions Framework from the World Health Organization (WHO).

The resulting CQI tools are based on evidence, nationally applicable and realistic for use in a variety of PHC settings. Box 9.1 describes how PHC teams use the tools.

Box 9.1 How PHC teams use clinical audit and systems assessment tools

The ABCD clinical audit tools and processes cover major chronic conditions (diabetes, hypertension, coronary heart disease and renal disease), maternal health care, child health care, preventive services, mental health, sexual health, rheumatic heart disease and youth health. The clinical audit tools are used to retrospectively measure the quality of care documented in client records: they gather data on clinical performance to identify strengths in service delivery and important evidence-to-practice gaps. The ABCD system assessment tool enables PHC teams to undertake a structured assessment of the strengths and weaknesses of the organisational systems that support client care in each of these clinical areas. Each tool has a detailed protocol, which guides staff in using the tool and supports the generation of consistent data for comparison across consecutive audit cycles.

Within health services, PHC teams have used the tools for annual cycles of assessment and feedback. Data about "quality gaps" in clinical care and in health service systems have been used in conjunction with knowledge about the health service infrastructure, resources, staffing, community context and client population to inform goal setting and to plan and implement improvement. The effectiveness of improvement strategies is measured in the following audit cycle.

The ABCD tools provide PHC teams with data that can be presented in different formats to aid analysis and interpretation.

Using aggregated data for system improvement

Between 2005 and 2014, over 250 health services across five Australian jurisdictions used the same CQI tools to audit client records and assess system function. With consent from 175 of these services, de-identified data were brought together to provide information about the quality of care provided across a wider Aboriginal and Torres Strait Islander population living in urban, regional and remote areas. By aggregating and analysing these CQI data, it has been possible to establish patterns, variations, gaps and improvements in key areas of clinical PHC. Many of the examples in this part of the book report these results.

Aggregated CQI data can be used at different health system levels. Individual local PHC services and teams can use the data to benchmark the quality of care they provide against regional or national standards. Policymakers, government departments and large health organisations can use aggregated CQI data to compare service delivery between local health services or regions, to explore factors that contribute to variations in care, and to establish baselines for measuring the effect of their improvement policies and strategies. At all levels, aggregated CQI data can help to identify shared priorities for strengthening systems and policies to improve care. There has been very little CQI data available to date for these purposes. The data on clinical performance in PHC arising from the ABCD program is a unique resource in terms of its scale (number and geographic spread of PHC services), and its scope (range of important aspects of PHC care and service and system development). The data has ongoing relevance for meeting challenges in PHC equity.

International relevance of the ABCD research program

The knowledge gained from this work in Aboriginal and Torres Strait Islander PHC settings has wider relevance for implementing CQI. Although population needs and characteristics, health service structures and resources, PHC teams, settings and policy contexts differ, similar PHC improvement challenges prevail across settings and countries. In addition, these internationally accepted principles for the effective implementation of CQI underpin our approach and are reflected in:

- the use of CQI tools that are based on the best available evidence about what constitutes best practice
- the use of accurate, context-relevant data
- the participation of people in a range of roles relevant to care and service delivery
- the importance of contextual knowledge in data interpretation and intervention planning.

In the following chapters, we describe the implementation of CQI in 10 key areas of clinical PHC. These areas are considered key because they are important for the delivery of comprehensive PHC across the life span; they reflect Australian and international priorities for improving primary care for First Nations peoples; and they are important for improving health equity. In Australia, Aboriginal and Torres Strait Islander peoples continue to experience unequal access to health care, shorter life expectancy and an unequal burden of ill health compared with the general population. Many people experience health conditions associated with low-resource settings, including otitis media in children, trachoma and rheumatic heart disease. The topics of the next 10 chapters reflect these PHC challenges and CQI priorities.

Presentation of research findings

For each chapter topic, we provide background information, key aspects of recommended care, data and findings from our CQI research in Aboriginal and Torres Strait Islander PHC. Drawing on these findings, and research and experience in broader PHC contexts, we offer general messages for improving PHC delivery relevant to that condition or aspect of clinical care. Specific considerations for improving care for Aboriginal and Torres Strait Islander peoples are also included. As colonisation is a fundamental determinant of Indigenous peoples' health worldwide, these considerations have relevance for improving care for other First Nations populations.

How to interpret the graphs in these chapters

The results of CQI research are presented using bar graphs and box and whisker plots. Here are some tips for interpreting the box and whisker plots in these chapters (Figure 9.1).

Box and whisker plots are used to show variation in PHC delivery between health centres, such as these examples:

- health centres with the minimum and maximum mean percentage in recorded delivery of care in accordance with best-practice guidelines (ends of whiskers show highest value if no outliers)
- outliers – health centres that are far away from most others in the dataset (or a distance that is greater than 1.5 times the length of the box)
- the level of variation between health centres in recorded delivery of care by dividing scores into quarters:
  - the box represents the middle 50 per cent of health centres, and the line within the box represents the median (or middle health centre)
  - the "whisker" at the top of the box (and outliers if present) represents the top 25 per cent of health centres
  - the "whisker" at the bottom of the box (and outliers if present) represents the bottom 25 per cent of health centres
  - the longer the box plot, the greater the range of care delivery (or variation) between health centres.

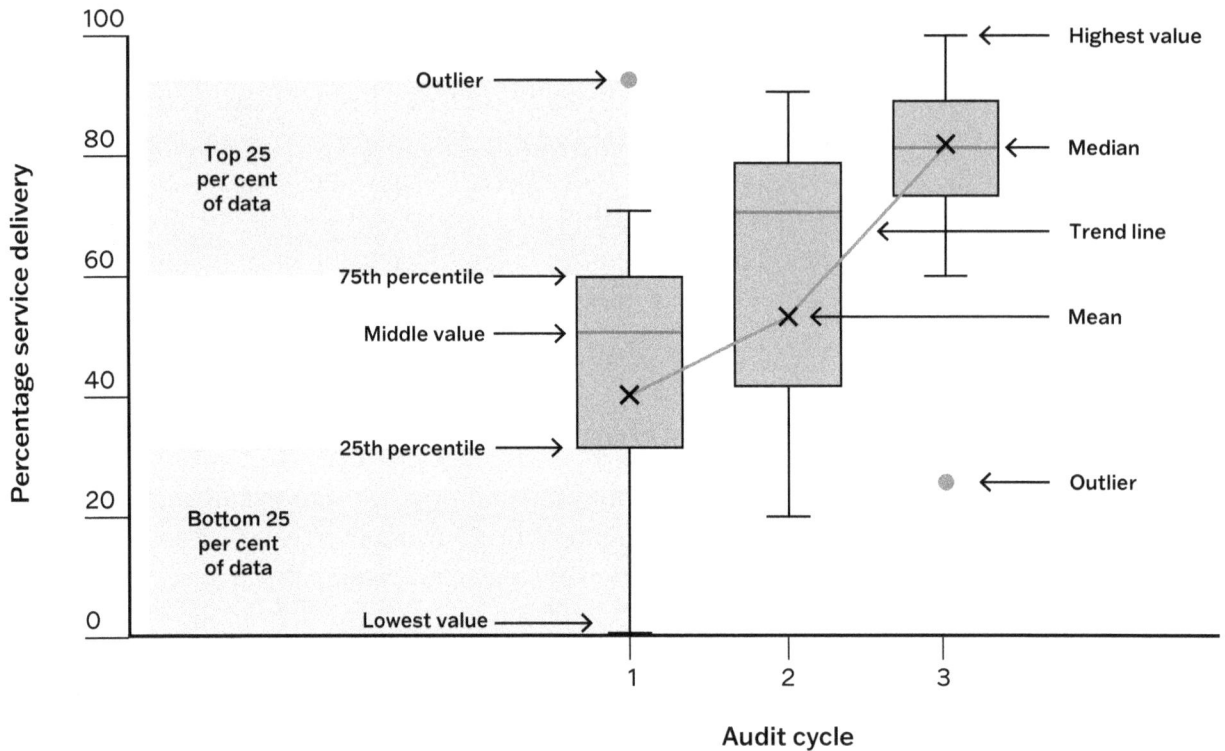

Figure 9.1 How to interpret box and whisker plots.

In assessing data trends, it is helpful to focus on:

- the trend for the mean (average) and median (middle) values for health centres – in particular, whether the mean and median are increasing, staying steady or decreasing
- the trend in the variation between health centres – in particular, whether the variation is getting less (shorter boxes, shorter whiskers) and, importantly, whether there is an improvement in the values for the health centres at the lower end of the range (higher level for the bottom end of whiskers under boxes).

References

Bailie, J., A. Laycock, D. Peiris, R. Bainbridge, V. Matthews, F. Cunningham et al. (2020). Using developmental evaluation to enhance continuous reflection, learning and adaptation of an innovation platform in Australian Indigenous primary health care. *Health Research Policy and Systems* 18(1): 45. DOI: 10.1186/s12961-020-00562-4.

Bailie, R., J. Bailie, S. Larkins and E. Broughton (2017). Editorial: Continuous quality improvement (CQI)—advancing understanding of design, application, impact, and evaluation of CQI approaches. *Frontiers in Public Health* 5(306). DOI: 10.3389/fpubh.2017.00306.

Bailie, R., D. Si, C. Connors, T. Weeramanthri, L. Clark, M. Dowden et al. (2008). Study protocol: Audit and Best Practice for Chronic Disease Extension (ABCDE) Project. *BMC Health Services Research* 8: 184. DOI: 10.1186/1472-6963-8-184.

Bailie, R., D. Si, C. Shannon, J. Semmens, K. Rowley, D.J. Scrimgeour et al. (2010). Study protocol: national research partnership to improve primary health care performance and outcomes for Indigenous peoples. *BMC Health Services Research* 10(129): 1–11. DOI: 10.1186/1472-6963-10-129.

Bailie, R., D. Si, S. Togni, G. Robinson and P. d'Abbs (2004). A multifaceted health-service intervention in remote Aboriginal communities: 3-year follow-up of the impact on diabetes care. *Medical Journal of Australia* 181(4): 195–200. DOI: 10.5694/j.1326-5377.2004.tb06235.x.

CRE-STRIDE (n.d.). *Strengthening systems for Indigenous health care equity*. http://cre-stride.org.

Cunningham, F., S. Ferguson-Hill, V. Matthews and R. Bailie (2016). Leveraging quality improvement through use of the Systems Assessment Tool in Indigenous primary health care services: a mixed methods study. *BMC Health Services Research* 16(1): 583. DOI: 10.1186/s12913-016-1810-y.

Laycock, A., K. Conte, K. Harkin, J. Bailie, V. Matthews, F. Cunningham et al. (2020). *Improving the quality of primary health care for Aboriginal and Torres Strait Islander Australians: Messages for Action, Impact and Research*. Centre for Research Excellence in Integrated Quality Improvement 2015–2019. Lismore, NSW: University Centre for Rural Health, University of Sydney.

10
Improving diabetes care

Diabetes

Diabetes is a chronic condition marked by high levels of glucose in the blood. It is caused by the body's inability to effectively produce or use insulin, a hormone that regulates blood glucose. Undiagnosed or poorly managed diabetes leads to serious damage to many of the body's systems over time, and to premature death. Adults with diabetes have two to three times the risk of heart attacks and strokes. Reduced blood flow and nerve damage from uncontrolled diabetes increase the risk of ulcers, infection and limb amputation. Diabetes is among the leading causes of kidney failure and causes 2.6 per cent of global blindness.[1]

Diabetes is the world's fastest growing chronic condition. The global prevalence of diabetes among adults rose from 4.7 per cent (108 million) in 1980 to 8.5 per cent (422 million) in 2014,[2] and was estimated to be 9.3 per cent (463 million people) in 2019, and projected to rise to 10.2 per cent (578 million) by 2030.[3] The International Diabetes Federation reported that diabetes caused 6.7 million deaths in 2021, with 75 per cent of people with diabetes living in low- and middle-income countries and almost half of people with diabetes not diagnosed.[4]

Type 2 diabetes is the most common form of diabetes and results from a combination of genetic and environmental factors. Although genetics play a major role, the risk of developing type 2 diabetes increases with factors such as high blood pressure, high blood cholesterol, overweight or obesity, poor diet and insufficient physical activity. Multiple risk factors increase the chances of developing diabetes, including historical, social and cultural factors that have resulted in health, social and economic inequities. These factors also challenge effective disease management.[5] Indigenous Peoples and other racial or ethnic minorities who experience oppression have comparatively higher rates of diabetes, and diabetes-related complications and mortality.[6] Until recently, type 2 diabetes was mostly seen in adults, but incidence among children is rising. Women who develop gestational diabetes, and their children, have increased

---

1   World Health Organization 2021.
2   World Health Organization 2021.
3   Saeedi, Petersohn et al. 2019.
4   International Diabetes Federation 2021.
5   Gaskin, Thorpe et al. 2014; Naqshbandi, Harris et al. 2008.
6   Australian Institute of Health and Welfare 2015; Gaskin, Thorpe et al. 2014; Naqshbandi, Harris et al. 2008.

risk of developing type 2 diabetes in the future. Type 1 diabetes, which is managed with insulin, generally occurs from childhood and is not preventable with current knowledge.[7]

Aboriginal and Torres Strait Islander peoples

Type 2 diabetes contributes significantly to the disease burden of Aboriginal and Torres Strait Islander peoples, with cardiovascular and metabolic diseases responsible for most of the gap in life expectancy compared with the non-Indigenous population. Diabetes risk factors are higher for Aboriginal and Torres Strait Islander peoples and prevalence is increasing.[8] In 2018–19, 13 per cent of Aboriginal and Torres Strait Islander adults reported having diabetes or high sugar levels. This increased with age, from 0.8 per cent for those aged 18–24, to more than one-third of those aged 55 and over (36 per cent).[9] The age of onset is younger than for non-Indigenous Australians, and the rate of new diagnoses among young people is rising.[10]

The evidence of severe and increasing impact of diabetes has led to development of programs and strategies to improve diabetes health outcomes, including through holistic, culturally appropriate care tailored to meet the needs of communities. The above statistics highlight the critical importance of effective diabetes prevention and management. Programs and services need to be supported by broader actions that address the historical and social causes of Aboriginal and Torres Strait Islander health inequity – colonisation, land dispossession, displacement, disempowerment, social and economic exclusion, and systemic racism[11] – and that embrace Indigenous values and concepts of health and wellbeing.

Recommended clinical care

A comprehensive PHC approach

Recommendations for improving diabetes prevention and management apply across populations and settings. Diabetes prevention programs need to work across the life cycle. Effective diabetes management requires earlier detection of undiagnosed diabetes, good quality care including management of comorbidities and service integration, social and emotional wellbeing support for clients, access to medications, self-management education and specialist treatment when complications develop.

Diabetes prevention

A holistic approach can help people to reduce their risk of developing type 2 diabetes. Prevention measures should include public health approaches (for example, ensuring access to affordable healthy foods, appropriate services and resources); community health promotion programs (for example, supporting communities and groups to develop and deliver prevention programs); and individual approaches that identify people at high risk using risk assessment tools, provide clients with education, and support people to increase physical activity, reduce obesity, eat healthy foods and avoid tobacco use.

---

7   World Health Organization 2021.
8   Australian Institute of Health and Welfare 2015.
9   Australian Institute of Health and Welfare 2023.
10   Titmuss, Davis et al. 2019; Titmuss, Davis et al. 2022.
11   Durey and Thompson 2012; Ride and Burrow 2016.

Identifying risk – early detection

Australian guidelines recommend screening people for risk of type 2 diabetes every three years from 40 years of age, and from 18 years for Aboriginal and Torres Strait Islander peoples.[12] The CARPA Standard Treatment Manual recommends a preventive health check, which includes diabetes screening, every two years for Aboriginal and Torres Strait Islander peoples 15 years and older, or annually for people with identified risk factors.[13]

Anyone who is identified with high risk factors for diabetes should be screened with fasting blood glucose (or glycated haemoglobin) every three years. People with an impaired glucose tolerance or fasting glucose test (not limited by age) should be screened every 12 months.

Managing comorbidities

Most clients with diabetes have at least one other chronic condition, which may or may not be diabetes related but which influences clinical management. Common comorbidities are high blood pressure, dyslipidaemia (abnormally high levels of fat in the blood), obesity, chronic kidney disease, chronic obstructive pulmonary disease and mental health problems.

Complications of diabetes

Having diabetes causes other health problems over time, making good diabetes management even more important. These other problems commonly include circulatory complications (coronary heart disease, stroke and peripheral vascular disease, which increases the risk of developing foot complications and can lead to amputations); renal complications (diabetic nephropathy or kidney damage, and chronic kidney failure); eye health complications (retinopathy, cataracts and glaucoma); nerve damage (peripheral neuropathy and autonomic neuropathy, which can affect organ function); depression and "diabetes distress" (a response to the emotional burden of managing diabetes).[14]

Care and management

Client-centred diabetes care aims to improve the person's health and quality of life. Treatment decisions need to be based on best-practice clinical guidelines and be made from a position of understanding the client's thoughts, fears, preferences and expectations, and their social, cultural, family and community context. Does the client have the resources needed for treatment and self-care? Do you need to link them with other agencies and support networks? Providing culturally safe care is essential (for example, engaging translators when required, responding to cultural values, involving staff with the same cultural or ethnic background in care delivery).

High-quality diabetes care includes cardiovascular risk assessment, visual acuity check, dilated eye check and foot check at least every 12 months, with appropriate follow-up and referral for specialist care as required. Up-to-date influenza and pneumococcal vaccinations are also recommended. Planning disease management in partnership with clients and organising multidisciplinary team care take account of many important factors: biomedical, medications, any complications of diabetes, cultural factors, social and emotional wellbeing, health literacy and available resources.

---

12   Royal Australian College of General Practitioners 2020.
13   Remote Primary Health Care Manuals 2022.
14   Ride and Burrow 2016.

Chronic disease management plans should be developed and regularly reviewed in consultation with clients and their families or carers as appropriate. An initial review should be done within the first month after diagnosis, and then every three to six months, depending on the therapies used and the complexity of health issues.[15] Regular review of management plans can result in improved care processes and clinical outcomes.[16]

Meeting the complex clinical care needs of all people diagnosed with diabetes requires well-functioning systems at different health system levels and coordination amongst different providers. PHC systems should support team-based care, community involvement, patient registries and embedded decision-support tools. PHC systems should also support the integration of clinical consultations by PHC teams, laboratory tests, specialist services, and community programs that protect and promote health and wellbeing.

Findings: quality of diabetes care

The data presented below on the quality of diabetes care come mainly from six research papers and key reports published by the ABCD CQI research program between 2007 and 2016. These are the most recent audit data available for analysis. Studies analysed more than 17,879 client records from 160 PHC centres between 2005 and 2014. Approximately half of the centres were in geographically remote locations; urban and regional PHC centres were also represented. PHC stakeholders participated in data interpretation to identify priority evidence-to-practice gaps and factors influencing improvement.

Clinical care: testing and control of blood glucose levels

Blood glucose (glycated haemoglobin or HbA1c) measurement is used to assess long-term blood glucose control. Good blood glucose control substantially reduces the risk of microvascular disease in diabetes, including kidney disease, retinopathy and neuropathy.

- Goals for HbA1c levels vary according to client circumstances; the general aim is for a level of 6.5–7.5 per cent (or 48–58 millimole per mole).
- Checks are recommended every three to six months (HbA1c readings assess blood glucose levels over the past three months).
- Follow-up action for an abnormal HbA1c reading should involve counselling about blood glucose control and closer monitoring. People with repeated or especially high readings need referral to a doctor for assessment and action, which may involve multiple interventions and medication adjustment.

Clinical audit and interpretation of the HbA1c data from the audits found several key points for CQI:

- Improvement was needed in regular monitoring of HbA1c, and in follow-up of abnormal HbA1c results and review of medication.
- Over time, the median rate of six-monthly HbA1c checks for clients with diabetes was relatively high (around 75 per cent) (Figure 10.1). There was consistently wide variation

15   Royal Australian College of General Practitioners 2020.
16   Wickramasinghe, Schattner et al. 2013.

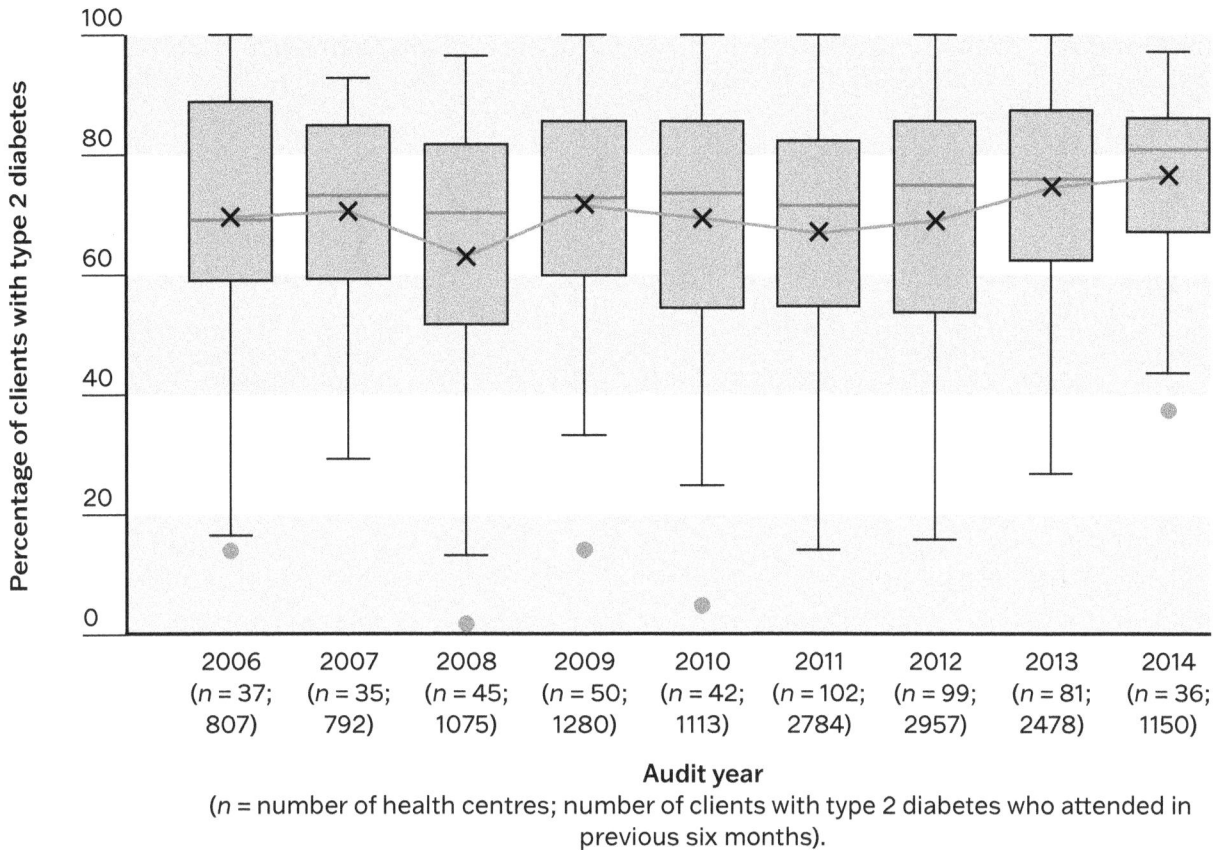

Figure 10.1 Mean health centre delivery of HbA1c checks within six months, by audit year for all health centres. Source: Matthews, Connors et al. 2015.

across health centres, which did not appear to improve over time for those health centres at the lower end of the range.

- Follow-up action for abnormal HbA1c results showed an improving trend in medication review across audit cycles. Median rates increased from 25 per cent to 60 per cent between cycles 1 and 4, but the variation in rates between health centres was consistently wide, ranging from 0 to 100 per cent in audit cycles 1 to 4 (Figure 10.2).[17]

Cardiovascular disease risk assessment and blood pressure control

People who have diabetes and pre-existing cardiovascular disease are at high risk of a cardiovascular event (see Chapter 16). The risk is also high if people with diabetes are older than 60 years, or if they have microalbuminuria (a high level of protein in the urine), moderate or severe chronic kidney disease, high blood cholesterol (serum total cholesterol over 7.5 mmol/L), or high blood pressure (more than or equal to 140/90 mmHg).[18] Good blood pressure control is important for good diabetes care. Blood pressure targets are based on informed decision-making between clients and clinicians, considering the benefits and harms.

---

17   Matthews, Connors et al. 2015.
18   National Heart Foundation of Australia 2016.

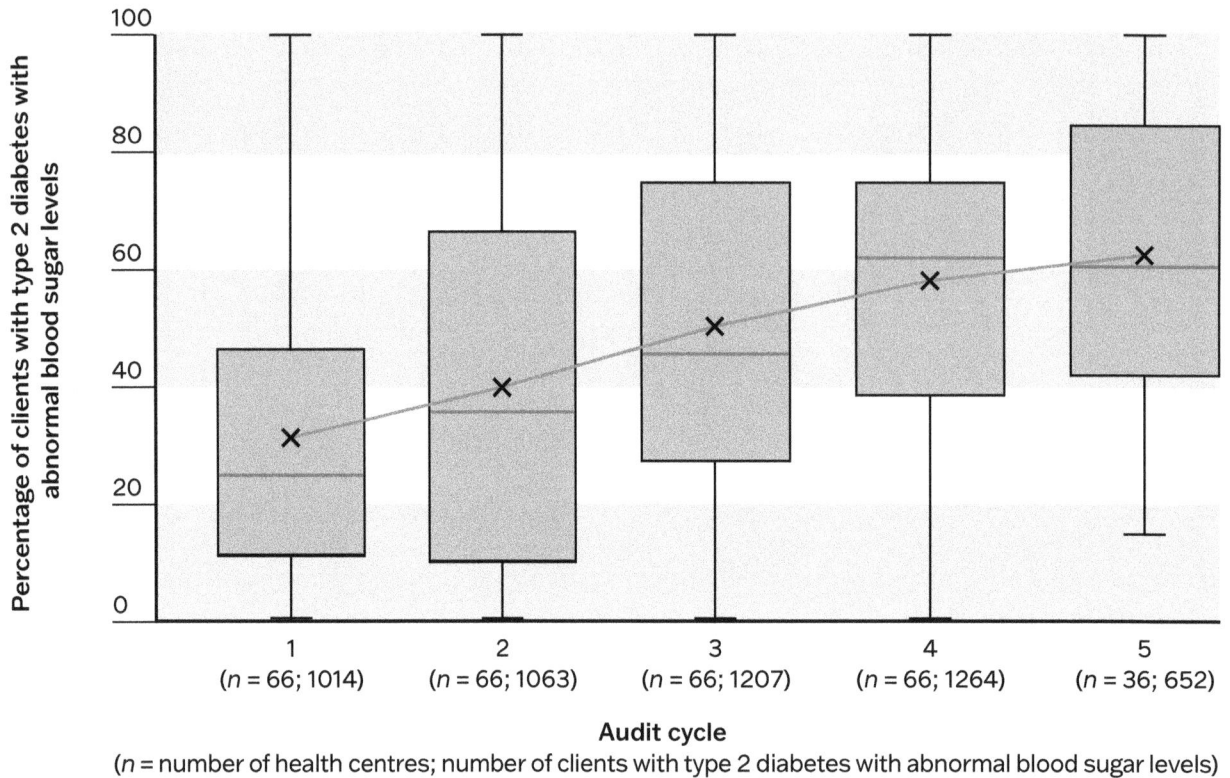

Figure 10.2 Mean health centre rates of medication review or adjustment for patients with abnormal HbA1c, by audit cycle for health centres that have at least three years of audit data. Source: Matthews, Connors et al. 2015.

- Target blood pressure for people with diabetes depends on comorbidities and complications. The general target is less than or equal to 130/80 mmHg.[19] Therapy is strongly recommended for clients with diabetes and systolic blood pressure more than or equal to 140 mmHg. A blood pressure target less than 140/90 mmHg is recommended for people with diabetes and hypertension. A systolic blood pressure target less than 120 mmHg may be considered when the priority is to prevent stroke.[20]
- When a client has a high blood pressure reading, it is important that appropriate follow-up action is taken: at least counselling the client about blood pressure control and frequent monitoring.
- A client with a repeated or especially high reading should be referred to a doctor for assessment and action, which may involve adjustment of medications and therapy to lower blood pressure (for example, angiotensin converting enzyme inhibitor or angiotensin receptor blocker) and should include discussion about lifestyle.
- Once control is achieved, blood pressure should be measured every three–six months.[21]

---

19   Australian Chronic Disease Prevention Alliance: National Vascular Disease Prevention Alliance 2012.

20   Gabb, Mangoni et al. 2016.

21   Remote Primary Health Care Manuals 2022; Royal Australian College of General Practitioners 2020.

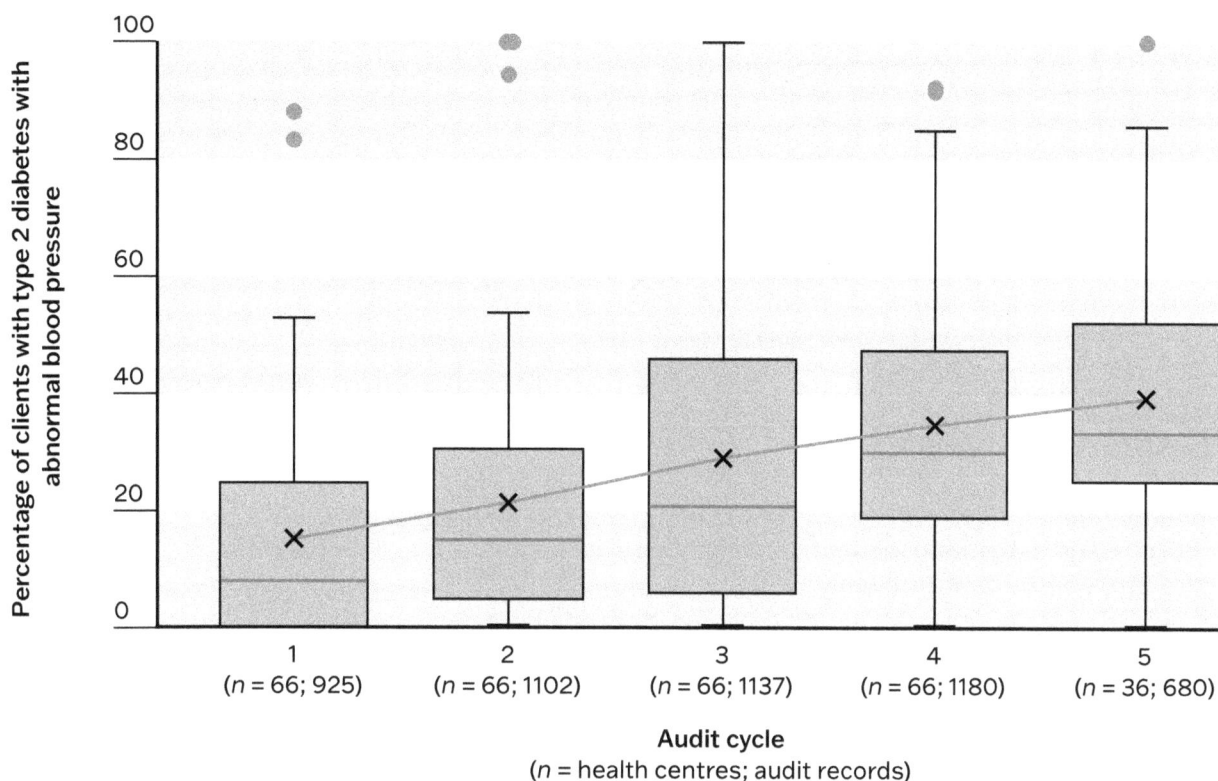

Figure 10.3 Mean health centre rates of medication review or adjustment for clients with abnormal blood pressure, by audit cycle for health centres that have at least three years of audit data. Source: Matthews, Connors et al. 2015.

Clinical audit and interpretation of the data from the audits found several key points for CQI:

- Improvement was needed in regular monitoring of blood pressure, and in follow-up of abnormal blood pressure results and review of medication.
- Rates of medication review or adjustment for clients with abnormal blood pressure was generally low but improved over successive audit cycles. Median rates increased from 7 per cent to more than 30 per cent over four cycles (Figure 10.3).
- There was wide variation in blood pressure control and rates of medication review or adjustment between health centres.[22]

Follow-up of abnormal total cholesterol showed similar results and trends.

Risk factors, brief intervention, counselling and education

Routine diabetes care involves identifying factors that are likely to progress disease severity and complications, and supporting clients to reduce these risks and self-manage their illness. Screening, brief intervention and, when necessary, counselling and referral may focus on social risk factors (food security, housing condition, financial support, family environment, experiences of trauma), or behavioural risk factors (for example, smoking, alcohol intake, other drug use, weight management, nutrition, exercise needs and social and emotional wellbeing).

---

22   Matthews, Connors et al. 2015.

Data from over 15,000 clinical audit records of clients with type 2 diabetes were collected from 162 PHC centres between 2005 and 2014. Analysis over nine audit cycles showed the following information:

- Delivery of brief intervention, counselling and education about risk factors showed improvement in early audit cycles, which then plateaued.
- Variation in these care processes for nutrition, physical activity and high-risk alcohol and other drug use may be influenced by the composition of PHC teams, allocation of work within teams, staff perceptions about the effectiveness and accessibility of support services, and different policies and practices for recording these care processes in client records.[23]

Diabetes and depression

Having diabetes more than doubles a person's risk of developing depression.[24] The combination of diabetes and depression presents a major clinical challenge as the outcomes of both conditions are generally worsened by the presence of the other: quality of life is poorer, diabetes self-management is impaired, the risk of diabetes complications is increased, and life expectancy is reduced.[25] Coexisting diabetes and depression is associated with a 50 per cent increase in mortality risk.[26] Despite this knowledge and the availability of effective screening tools, depression is frequently missed in people with diabetes.[27] (See also Chapter 15, Improving mental health and wellbeing care.)

The high prevalence of diabetes in Aboriginal and Torres Strait Islander peoples and their reported high or very high levels of psychological distress and mental illness[28] indicate that a high percentage of Aboriginal and Torres Strait Islander peoples who have diabetes experience depression.

The CQI research found low rates of screening for social and emotional wellbeing amongst people with diabetes. Screening and diagnosed depression were even lower for people with severe disease. Analysis of data from 62 PHC centres and 1,592 clinical audit records of clients with type 2 diabetes resulted in these findings:

- 14 health centres (23 per cent) had no documented depression in the records of clients with diabetes. For the remaining 48 health centres, documented depression varied between 3.3 and 36.7 per cent.
- One-third of the clients (45 of 140) with documented depression in their medical records had no recorded diagnosis of depression but had been prescribed a medication commonly used to treat depression.[29]

A later study of 1,174 clinical audit records of clients with type 2 diabetes from 44 PHC centres resulted in these findings:

- Documentation of screening for depression and of diagnosed depression was low overall (5 per cent and 6 per cent respectively) and even lower for clients with renal disease and with poorly controlled diabetes.

---

23   Schierhout, Matthews et al. 2016.
24   Diabetes Australia n.d.
25   Holt and Katon 2012.
26   Lin, Heckbert et al. 2009.
27   Holt and Katon 2012.
28   Australian Institute of Health and Welfare 2022.
29   Si, Dowden et al. 2011.

- Screening for depression was lower for those on medication for blood glucose control compared to those not on glucose-lowering medication.
- Antidepressant prescription was not associated with level of diabetes control or disease severity.[30]

Comprehensive diabetes care

Audit and systems assessment data for various aspects of diabetes care were brought together to analyse the overall quality of type 2 diabetes care (17,879 client records, 162 PHC centres). The audit tool used to collect the data included 22 best-practice indicators for type 2 diabetes care.[31] The systems assessment tool included 5 key components and 18 scored items relating to PHC system support.[32]

The importance of continuous quality improvement work was reinforced by the findings, which enabled diabetes care to improve. Over the course of the audit years, these were the findings that emerged:

- The mean and median levels of care ranged between 60 and 80 per cent of service items, with some health centres delivering fewer than 40 per cent of the elements of best-practice care. There was an improvement trend and reducing variation between health centres over the final four years of data collection (Figure 10.4).
- Health centres with longer participation in CQI were more likely to be in the top quartile of delivery for all aspects of diabetes care.[33]
- There were different patterns of improvement for different aspects of diabetes care. While follow-up of abnormal results, screening for emotional wellbeing, recording of risk factors and brief interventions improved, there was no clear improvement for six-monthly checks of HbA1c, medication prescription, emotional wellbeing support and adult vaccinations.[34]
- Variation between health centres was less in the areas of medication prescriptions and medication review following abnormal findings, brief interventions and health centre systems. Variation did not reduce for six-monthly HbA1c checks, documentation of follow-up plan for abnormal blood pressure, emotional wellbeing screening and support, recording of risk factors and adult vaccinations.[35]
- Adherence to best-practice guidelines was linked to geographical remoteness of health centres (the more remote, the greater the adherence) and regularity of client attendance. Clients were more likely to receive higher quality care with increasing age, disease severity, comorbidity or complications, or a combination of these. Health centre factors explained most of the differences in level of service delivery rather than client factors.[36]
- Systems assessments identified the need to strengthen systems for more effective links between PHC services and communities, and links with other services and resources.[37]

30   Schierhout, Nagel et al. 2013.
31   Menzies School of Health Research and One21seventy 2015.
32   Menzies School of Health Research and One21seventy 2012.
33   Matthews, Connors et al. 2015; Schierhout, Matthews et al. 2016.
34   Matthews, Connors et al. 2015; Schierhout, Matthews et al. 2016.
35   Matthews, Connors et al. 2015; Schierhout, Matthews et al. 2016.
36   Matthews, Schierhout et al. 2014.
37   Matthews, Connors et al. 2015.

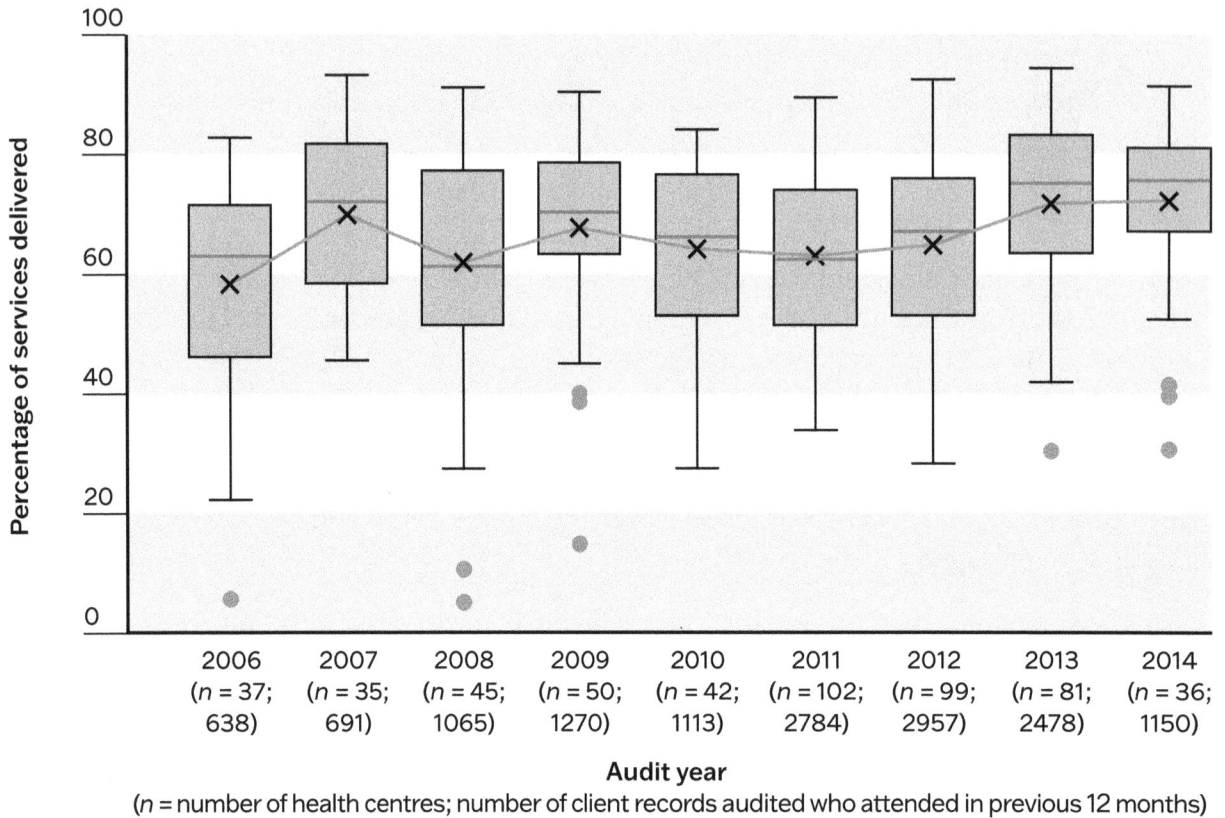

Figure 10.4 Trends in overall type 2 diabetes care. Source: Matthews, Connors et al. 2015.

Health centres with longer participation in CQI were more likely to be in the top quartile of delivery for all aspects of diabetes care.

Note: composite indicators include up to 22 best-practice indicators present in the type 2 diabetes audit tool: current chronic disease management plan; chronic disease management or medication discussion; influenza and pneumococcal vaccination; weight and waist circumference recorded (within six months); body mass index; blood pressure (within six months); visual acuity; dilated eye check; feet check; nutrition and physical activity advice; blood glucose level (within six months); urine albumin:creatinine ratio; estimated glomerular filtration rate; full lipid profile; total cholesterol; brief intervention if smoker or high risk alcohol user.

Across the studies, there was a need to strengthen systems and processes to support adherence to evidence-based clinical guidelines. Stakeholder input to data interpretation identified barriers and strategies for system improvement, as follows:

- staff recruitment and retention (for example, improving induction, training and mentoring programs; focusing on building a stable, qualified workforce)
- capacity to provide client-centred care (for example, modifying roles and career pathways for community health workers towards provision of comprehensive care; developing staff skills in holistic care; providing resources)

- community engagement and participation in the design of service delivery (for example, invest in strengthening health literacy and community leadership for quality improvement, develop staff skills in linking with the community)
- training and development of PHC teams and management (for example, in clinical skills, team building and collaboration, CQI knowledge and skills).[38]

Key messages for improving diabetes care

This CQI research identifies clear priorities and strategies for improving diabetes care in PHC and includes stakeholder interpretation of CQI data. Patterns of diabetes care delivery in Aboriginal and Torres Strait Islander PHC communities are likely to reflect, at least to some extent, care delivery in international settings.

There are common evidence-to-practice gaps in diabetes care that call for system-wide and local attention:

- follow-up of abnormal findings and review of medication, strengthening regular monitoring of blood glucose levels and reviewing and adjusting medication for clients with a recent abnormal blood glucose level, total cholesterol or blood pressure result

- adherence to evidence-based current treatment guidelines

- assessment and support regarding emotional wellbeing

- recording of risk factors, particularly cardiovascular risk assessment and healthy weight indicators, and recording of brief interventions and referrals (such as advice or referrals for physical activity and quit smoking programs)

- coverage of adult vaccinations

- development of systems for more effective links between PHC centres and communities.

There are several strategies that can be taken to improve the quality of diabetes care:

- At the local level, encourage regular attendance by clients with diabetes and those at high risk of developing diabetes.

- At different levels of the health system, focus on reducing systemic barriers and strengthening enablers for providing best-practice diabetes care. These are among the most important:

  - staff recruitment and retention

  - capacity to provide client-centred care

  - community engagement and participation in the design of service delivery

  - training and development of PHC teams and management.

---

38   Matthews, Connors et al. 2015.

> Success in tackling systemic barriers for diabetes care will have a positive effect on the delivery of best-practice care for other chronic conditions and for PHC more generally.
>
> - Involve a range of stakeholders in planning how to improve comprehensive diabetes care, including clients and carers or families, PHC practitioners and staff, health service and district and regional managers, support organisations and policymakers.
>
> Sustained commitment by everyone involved in CQI is required to realise and demonstrate improvement.

Improving diabetes care in Aboriginal and Torres Strait Islander PHC

Our research into the quality of diabetes care for Aboriginal and Torres Strait Islander peoples spans almost 15 years, and studies show persistent wide variation in performance between different aspects of diabetes care and between health services and centres. While many aspects of diabetes care are being done well in many health centres, there are important and consistent gaps between evidence and practice in some aspects of diabetes care. Our research indicates that these gaps are system-wide and likely to be due to deficiencies in the broader PHC system. Together with the growing prevalence of diabetes at earlier ages, this evidence reinforces, firstly, the critical importance of taking both system-level and local action to improve diabetes prevention and care for Aboriginal and Torres Strait Islander peoples, and, secondly, the need to shape these actions to meet the self-determined needs of Aboriginal and Torres Strait Islander communities.

The concept of comprehensive diabetes care aligns with the holistic nature of Aboriginal and Torres Strait Islander wellbeing. Our research on engaging stakeholders in interpreting quality-of-care data provides evidence that the PHC workforce has the collective knowledge to find practical solutions to improving diabetes care. Effective processes for engaging communities in planning service design, and culturally competent and well-prepared PHC teams are key.[39]

Best-practice type 2 diabetes care involves team care and dictates that clients receive certain services at regular intervals. It is unsurprising that health centres with a higher percentage of clients not attending in the previous six months were less likely to provide best-practice diabetes care,[40] but notable that health centre factors and jurisdiction-level support for CQI were more influential than client factors in adherence to best practice.[41] A focus on improving health centre systems, therefore, is crucial for improving diabetes care.

A focus on improving health centre systems is crucial for improving diabetes care.

Every care-delivery context provides challenges for PHC teams (for example, coordinating and monitoring comprehensive delivery by multiple service providers in urban locations;

---

39   Matthews, Connors et al. 2015.
40   Matthews, Schierhout et al. 2014.
41   Matthews, Connors et al. 2015; Matthews, Schierhout et al. 2014.

managing high staff turnover, dispersed populations and limited access to specialist services in remote PHC settings). Flexible models of care, well-functioning care systems, good documentation of client care and use of CQI can help in overcoming these challenges. Policy and infrastructure support and organisational commitment to CQI has been associated with steady improvements or maintenance of high-quality diabetes care for Aboriginal and Torres Strait Islander communities.[42]

References

Australian Chronic Disease Prevention Alliance: National Vascular Disease Prevention Alliance (2012). *Guidelines for the management of absolute cardiovascular disease risk*. Melbourne: National Stroke Foundation.

Australian Institute of Health and Welfare (2023). Aboriginal and Torres Strait Islander Health Performance Framework 1.09 Diabetes. *National Indigenous Australians Agency*. Canberra: Australian Government. https://www.indigenoushpf.gov.au/measures/1-09-diabetes.

Australian Institute of Health and Welfare (2022). *Australia's health 2022: First Nations People – Indigenous health and wellbeing*. Canberra: Australian Government. https://www.aihw.gov.au/reports/australias-health/indigenous-health-and-wellbeing.

Australian Institute of Health and Welfare (2015). *Cardiovascular disease, diabetes and chronic kidney disease – Australian facts: Aboriginal and Torres Strait Islander people*. Cardiovascular, Diabetes and Chronic Kidney Disease Series no. 5. Cat. no. CDK 5. Canberra: AIHW.

Bailie, R., V. Matthews, S. Larkins, S. Thompson, P. Burgess, T. Weeramanthri et al. (2017). Impact of policy support on uptake of evidence-based continuous quality improvement activities and the quality of care for Indigenous Australians: a comparative case study. *BMJ Open* 7. DOI: 10.1136/bmjopen-2017-016626.

Diabetes Australia (n.d.). Depression and mental health. *Diabetes Australia*. https://www.diabetesaustralia.com.au/living-with-diabetes/preventing-complications/depression-and-mental-health/.

Durey, A. and S. Thompson (2012). Reducing the health disparities of Indigenous Australians: time to change focus. *BMC Health Services Research* 12: 151. DOI: 10.1186/1472-6963-12-151.

Gabb, G., A. Mangoni, C. Anderson, D. Cowley, J. Dowden, J. Golledge et al. (2016). Guideline for the diagnosis and management of hypertension in adults – 2016. *Medical Journal of Australia* 205(2): 85–9. DOI: 10.5694/mja16.00526.

Gaskin, D., R. Thorpe, E. McGinty, K. Bower, C. Rohde, J. Young et al. (2014). Disparities in diabetes: the nexus of race, poverty, and place. *American Journal of Public Health* 104(11): 2147–55. DOI: 10.2105/AJPH.2013.301420.

Holt, R. and W. Katon (2012). Dialogue on diabetes and depression: dealing with the double burden of co-morbidity. *Journal of Affective Disorders* 142: S1–S3. DOI: 10.1016/S0165-0327(12)00632-5.

International Diabetes Federation (2021). Facts and Figures. *International Diabetes Federation*. https://www.idf.org/aboutdiabetes/what-is-diabetes/facts-Figures.html.

Lin, E., S. Heckbert, C. Rutter, W. Katon, P. Ciechanowski, E. Ludman et al. (2009). Depression and increased mortality in diabetes: unexpected causes of death. *Annals of Family Medicine* 7(5): 414–21. DOI: 10.1370/afm.998.

Matthews, V., C. Connors, A. Laycock, J. Bailie and R. Bailie (2015). *Chronic illness care for Aboriginal and Torres Strait Islander people: final report*. ESP Project: Priority Evidence-Practice Gaps and Stakeholder Views on Barriers and Strategies for Improvement. Brisbane: Menzies School of Health Research.

Matthews, V., G. Schierhout, J. McBroom, C. Connors, C. Kennedy, R. Kwedza et al. (2014). Duration of participation in continuous quality improvement: a key factor explaining improved delivery of type 2 diabetes services. *BMC Health Services Research* 14(1): 578. DOI: 10.1186/s12913-014-0578-1.

42　Bailie, Matthews et al. 2017.

Menzies School of Health Research and One21seventy (2015). *Vascular and metabolic syndrome management clinical audit tool.* Brisbane: Menzies School of Health Research.

Menzies School of Health Research and One21seventy (2012). *Systems assessment tool – all client groups.* Darwin: Menzies School of Health Research.

Naqshbandi, M., S. Harris, J. Esler and F. Antwi-Nsiah (2008). Global complication rates of type 2 diabetes in Indigenous peoples: A comprehensive review. *Diabetes Research and Clinical Practice* 82(1): 1–17. DOI: https://doi.org/10.1016/j.diabres.2008.07.017.

National Heart Foundation of Australia (2016). *Guidelines for the diagnosis and management of hypertension in adults – 2016.* Melbourne: National Heart Foundation of Australia.

Remote Primary Health Care Manuals, ed. (2022). *CARPA standard treatment manual for remote and rural practice.* Alice Springs, NT: Flinders University. https://www.remotephcmanuals.com.au/home.html.

Ride, K. and S. Burrow (2016). Review of diabetes among Aboriginal and Torres Strait Islander people. Australian Indigenous HealthInfoNet. Western Australia: Edith Cowan University.

Royal Australian College of General Practitioners (2020). *Management of type 2 diabetes: a handbook for general practice.* Melbourne: RACGP.

Saeedi, P., I. Petersohn, P. Salpea, B. Malanda, S. Karuranga, N. Unwin et al. (2019). Global and regional diabetes prevalence estimates for 2019 and projections for 2030 and 2045: results from the *International Diabetes Federation Diabetes Atlas,* 9th edn. *Diabetes Research and Clinical Practice* 157: 107843-43. DOI: 10.1016/j.diabres.2019.107843.

Schierhout, G., V. Matthews, C. Connors, S. Thompson, R. Kwedza, C. Kennedy et al. (2016). Improvement in delivery of type 2 diabetes services differs by mode of care: a retrospective longitudinal analysis in the Aboriginal and Torres Strait Islander primary health care setting. *BMC Health Services Research* 16(1): 560. DOI: 10.1186/s12913-016-1812-9.

Schierhout, G., T. Nagel, D. Si, C. Connors, A. Brown and R. Bailie (2013). Do competing demands of physical illness in type 2 diabetes influence depression screening, documentation and management in primary care: a cross-sectional analytic study in Aboriginal and Torres Strait Islander primary health care settings. *International Journal of Mental Health Systems* 7(1): 16. DOI: 10.1186/1752-4458-7-16.

Si, D., M. Dowden, C. Kennedy, R. Cox, L. O'Donoghue, H. Liddle et al. (2011). Indigenous community care: documented depression in patients with diabetes. *Australian Family Physician* 40(5): 331–3.

Titmuss, A., E. Davis, A. Brown and L. Maple-Brown (2019). Emerging diabetes and metabolic conditions among Aboriginal and Torres Strait Islander young people. *Medical Journal of Australia* 210(3): 111113.e1. DOI: 10.5694/mja2.13002.

Titmuss, A., E. Davis, V. O'Donnell, M. Wenitong, L. Maple-Brown, A. Haynes et al. (2022). Youth-onset type 2 diabetes among First Nations young people in northern Australia: a retrospective, cross-sectional study. *Lancet. Diabetes and Endocrinology* 10(1): 11–13. DOI: 10.1016/S2213-8587(21)00286-2.

Wickramasinghe, L., P. Schattner, M. Hibbert, J. Enticott, M. Georgeff and G. Russell (2013). Impact on diabetes management of general practice management plans, team care arrangements and reviews. *Medical Journal of Australia* 199(4): 261–5. DOI: 10.5694/mja13.10161.

World Health Organization (2021, 10 November). Diabetes: key facts. *World Health Organization.* https://www.who.int/news-room/fact-sheets/detail/diabetes.

Improving preventive health care

Preventive health care

How health is defined influences how preventive care is approached. In a Western medical model, preventive care focuses on the prevention of illness to decrease disease and associated risk factors, improve health outcomes and ease demand on health services. Preventive care is crucial for reducing the burden of chronic illnesses such as type 2 diabetes and for preventing diseases such as polio and rheumatic heart disease. Preventive measures can be applied at all stages of the life span and along a disease continuum, to prevent illness and further decline in health over time. When approached in a holistic way, preventive care is tailored to the health needs of individuals, communities and populations, and supports people to manage their own health. When such opportunities are missed, it leads to increased illness in the population, higher use of hospital care, higher healthcare costs and continuing health inequities for certain groups (for example, Indigenous peoples, refugees, people with disabilities).

While the Western medical model is dominant in many parts of the world, other models and knowledges are important for preventing illness and promoting health, including in specific populations within "Western" countries. Preventive approaches grounded in Indigenous worldviews, for example, may challenge the person-centred approach prevalent in Western approaches, centralising the connections between people, their lived experiences, histories, cultures and environments that protect health and enable wellbeing.[1] Chinese medicine and India's Ayurveda centralise individualised lifestyle practices and integrated preventive strategies.[2] In various approaches, good preventive care is critical in the shift towards primary health care (PHC) that reflects the values and cultures of consumers, aims for better quality of life and outcomes, and uses healthcare resources effectively.

A Western approach to preventive care is widely adopted in PHC services and defines four levels of prevention.

- *Primordial prevention* – action taken to prevent future hazards to health and to decrease factors known to increase disease risks. Examples are promoting healthy behaviours in childhood, improving housing and sanitation, tackling systemic racism, reducing air pollution and taking action on climate change.
- *Primary prevention* – aims to avoid the development of disease or disability in healthy people and generally focuses on specific risk factors for certain diseases or injuries.

---

1   Durey and Thompson 2012; Heke, Rees et al. 2018.
2   Bodeker 2020.

Examples in PHC settings are immunisation against infectious diseases (for example, childhood and Covid-19 vaccines), health education, interventions supporting behaviour change (for example, healthy eating, not smoking) and community programs to protect health (for example, by strengthening cultural practices). Primary prevention may include "passive" strategies (for example, nutrient-enriched foods) and legislation to reduce harm (for example, restricting the sale of tobacco and alcohol, mandating the use of seatbelts in vehicles).

- *Secondary prevention* – aims to reduce the effect of a condition or injury by detecting it and halting or slowing its progress. Examples are screening people for risk factors and early detection of diseases (for example, assessing cardiovascular risk), and interventions to reduce risks (for example, changes to diet, preventive drug therapies). Screening and early detection has limited value unless systems and resources are available to follow up people "at risk". Providing affordable treatment is a key challenge in low-resource settings.[3]

- *Tertiary prevention* – aims to reduce the effect of an ongoing illness or an injury with lasting effects. An example is helping people to manage long-term, complex health problems (for example, chronic illness, brain injury) so their ability to function, quality of life and life expectancy are improved. Clients who need this level of preventive care have considerable contact with healthcare providers.[4]

Prevention and public health were elevated during the Covid-19 pandemic. Data has shown that people with preventable chronic conditions, health vulnerabilities (for example, smoking, some disabilities), poor and elderly people and those not traditionally well served by health systems (for example, Indigenous peoples, people living in rural and remote areas) are at greater risk of adverse outcomes linked to Covid-19. The data has provided evidence that more needs to be invested in keeping people healthy and reducing health inequities.[5]

Clinical PHC teams generally deliver primary, secondary and tertiary prevention. A comprehensive approach to PHC addresses the clinical, social, cultural and environmental determinants of health as part of prevention and health promotion. The main focus of this chapter is the quality of preventive clinical care provided to individuals and populations, rather than the prevention of health issues from a public health, population health or health promotion perspective.

Preventive health and Aboriginal and Torres Strait Islander peoples

Preventable chronic disease is the largest contributor to the difference in health status between Aboriginal and Torres Strait Islander peoples and non-Indigenous Australians. While important gains are being made (for example, through Indigenous-led strengths-based prevention programs), two-thirds of 2018–19 National Aboriginal and Torres Strait Islander Health Survey respondents reported at least one chronic condition, and 36 per cent reported 3 or more.[6] It is not the same for everyone everywhere, but overall, rates of diabetes are higher compared

---

3   Oti, van de Vijver et al. 2016.
4   Institute for Work and Health 2015; World Health Organization 2020.
5   Department of Health 2021; Yashadhana, Pollard-Wharton et al. 2020.
6   Australian Institute of Health and Welfare 2024b.

with non-Indigenous Australians[7] and type 2 diabetes occurs at earlier ages.[8] Aboriginal and Torres Strait Islander peoples are more likely to report cardiovascular disease,[9] and in 2018 the burden of chronic kidney disease was almost eight times as high among First Nations people as non-Indigenous people.[10] Self-reported experience of psychological distress was 2.7 times the rate of other Australians[11] and rates of hospital admission for most health problems were higher.[12] These health inequities provide clear evidence of the need for best-practice preventive health care with broad population coverage at all levels, and culturally safe services that build on Aboriginal and Torres Strait Islander knowledge, resilience and strengths to improve outcomes. Strong cultural, family and community connections, continuing cultural practices and a holistic approach to wellness are linked with positive health and wellbeing.[13]

This chapter reports on clinical preventive care. However, the social determinants of health account for a third of the health gap and result in differences in health risks, exposures, access to services and health outcomes throughout a person's life.[14] Clinical preventive care is important but does not adequately address the social determinants and further actions are needed across the health system and other sectors. Action is needed to improve poor housing, health hardware and living conditions that increase the risk of preventable conditions, including infectious diseases and chronic illnesses, for many communities.[15] Tackling racism and economic exclusion,[16] and supporting Aboriginal and Torres Strait Islander peoples' rights to self-determine how services and programs are designed, delivered and managed are also essential for protecting and improving health.

Since the introduction of Medicare-funded Indigenous-specific health assessments in 1999, clinical preventive care services have been progressively expanded for Aboriginal and Torres Strait Islander peoples of all ages. There has been a substantial increase in the delivery of health assessments, but it is difficult to assess the effect of this expansion on improving health outcomes. Research shows that health assessments may not be reaching those most in need, thereby reducing the potential benefits at a population level,[17] and that the rate of follow-up of health assessments has been low.[18]

Recommended preventive health care

A comprehensive PHC approach

Clinical preventive care should follow a life-course approach. Screening and illness prevention services for child and youth health should continue into adulthood. General prevention measures for adults are consistent with the measures identified for preventing diabetes in

---

7   Australian Institute of Health and Welfare 2024d.
8   Titmuss, Davis et al. 2019.
9   Australian Institute of Health and Welfare 2024a.
10   Australian Institute of Health and Welfare 2024c.
11   Australian Institute of Health and Welfare 2018; Dudgeon, Wright et al. 2014.
12   Australian Institute of Health and Welfare 2024a.
13   Verbunt, Luke et al. 2021.
14   Australian Institute of Health and Welfare 2018.
15   Verbunt, Luke et al. 2021.
16   Durey and Thompson 2012; Ride and Burrow 2016.
17   J. Bailie, Schierhout et al. 2014; R. Bailie, Griffin et al. 2013; Russell 2010; Si, Moss et al. 2014.
18   J. Bailie, Schierhout et al. 2014; R. Bailie, Griffin et al. 2013.

the previous chapter. They include community health promotion programs, identifying people at high risk using recommended assessment tools, providing client education and promoting changes that reduce health risks as needed (for example, focusing on exercise, weight reduction, diet, smoking, alcohol intake, emotional wellbeing), and appropriate therapies to reduce the effects of illness and to improve health.

Preventive health assessments and other preventive interventions

These types of interventions may be delivered opportunistically during clinical encounters in PHC settings, or through integrated approaches between PHC providers and other services (for example, breast cancer screening). Strategies for increasing the delivery of prevention services might include electronic reminders in clinical information systems when screening is due, doing health assessments incrementally over multiple sessions and offering outreach programs (for example, to deliver vaccinations in work and community settings).

Follow-up of abnormal results

PHC teams or practitioners should always plan to follow up people who have had preventive health assessments and screening, so that abnormalities found during assessments can be addressed. Clients' social and emotional wellbeing can also be affected by the outcomes of screening, especially when a new condition is diagnosed. Counselling should be available.

Client-centred preventive care

Regardless of where or how prevention services are delivered, they should support holistic assessment of the client's health, recognising the interdependence of many risk factors and determinants of disease. The person's strengths and potential to change high-risk health behaviours, their health literacy, life circumstances, family and community support are considered when planning strategies to reduce health risks and provide ongoing care. Continuing engagement with PHC services needs to be encouraged. Cultural safety should be a priority, and may involve, for example, the engagement of Aboriginal and Torres Strait Islander health practitioners and other culturally specific support services.

Findings: quality of preventive care

The data presented below on the quality of preventive care come mainly from nine research papers and key reports published by the ABCD CQI research program between 2003 and 2019. Studies analysed more than 17,108 records of people aged between 15 and 55 years who had not been diagnosed with a chronic illness. The ABCD Preventive services audit tool[19] was used to collect data from 137 PHC centres between 2005 and 2014 (the most recent audit data available for analysis). The majority of health centres (almost 80 per cent) were located in geographically remote locations and 73 per cent were government managed. Stakeholders participated in data interpretation to identify priority evidence-to-practice gaps and factors influencing improvement.

---

19   Menzies School of Health Research and One21seventy 2013.

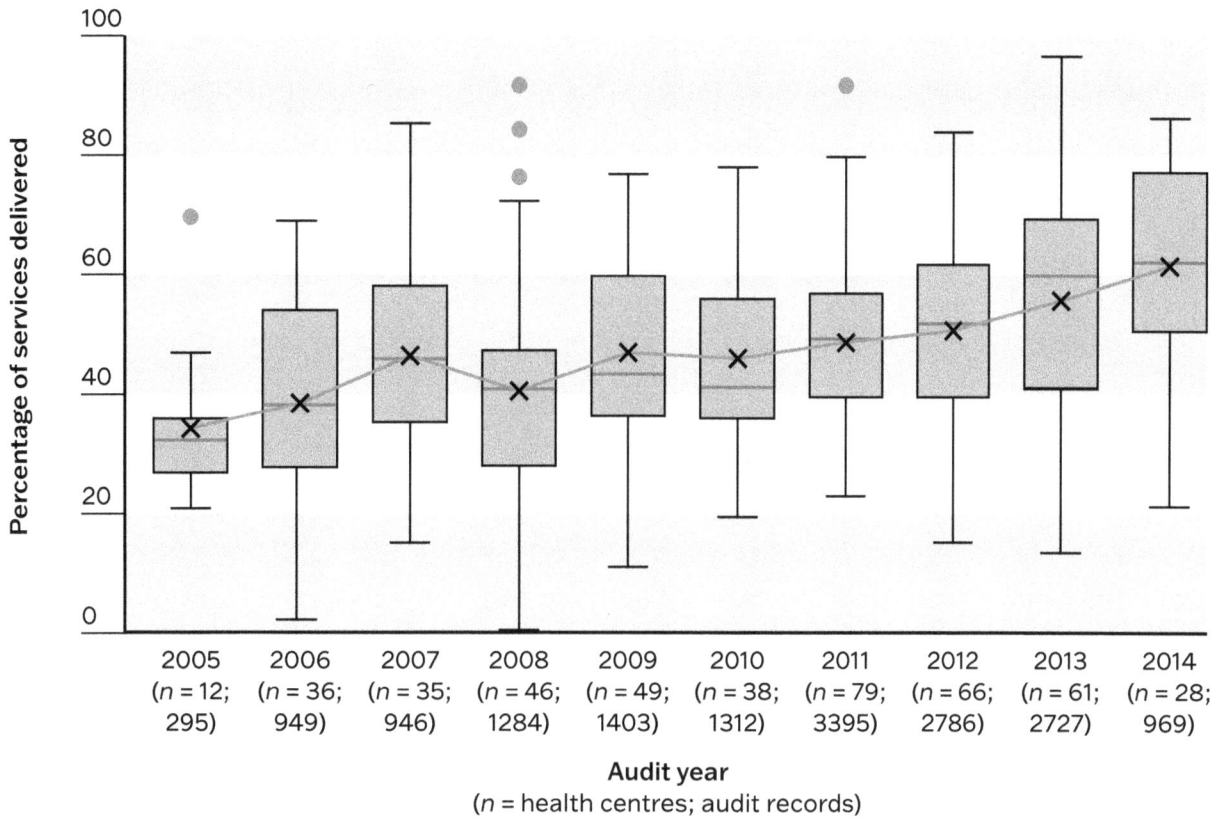

Figure 11.1 Trends in overall service delivery to well clients. Source: J. Bailie, V. Matthews et al. 2017.

Comprehensive preventive care

Audit data relating to 26 best practice indicators for preventive care were brought together to analyse the overall quality of preventive health care from 2005 to 2014 (17,108 client records, 137 PHC centres).

Clinical audit and interpretation of the data from the audits found several key points for continuous quality improvement.

- Delivery of recommended preventive care varied widely between service items.[20]
- Clear improvements were made in overall adherence to recommended preventive care. The mean and median levels of care delivery improved from 30 to 35 per cent in 2005 to about 60 per cent in 2014 (Figure 11.1).[21]
- A smaller PHC centre service population was associated with greater adherence to best practice guidelines.[22]
- No reduction occurred in the variation in the level of preventive care delivery between health centres. Variation increased over the four consecutive audit cycles 2011–2014 (Figure 11.1).[23]

---

20   C. Bailie, Matthews et al. 2016.
21   J. Bailie, Matthews et al. 2016.
22   C. Bailie, Matthews et al. 2016.
23   J. Bailie, Matthews et al. 2016.

- Variation between PHC centres in the level of delivery of preventive care may be partly explained by community–PHC centre linkages, organisational culture, effectiveness of team structure and function, degree of staff turnover, availability of community health workers (for example, Aboriginal and Torres Strait Islander health practitioners), allied health professionals and other resources, and use of information technology systems for recall and reminders.[24]
- There was a small upward trend in the overall level of delivery of preventive care for services who participated in three or more CQI cycles. This suggests that a sustained commitment to CQI will result in improvements in the delivery of care for those services.[25]

> Over audit years there were clear improvements in the overall service delivery of preventive health care.

Note: the overall preventive care service delivery composite figure includes these checks and measurements: of weight, waist circumference, blood pressure, urinalysis, blood glucose level, sexually transmitted infections (gonorrhoea, chlamydia and syphilis), Pap smear, oral health, nutrition, physical activity, recording of smoking and alcohol status, brief intervention if smoker or high-risk alchohol user or both.

Planning for follow-up care: abnormal clinical results

Routine preventive care involves following up clients who have abnormal results from screening tests or risk factors for disease and chronic illnesses (or both). Follow-up care may include, for example, a plan for repeat measurement or the retesting of abnormal results, and may involve medical prescriptions, counselling, and referrals to medical specialists, allied health professionals or programs that support change (for example, to stop smoking or increase physical activity) as part of a management plan.

Analysis of data (17,108 audited records, 137 PHC centres, 2005–14) showed these results:

- The highest priority for improvement was the follow-up of clients with abnormal blood pressure, blood glucose levels and lipid profiles.
- Follow-up rates remained consistently low across the years, particularly for abnormal blood glucose and lipids testing (Figure 11.2a, b and c). This represents a significant missed opportunity for improving early intervention for chronic diseases.
- There was wide variation in follow-up between PHC centres across the years. A concerning proportion of clients had no plan for follow-up. This was the case for follow-up of abnormal tests for blood pressure, blood glucose levels and lipids (Figure 11.2a, b and c).
- Only a small proportion of "well" adults had records of, or plans for, follow-up of abnormal clinical findings in 2005–09 audits.[26] Audit data from 2012–14 showed similar results,[27] highlighting the need for more focus on this area of preventive care.

---

24   C. Bailie, Matthews et al. 2016.
25   J. Bailie, Matthews et al. 2016.
26   R. Bailie, Si et al. 2011.
27   J. Bailie, Matthews et al. 2016.

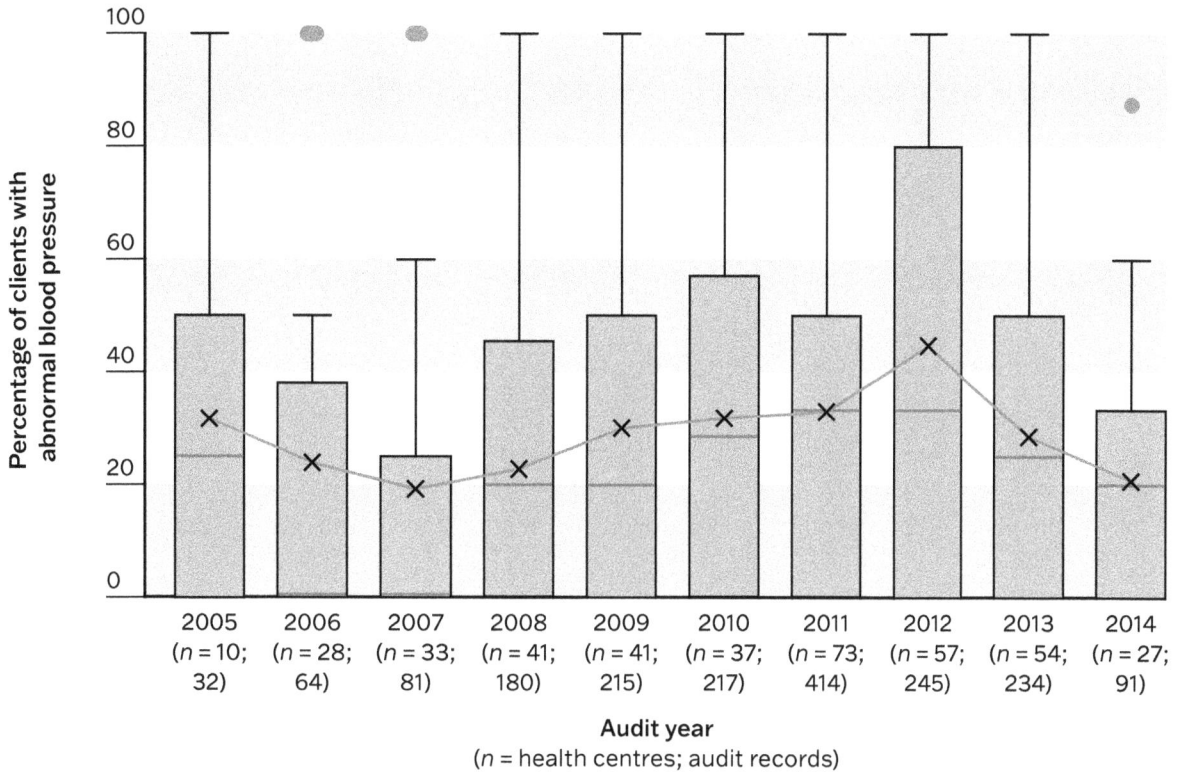

Figure 11.2a Mean health centre record of plan for follow-up by audit year for abnormal blood pressure. Source: J. Bailie, Matthews et al. 2017.

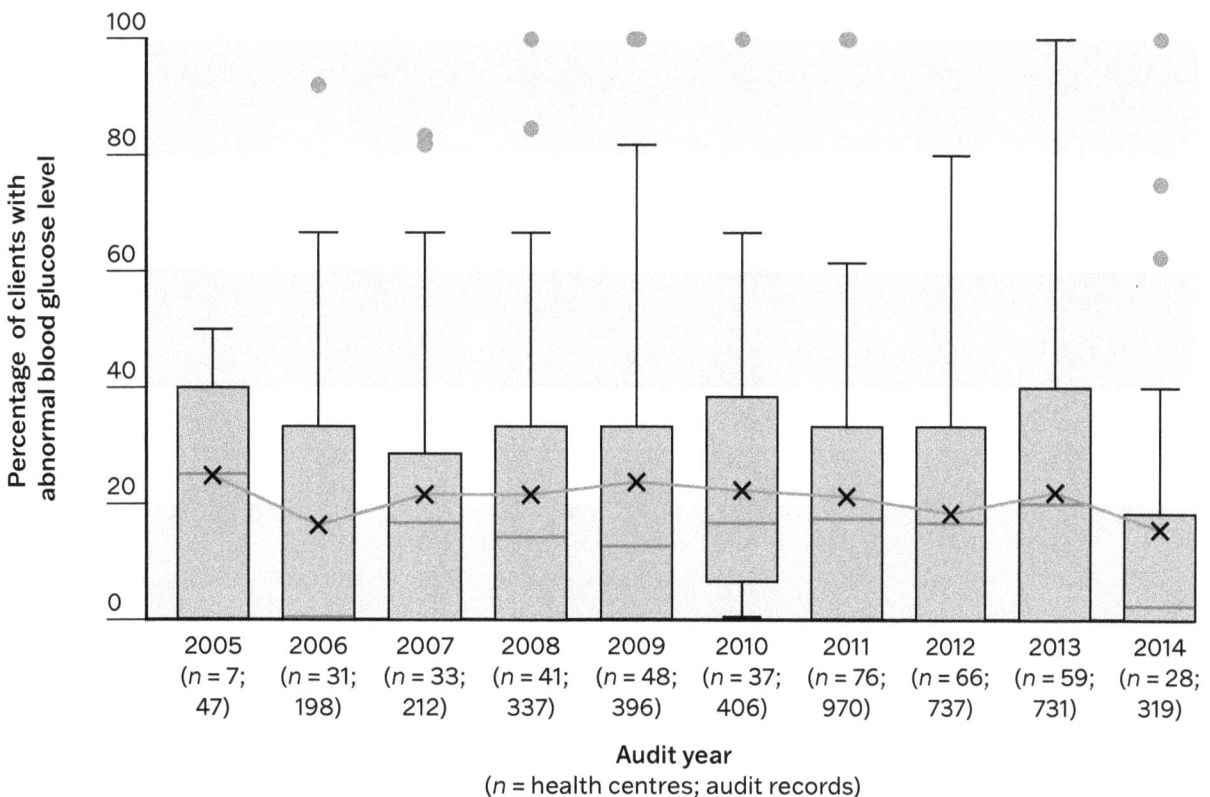

Figure 11.2b Mean health centre record of plan for follow-up by audit year for abnormal blood glucose level. Source: J. Bailie, Matthews et al. 2017.

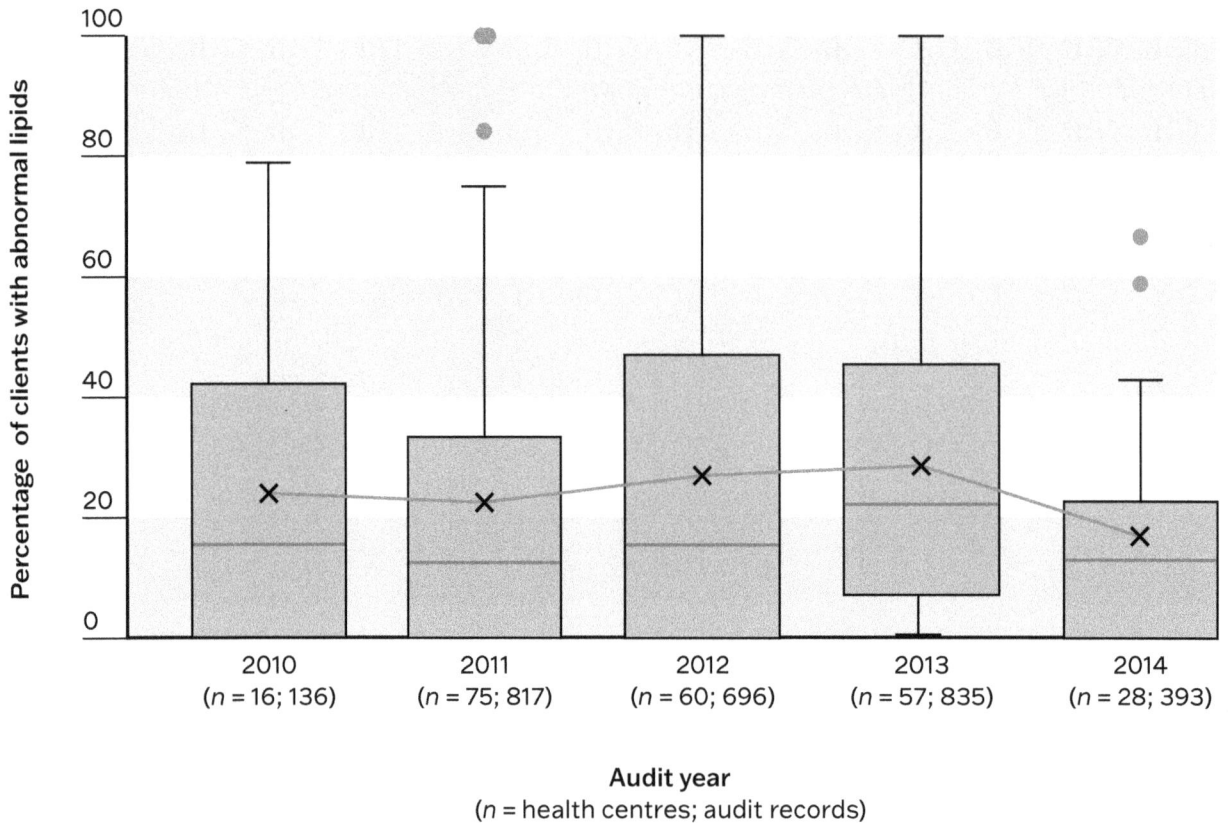

Figure 11.2c Mean health centre record of plan for follow-up by audit year for abnormal lipid profile. Source: J. Bailie, Matthews et al. 2017.

Emotional wellbeing screening, support and follow-up

Screening for emotional wellbeing and following best-practice pathways for those at risk are important parts of preventive care. They are particularly important for population groups experiencing high rates of illness and trauma, social and economic exclusion, or displacement.

Recommended care includes use of standard screening tools for emotional wellbeing (for example, Kessler 10; Patient Health Questionnaire 9). Social and emotional wellbeing assessment tools that have been culturally validated for use with Aboriginal and Torres Strait Islander adults include the Patient Health Questionnaire 9,[28] the Aboriginal Resilience and Recovery Questionnaire,[29] the Aboriginal and Islander Mental Health Initiative Northern Territory,[30] and the Here and Now Aboriginal Assessment.[31] Formal and informal discussions about emotional wellbeing (for example, guided by culturally specific resources[32]) can also be used to assess risk; discussions should be documented in client records. Options for follow-up action with clients assessed as at risk may include brief interventions, counselling, cognitive behaviour therapy, medication, strengths-based Indigenous programs (for example, Family

---

28   Getting it Right Collaborative Group, Hackett et al. 2019.
29   Gee 2016.
30   Download Aboriginal and Islander Mental Health Initiative (AIMhi) resources from Menzies School of Health Research n.d.
31   Janca, Lyons et al. 2015.
32   Such as resources available from Wellmob n.d.

Wellbeing Empowerment Program), and other types of support such as referral to housing and employment services.

There is a need to increase rates of emotional wellbeing screening, and to improve the ability of PHC services to provide appropriate support and follow-up for clients identified as being at risk, as part of preventive care.

- Analysis of audit data (3,571 client records, 95 PHC centres, 2012–14) found wide variation between PHC centres in the use of standard tools to assess emotional wellbeing, but low levels generally. In the majority of PHC centres this was being done for fewer than 20 per cent of clients.
- A small proportion of clients – less than 10 per cent in the majority of PHC centres – had a record of concern of being at risk for emotional wellbeing, but this is as high as 40 to 60 per cent in a few PHC centres.
- For clients assessed as being at risk, there was wide variation between PHC centres in referral or in provision of brief interventions, counselling or psychotropic medication, and no evidence of improvement in delivery of these follow-up services over time (Figure 11.3a, b and c).[33]
- Recording a subsequent review of clients who had been identified at risk, or having a report from an external service as a result of a referral, also varied widely between PHC centres.

Preventive health assessments

Best-practice guidelines for preventive health assessments for Aboriginal and Torres Strait Islander peoples include indicators of health risk across 17 topics: lifestyle; antenatal care; child health; health of young people; health of older people; eye health; hearing; oral health; respiratory health; acute rheumatic fever and rheumatic heart disease; cardiovascular disease; type 2 diabetes; kidney health; sexual health; cancer; family abuse; and mental health.[34] The focus of this chapter is preventive care for generally well adults. Separate ABCD CQI tools and processes are used to audit preventive health assessments for children and antenatal care (see Chapters 12 and 13.)

Preventive health assessments for adults were delivered at low levels. In the 2012–14 audit data, the mean rate of assessment using the recommended Adult Health Check assessment tool (Australian Medicare Benefits Schedule rebate item number 715) was just over 20 per cent and use of an alternative health check tool was even lower. The proportion of eligible clients receiving recommended preventive care ranged from 18 per cent to 85 per cent for individual preventive services.[35] Audit data showed that some aspects of screening and support for preventive care were being provided and documented at high levels by health centres. There was relatively better recording of these elements of care:

- up-to-date health summaries and immunisation records
- measurement of weight
- measurement of blood glucose level
- measurement of blood pressure, pulse rate and rhythm
- delivery of brief interventions for clients identified as drinking alcohol at high-risk levels, and for tobacco use.[36]

---

33 J. Bailie, Matthews et al. 2017.
34 National Aboriginal Community Controlled Health Organisation and Royal Australian College 2024.
35 C. Bailie, Matthews et al. 2016.
36 C. Bailie, Matthews et al. 2016; J. Bailie, Matthews et al. 2016; J. Bailie, Matthews et al. 2017.

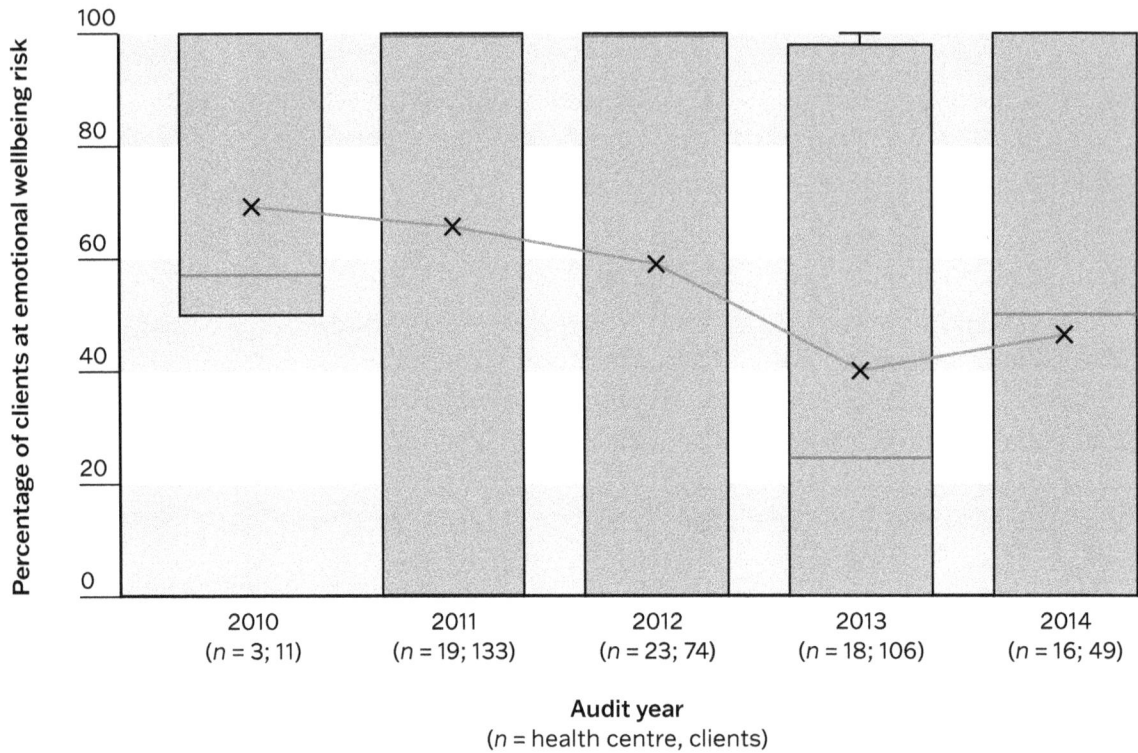

Figure 11.3a Mean health centre percentage (by audit year) of clients identified at social and emotional wellbeing risk using a standard tool, with a record of follow-up action: brief intervention. Source: J. Bailie, Matthews et al. 2017.

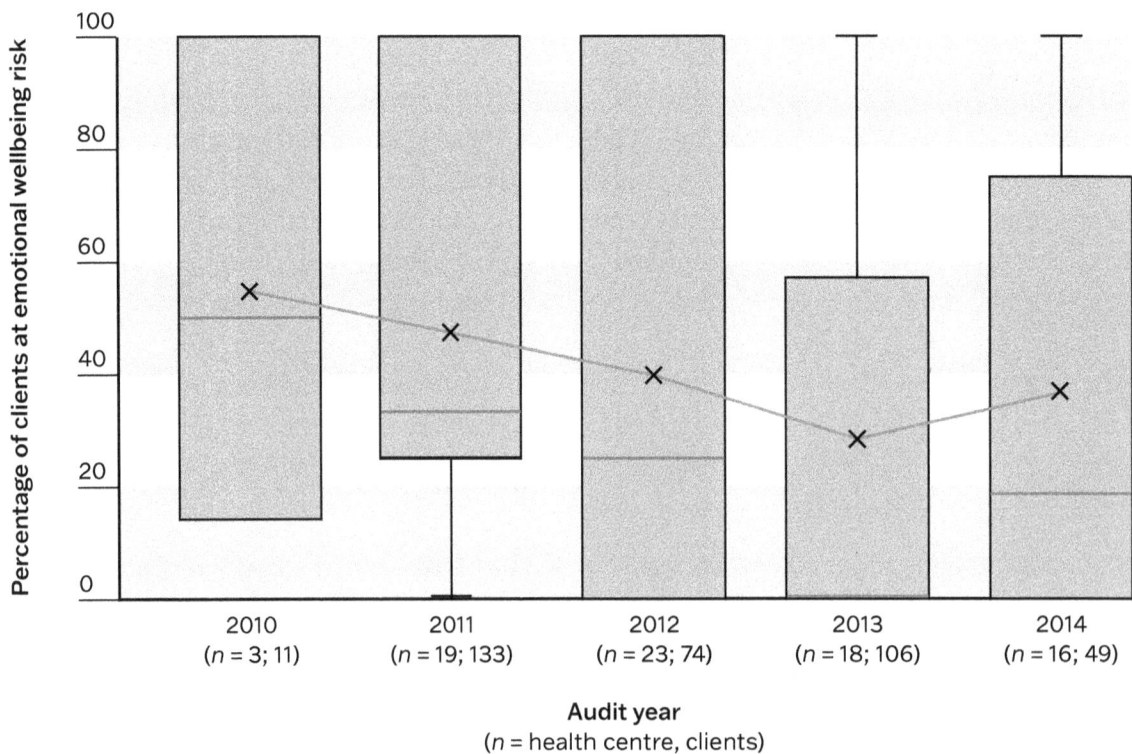

Figure 11.3b Mean health centre percentage (by audit year) of clients identified at social and emotional wellbeing risk using a standard tool, with a record of follow-up action: counselling. Source: J. Bailie, Matthews et al. 2017.

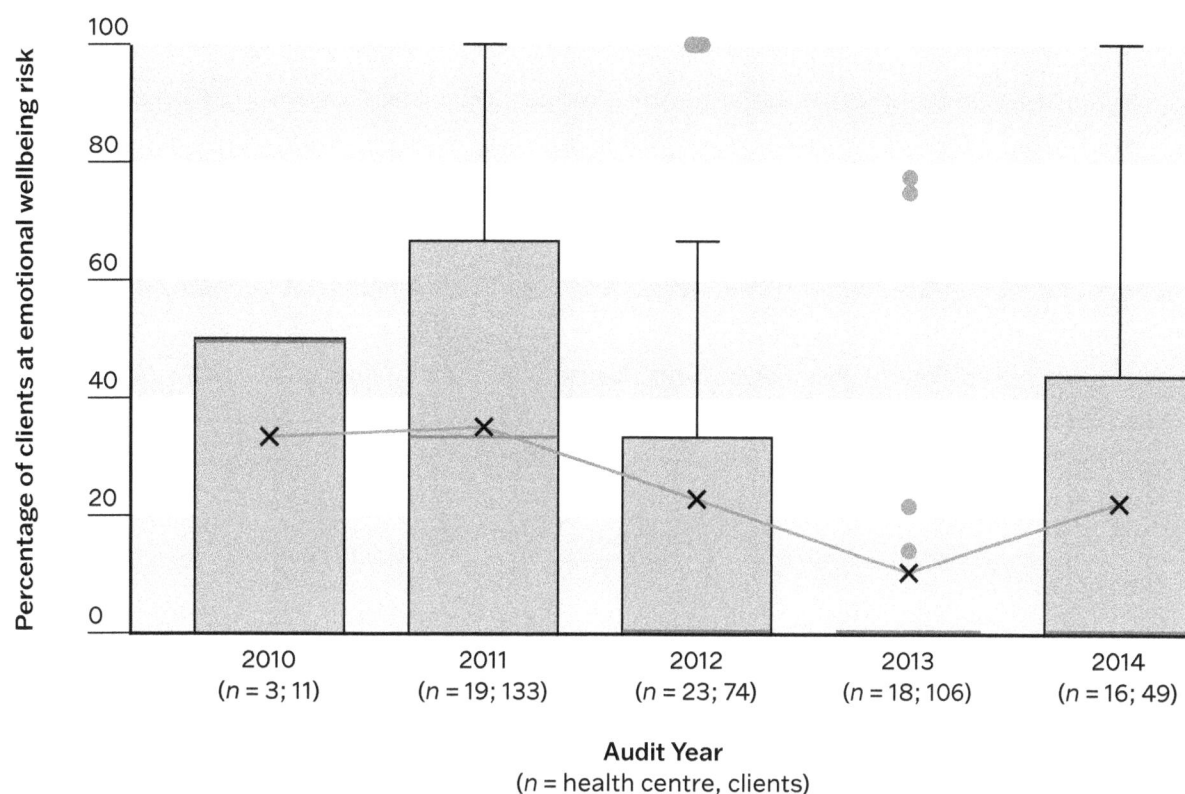

Figure 11.3c Mean health centre percentage (by audit year) of clients identified at social and emotional wellbeing risk using a standard tool, with a record of follow-up action: medication review. Source: J. Bailie, Matthews et al. 2017.

Better recording of care was needed for these elements:

- completing cardiovascular risk assessments – the mean across 92 health centres from 2012–2014 was 20 per cent
- urinalysis – the median level of delivery (95 PHC centres, 2012–14) was approximately 50 per cent
- lipid profile – the median level of delivery (95 PHC centres, 2012–14) was approximately 40 per cent
- inquiry or brief intervention about environmental and living conditions, family relationships and substance abuse – median rates for all three items ranged from 20 per cent to just over 30 per cent
- emotional wellbeing screening and support for clients identified as being at risk[37]
- oral health checks.[38]

---

37   J. Bailie, Matthews et al. 2016; J. Bailie, Matthews et al. 2017.
38   R. Bailie, Si et al. 2011.

Across the studies, there was a need to strengthen systems and processes to support preventive care. Stakeholder input to data interpretation identified drivers and strategies for system improvement, as follows:

- strong community participation in the local PHC service (for example, improve staff understanding of the culture, diversity and main features of the local population, involve community members in health service governance)
- appropriate PHC team structure and function to provide preventive care (for example, allocate resources and roles for preventive care with targeted recruitment; provide training, including to supporting client self-management; improve teamwork; establish links with other care providers for referral and care continuity)
- effective service delivery structures and supports (for example, adequate and flexible funding models for preventive care, incentives for delivering health assessments, employment of local community members in the PHC service)
- well-functioning clinical information systems and decision support tools (for example, adjust clinical information systems as needed to recall clients for health assessments and follow-up, record test results and follow-up action, calculate cardiovascular risk)
- PHC teams trained in using clinical information systems and documenting preventive care in client records
- use of data for CQI in preventive care (for example, allocate time and resources for CQI, bring in technical help to extract and interpret data if needed, plan and review improvement)
- improved client health literacy and strong links between preventive care and community health promotion programs.

Key messages for improving preventive health care

Patterns of preventive healthcare delivery in Aboriginal and Torres Strait Islander PHC communities are likely to reflect, at least to some extent, care delivery in international settings. This CQI research identifies clear priorities and strategies for improving preventive health care.

There are common evidence-to-practice gaps in preventive care that call for system-wide and local attention:

- planning for follow-up of clients with abnormal blood pressure, blood glucose levels and lipid profile

- completing cardiovascular risk assessments

- recording of urinalysis and lipid profiles

- recording of inquiry about environmental and living conditions, family relationships and substance use

- providing appropriate support and follow-up for clients identified as being at risk with respect to emotional wellbeing

- strengthening "PHC team structure and function" and "continuity of care".

There is a need to focus on the main drivers of best practice preventive care. These are the most important:

- strong community participation in the local PHC service

- appropriate PHC team structure and function to provide preventive care

- effective service delivery structures and supports

- well-functioning clinical information systems and decision support tools

- PHC teams trained in using clinical information systems and documenting preventive care in client records

- use of data for CQI in preventive care

- improved client health literacy and strong links between preventive care and community health promotion programs.

All involved in preventive care should aim to spread and continue improvement:

- taking action to improve systems for delivering preventive care will strengthen other areas of care (for example, chronic illness care)

- sustained commitment to CQI is needed to achieve and sustain improvement.

Sustained commitment to CQI is needed to achieve and sustain improvement.

Improving preventive care in Aboriginal and Torres Strait Islander PHC

Improving the delivery of preventive care for Indigenous Australians is crucial to closing the health gap between Aboriginal and Torres Strait Islander and non-Indigenous Australians. Despite efforts to improve preventive care at the PHC level and national policy initiatives, recommended best-practice preventive care is not consistently provided. Our research into the quality of preventive care for Aboriginal and Torres Strait Islander peoples since 2005 highlights major gaps in the delivery of recommended preventive care, particularly the recording of care provided, and a lack of follow-up of abnormal clinical findings. While many aspects of preventive care are being done well in many health centres, these common gaps and the persistent wide variation between health centres in the delivery of preventive services indicate deficiencies in the broader PHC system.[39]

This evidence reinforces the critical importance of taking both system-level and local action to improve preventive care, including effective processes for engaging Aboriginal and Torres Strait Islander communities in planning and delivering preventive services. There is need for, firstly, prevention activities based on needs identified by clients and communities; secondly, close collaboration between health promotion staff and clinicians within PHC teams;

---

39   C. Bailie, Matthews et al. 2016; J. Bailie, Matthews et al. 2016; J. Bailie, Matthews et al. 2017; R. Bailie, Si et al. 2011; Crinall, Boyle et al. 2017.

and, finally, a multi-sector, systems-wide approach that involves multiple service agencies and focuses the attention of funders towards all levels of prevention. A health system aimed at reducing the increasing burden of disease, reducing health inequity and preparing for emerging health threats will serve all Australians well.[40]

> A health system aimed at reducing the increasing burden of disease, reducing health inequity and preparing for emerging health threats will serve all Australians well.

Medicare rebates for annual preventive health assessments are available for all Aboriginal and Torres Strait Islander peoples of any age through the Medicare Benefits Schedule rebate item number 715. The rate of Aboriginal and Torres Strait Islander peoples who received an Indigenous-specific health check stabilised around 28 per cent in 2023, with people 65 years and older having the highest rates of health checks (42 per cent of the population in 2023), compared with 15- to 34-year-olds at 23 per cent. Older people also had the highest rates of follow-up (56 per cent), and women had higher rates of health checks and follow-up than men across all adult age groups.[41] The earlier onset of chronic diseases among the Aboriginal and Torres Strait Islander population indicates an urgent need to target younger people for health checks, and to increase the delivery of health assessments overall, as part of a holistic approach to PHC.

A key factor in improving preventive care for Aboriginal and Torres Strait Islander clients is the availability of appropriate services for client referral. Remote practitioners may reasonably be reluctant to carry out services such as visual acuity testing and oral health checks where there are limited options for referral for treatment. Client care can also be compromised in urban settings if services make strategic decisions to increase service remuneration through Medicare-funded health assessments without adequate resources to provide follow-up care.[42]

Our studies indicate that PHC teams generally know the content and objectives of best-practice preventive healthcare delivery, but high demand for acute care, competing demands on staff time and inadequate staffing levels in PHC services present barriers to delivering preventive care. This is borne out in audit data, which show that 48 per cent of clients last attended their health service for acute care and only 11 per cent for a preventive health assessment. Dedicated preventive care resources, workflow strategies that enable delivery of preventive care and clear role definitions help PHC teams to provide recommended preventive services.[43] Clinical services need to complement community-led programs that use strengths-based and culturally based approaches to protect health. CQI offers opportunities to reflect on the context in which PHC is operating and to seek input from different stakeholders about how to improve care. It provides data that can be used to advocate for public health measures and policy change.

The upward trend in overall delivery of preventive care for services that participated in three or more CQI cycles suggests that a sustained commitment to CQI will result in improvements

---

40   Department of Health 2021.
41   Australian Institute of Health and Welfare 2024e.
42   C. Bailie, Matthews et al. 2016.
43   J. Bailie, Matthews et al. 2016; J. Bailie, Matthews et al. 2017.

in the delivery of care for those services.[44] At higher levels of the health system, policy and infrastructure support and organisational commitment to CQI have been associated with steady improvements or maintenance of high-quality preventive care for Aboriginal and Torres Strait Islander communities.[45]

> Policy and infrastructure support and organisational commitment to CQI have been associated with steady improvements in preventive care.

References

Australian Institute of Health and Welfare (2024a). *Aboriginal and Torres Strait Islander Health Performance Framework: summary report August 2024*. Canberra: AIHW. https://www.indigenoushpf. gov.au/report-overview/overview/summary-report.

Australian Institute of Health and Welfare (2024b) *Australia's health 2024: health and wellbeing of First Nations people*. Canberra: Australian Government. https://www.aihw.gov.au/reports/ australias-health/indigenous-health-and-wellbeing.

Australian Institute of Health and Welfare (2024c). *Chronic kidney disease: Australian facts*. Cat. no. CDK 2024. Canberra: AIHW. https://www.aihw.gov.au/reports/chronic-kidney-disease/ chronic-kidney-disease/contents/about.

Australian Institute of Health and Welfare (2024d). *Diabetes*. Cat. no. CVD 96. Canberra: Australian Government. https://www.aihw.gov.au/reports/diabetes/diabetes/contents/summary.

Australian Institute of Health and Welfare (2024e). *Health checks and follow-ups for Aboriginal and Torres Strait Islander people*. Cat. no. IHW 209https://www.aihw.gov.au/reports/indigenous-australians/ indigenous-health-checks-follow-ups/contents/summary.

Australian Institute of Health and Welfare (2018). *Australia's health 2018*. Cat. no. AUS 221. Canberra: AIHW.

Bailie, C., V. Matthews, J. Bailie, P. Burgess, K. Copley, C. Kennedy et al. (2016). Determinants and gaps in preventive care delivery for Indigenous Australians: a cross-sectional analysis. *Frontiers in Public Health* 4: 34. DOI: 10.3389/fpubh.2016.00034.

Bailie, J., V. Matthews, A. Laycock, R. Schultz and R. Bailie (2016). *Preventive health care for Aboriginal and Torres Strait Islander people: final report*. ESP Project: Priority Evidence-Practice Gaps and Stakeholder Views on Barriers and Strategies for Improvement. Brisbane: Menzies School of Health Research.

Bailie, J., V. Matthews, A. Laycock, R. Schultz, C. Burgess, D. Peiris et al. (2017). Improving preventive health care in Aboriginal and Torres Strait Islander primary care settings. *Globalization and Health* 13(1). DOI: 10.1186/s12992-017-0267-z.

Bailie, J., G. Schierhout, M. Kelaher, A. Laycock, N. Percival, L. O'Donoghue et al. (2014). Follow-up of Indigenous-specific health assessments – a socioecological analysis. *Medical Journal of Australia* 200(11): 653–7. DOI: 10.5694/mja13.00256.

Bailie R., J. Griffin, M. Kelaher, T. McNeair, N. Percival, A. Laycock et al. (2013). *Sentinel sites evaluation: final report*. Canberra: Report prepared by Menzies School of Health Research for the Australian Government Department of Health.

Bailie, R., V. Matthews, S. Larkins, S. Thompson, P. Burgess, T. Weeramanthri et al. (2017). Impact of policy support on uptake of evidence-based continuous quality improvement activities and the quality of care for Indigenous Australians: a comparative case study. *BMJ Open* 7(10). DOI: 10.1136/ bmjopen-2017-016626.

---

44   J. Bailie, Matthews et al. 2016.
45   J. Bailie, Matthews et al. 2017.

Bailie, R., D. Si, C. Connors, R. Kwedza, L. O'Donoghue, C. Kennedy et al. (2011). Variation in quality of preventive care for well adults in Indigenous community health centres in Australia. *BMC Health Services Research* 11: 139. DOI: 10.1186/1472-6963-11-139.

Bodeker, G. (2020). Asian traditions of wellness: background paper. *Asian Development Outlook 2020 Update: Wellness in Worrying Times.* Manila: Asian Development Bank.

Crinall, B., J. Boyle, M. Gibson-Helm, D. Esler, S. Larkins and R. Bailie (2017). Cardiovascular disease risk in young Indigenous Australians: a snapshot of current preventive health care. *Australian and New Zealand Journal of Public Health* 41(5): 460–6. DOI: 10.1111/1753-6405.12547.

Department of Health (2021). *National Preventive Health Strategy 2021–2030.* Canberra: Commonwealth of Australia.

Dudgeon, P., M. Wright, Y. Paradies, D. Garvey and I. Walker (2014). Aboriginal social, cultural and historical contexts. In *Working Together: Aboriginal and Torres Strait Islander Mental Health and Well-being Principles and Practice.* Dudgeon P., Milroy H. and Walker R. Canberra: Commonwealth Government 3–24.

Durey, A. and S. Thompson (2012). Reducing the health disparities of Indigenous Australians: time to change focus. *BMC Health Services Research* 12: 151. DOI: 10.1186/1472-6963-12-151.

Gee, G. (2016). Resilience and recovery from trauma among Aboriginal help seeking clients in an urban Aboriginal community controlled organisation. PhD thesis, University of Melbourne.

Getting it Right Collaborative Group, M. Hackett, A. Teixeira-Pinto, S. Farnbach, N. Glozier, T. Skinner et al. (2019). Getting it Right: validating a culturally specific screening tool for depression (aPHQ- 9) in Aboriginal and Torres Strait Islander Australians. *Medical Journal of Australia* 211(1): 24–30. DOI: 10.5694/mja2.50212.

Heke, I., D. Rees, B. Swinburn, R.T. Waititi and A. Stewart (2018). Systems thinking and indigenous systems: native contributions to obesity prevention. *AlterNative: An International Journal of Indigenous Peoples* 15(1): 22–30. DOI: 10.1177/1177180118806383.

Institute for Work and Health (2015). *What researchers mean by primary, secondary and tertiary prevention.* https://www.iwh.on.ca/what-researchers-mean-by/primary-secondary-and-tertiary-prevention.

Janca, A., Z. Lyons, S. Balaratnasingam, D. Parfitt, S. Davison and J. Laugharne (2015). Here and Now Aboriginal Assessment: background, development and preliminary evaluation of a culturally appropriate screening tool. *Australasian Psychiatry* 23(3): 287–92. DOI: 10.1177/1039856215584514.

Menzies School of Health Research (n.d). Resources. *Menzies School of Health Research.* https://www.menzies.edu.au/Resources.

Menzies School of Health Research and One21seventy (2013). *Preventive services clinical audit tool.* Brisbane: Menzies School of Health Research.

National Aboriginal Community Controlled Health Organisation and Royal Australian College of General Practitioners (2024). *National guide to a preventative health assessment for Aboriginal and Torres Strait Islander people,* 4th edn. Melbourne: RACGP.

Oti, S., S. van de Vijver, G. Gomez, C. Agyemang, T. Egondi, C. Kyobutungi et al. (2016). Outcomes and costs of implementing a community-based intervention for hypertension in an urban slum in Kenya. *Bulletin of the World Health Organization* 94(7): 501–09. DOI: 10.2471/BLT.15.156513.

Ride, K. and S. Burrow (2016). Review of diabetes among Aboriginal and Torres Strait Islander people. Australian Indigenous HealthInfoNet. Western Australia: Edith Cowan University.

Russell, L. (2010). Indigenous health checks: a failed policy in need of scrutiny. Menzies Centre for Health Policy: University of Sydney. https://ses.library.usyd.edu.au/bitstream/2123/11447/1/atsihealthchecks2.pdf.

Si, S., J. Moss, T. Sullivan, S. Newton and N. Stocks (2014). Effectiveness of general practice-based health checks: a systematic review and meta-analysis. *British Journal of General Practice* 64(618): e47–e53. DOI: 10.3399/bjgp14X676456.

Titmuss, A., E. Davis, A. Brown and L. Maple-Brown (2019). Emerging diabetes and metabolic conditions among Aboriginal and Torres Strait Islander young people. *Medical Journal of Australia* 210(3). DOI: 10.5694/mja2.13002

Verbunt, E., J. Luke, Y. Paradies, M. Bamblett, C. Salamone, A. Jones et al. (2021). Cultural determinants of health for Aboriginal and Torres Strait Islander people – a narrative overview of reviews. *International Journal for Equity in Health* 20(1): 1–181. DOI: 10.1186/s12939-021-01514-2.

Wellmob (n.d.). *Wellmob: healing our way.* Social, emotional and cultural wellbeing online resources for Aboriginal and Torres Strait Islander people. https://wellmob.org.au.

World Health Organization (2020). *Health promotion and disease prevention through population-based interventions, including action to address social determinants and health inequity.* http://www.emro.who.int/about-who/public-health-functions/health-promotion-disease-prevention.html.

Yashadhana, A., N. Pollard-Wharton, A. Zwi and B. Biles (2020). Indigenous Australians at increased risk of COVID-19 due to existing health and socioeconomic inequities. *Lancet Regional Health. Western Pacific* 1: 100007-07. DOI: 10.1016/j.lanwpc.2020.100007.

Improving child health

Children's health

There is strong evidence of the vital role of health care in the early years to ensure that health throughout the life course is the best it can be.[1] Primary health care (PHC) can play an important role, particularly during pregnancy when the foundations are laid and in the early years that set the beginning of health trajectories that may be difficult to shift.[2]

Over the past quarter century, child mortality globally has more than halved, yet in 2018 an estimated 6.2 million children and adolescents under the age of 15 years died, mostly from preventable causes. Of these deaths, 5.3 million occurred in the first five years of life, with almost half of these in the first month of life. Among the leading causes of death are congenital anomalies, pneumonia, diarrhoea and malaria. More than half of early child deaths are preventable or can be treated with simple, affordable interventions including immunisation, adequate nutrition, safe water and food, and appropriate health care.[3]

High-quality preventive care for babies and children should begin a continuum of preventive PHC services that extends into youth and adulthood. Good preventive care in childhood can have long-term positive effects on individual and population health, and focuses on increasing protective factors and reducing risks that affect children's health and wellbeing. It involves monitoring growth and development, decreasing the risk of diseases (for example, through immunisation, prompt treatment of infection or illness and education to prevent chronic illnesses in adulthood), early identification and referral for children and families who need targeted specialist services, and protecting children who are at risk (for example, from poverty, violence or abuse). Holistic child health care also involves acute care and general clinical management of health and wellbeing needs.

Globally, 10 to 15 per cent of all children and 40 per cent of disadvantaged children under five years of age are estimated to have developmental problems that affect their long-term social, emotional and educational outcomes.[4] These developmental problems may be experienced in fine or gross motor skills, communication, play, speech, language, hearing, vision, learning and cognition. In many places, PHC staff are the only service providers who reach young children and their families. Globally, PHC staff provide more than 90 per cent of health care

---

1   Barker, Eriksson et al. 2002.
2   Hertzman and Power 2004.
3   World Health Organization 2020.
4   Engle, Fernald et al. 2011; Grantham-McGregor, Cheung et al. 2007; Walker, Wachs et al. 2011.

for families during a child's first five years of life and are in a unique position to improve child developmental outcomes through early detection and management of developmental problems.[5]

Child health screening and intervention in PHC settings require that health professionals have access to concise, context-specific, evidence-based clinical guidance and continuously evaluate their practice against it.[6] Effective delivery systems and resources to follow up at-risk children and their families, and provide interventions when needed, are also essential. These are key challenges for improving child health, particularly in settings with a low level of resources.

> PHC staff are in a unique position to improve child developmental outcomes.

Health of Aboriginal and Torres Strait Islander children

Aboriginal and Torres Strait Islander families and communities have taken important action to achieve improvements in children's health and wellbeing, and there are positive trends in measures for birth weight, infant mortality, early childhood education, ear health, and basic skills for life and learning.[7] The proportion of mothers who smoke at any time during pregnancy fell from 52 per cent in 2009 to 44 per cent in 2019.[8] Indigenous children were first to reach the target of 95 per cent for national immunisation coverage.[9] In 2022, 99 per cent of Indigenous children were enrolled in a preschool program in the year before full-time schooling age and the percentage of Indigenous children completing the final year of secondary school has improved.[10]

In addition to families and carers, many people and organisations are working to enable Aboriginal and Torres Strait Islander children to grow up healthy, happy and safe, but significant health inequities persist. There was little improvement in the Aboriginal and Torres Strait Islander infant mortality rate in the decade to 2019[11] and no improvement in the percentage of children assessed as being developmentally on track between 2018 (baseline) and 2021.[12] While rates of ear disease among Aboriginal and Torres Strait Islander children are decreasing, the 2018–19 National Aboriginal and Torres Strait Islander Health Survey found 3 in 10 (29 per cent) children aged 7–14 had measurable hearing loss.[13] In 2014–15, among Indigenous children aged 4–14 years, 67 per cent had experienced at least one significant stressor in the previous 12 months.[14]

---

5   Blair and Hall 2006; Sabanathan, Wills and Gladstone 2015.
6   Siddiqi and Newell 2005.
7   Productivity Commission 2020.
8   Australian Institute of Health and Welfare 2023.
9   Department of Health 2019.
10   Productivity Commission 2023.
11   Australian Institute of Health and Welfare 2023.
12   Productivity Commission 2023.
13   Australian Bureau of Statistics 2019.
14   Australian Bureau of Statistics 2017.

In addition to families and carers, many people and organisations are working to enable Aboriginal and Torres Strait Islander children to grow up healthy, happy and safe.

A limitation of data about Aboriginal and Torres Strait Islander children's health is that much data comes from remote communities, whereas most Indigenous children live in urban settings.[15] Living in remote areas also presents particular health challenges. For example, a relatively recent study across six Aboriginal communities in northern Australia found 42 per cent of children aged 6–24 months were anaemic.[16] Anaemia is linked with poor cognitive development and educational outcomes,[17] and is caused mainly by iron deficiency, and by poverty, poor environmental conditions and chronic infection. Social and environmental factors also underlie the development of acute rheumatic fever (ARF) in childhood – the incidence of ARF and rheumatic heart disease in some Aboriginal and Torres Strait Islander communities is among the highest documented globally (see Chapter 17). Trachoma persists among children living in at-risk areas (Chapter 19). A high proportion of children living in remote communities experience chronic otitis media in their developmental years, which causes hearing loss that is associated with developmental delays and effects on education outcomes. Education, social, environmental and clinical interventions are needed to improve children's health in these settings, as part of comprehensive PHC.[18]

Indigenous Australians experience widespread socio-economic challenges. Aboriginal and Torres Strait Islander children are over-represented in the homelessness, child protection and youth justice systems.[19] These factors link directly to the trauma of colonisation, racism and oppression, and highlight the importance of tackling the social and structural determinants of health. They also highlight the resilience of Aboriginal and Torres Strait Islander communities. A 2016 study of factors linked with good mental health among 1,005 urban Aboriginal children aged 4–17 years in New South Wales found 72 per cent were not at high risk for emotional or behavioural problems. Healthy eating, not suffering from frequent infections and having a carer who was not highly psychologically distressed were contributing factors, while being raised in foster care or in four or more homes since birth increased risk.[20] A study of 725 urban Aboriginal children younger than 8 years found 32 per cent were at high, 28 per cent at moderate, and 40 per cent at low or no developmental risk.[21]

Policy initiatives such as "Closing the Gap",[22] Commonwealth funding under the Medical Benefits Scheme for health checks[23] for Aboriginal and Torres Strait Islander peoples, improvement in data surveillance systems and use of CQI are important for monitoring and improving child health. Regardless of the setting or circumstances in which children live,

15   Priest, Mackean et al. 2009.
16   Aquino, Leonard et al. 2018.
17   Grantham-McGregor and Ani 2001.
18   McDonald, R. Bailie et al. 2008.
19   Australian Institute of Health and Welfare 2021.
20   Williamson, D'Este et al. 2016.
21   Chando, Craig et al. 2020.
22   See Closing the Gap n.d.
23   See Department of Health and Aged Care 2022.

high-quality PHC with integrated service approaches and strengths-based, community-led responses that affirm cultural connections are needed for improving child health and wellbeing.[24]

Findings: quality of child health care

Comprehensive child health care includes prevention, detection of developmental problems, early intervention, care and support for children living in a range of geographical settings and circumstances. On-target child growth and development are important signs that a child is physically, emotionally, culturally and spiritually healthy. Important information to track a child's development includes a growth chart and a current completed health check. For example, the Australian government advises PHC providers to administer a "child health check" annually to each Indigenous child across the country. Child health checks are used to plan and track the management of care, through regular checking of risk factors, scheduled services, required pathology tests, immunisations and specialist care, brief interventions and conversations with the family and child about health and wellbeing. These items, episodes of acute care, management of illnesses and disabilities, and referrals are documented in a child's health record to provide an overall picture of the care delivered. PHC services should use a recall system for recommended child health checks, immunisations, follow-up of abnormal results and treatments.

The data presented below on the quality of care provided to children come mainly from 14 research papers and key reports published by the ABCD CQI research program between 2008 and 2018. Studies analysed more than 10,405 records of children aged between 3 months and 15 years, and 265 systems assessments completed by PHC teams. Audit data were collected from 132 PHC centres between 2007 and 2013. Stakeholders participated in data interpretation to identify priority evidence-to-practice gaps and factors influencing improvement.

Comprehensive PHC for children

The ABCD child health audit tool[25] (see Table 12.2) was used to collect data about the delivery of child health services, to assess the quality of overall adherence to child health care in accordance with best-practice guidelines. Over five consecutive audit cycles these findings were made:

- significant improvements in quality of care, which appear to be related to PHC services participating in regular CQI activities[26]
- evidence of improvement for most indicators, including overall child health care; measles, mumps and rubella vaccination at 4 years; clinical examinations (recording of weight, ear checks, developmental milestones); follow-up of children with growth faltering; records of advice, brief interventions and improvement in health centre systems[27]

---

24   Chando, Craig et al. 2020; McCalman, R. Bailie et al. 2018.
25   Menzies School of Health Research and One21seventy 2015.
26   McAullay, McAuley et al. 2018.
27   R. Bailie, Matthews et al. 2014.

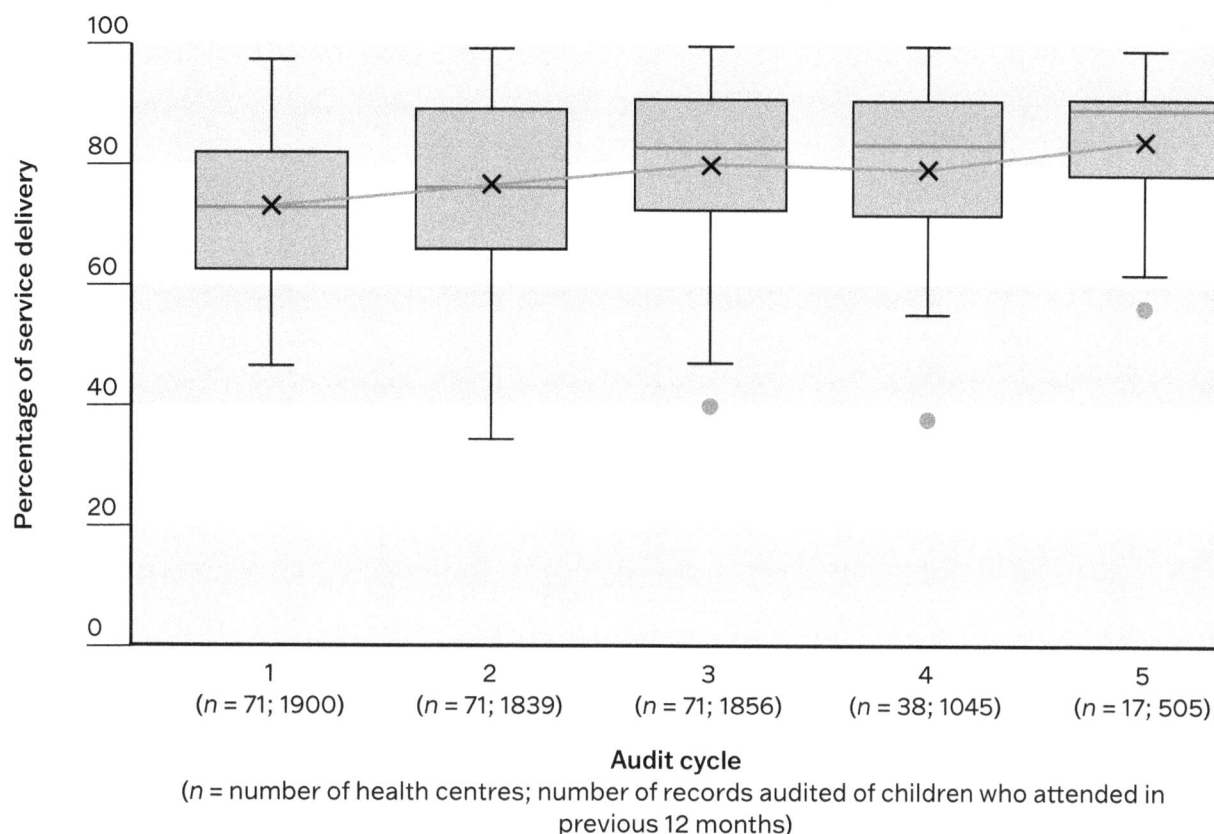

Figure 12.1 Trends in overall child health service delivery. Source: R. Bailie, Matthews et al. 2014.

- reduced variation between PHC centres for most indicators, including overall child health, most clinical examinations, and health centre systems assessment scores[28]
- no clear evidence of improvement in having immunisation charts in children's health files, or a record of a haemoglobin check or follow-up of children with anaemia[29]
- no reduction in variation for recording of Hepatitis B immunisation at birth, haemoglobin check or follow-up of children with anaemia.[30]

Figure 12.1 shows trends in the quality of overall child health service delivery, based on 10 indicators or items of care: weight, height, head circumference, hip exam, testes check, ear exam, breastfeeding, nutrition advice, sudden infant death syndrome prevention, and developmental check. Successive audit cycles showed evidence of improvement for overall child health care, and variation in the delivery of child health services reduced between health centres. There was also less variation across health centres in the fourth and fifth audit cycles; PHC centres with the lowest levels of overall delivery of care improved their performance.[31]

---

28   R. Bailie, Matthews et al. 2014.
29   R. Bailie, Matthews et al. 2014.
30   R. Bailie, Matthews et al. 2014.
31   R. Bailie, Matthews et al. 2014.

Monitoring and recording of growth and development measures and follow-up of abnormal findings

Growth and development checks should be delivered at specific ages and intervals, according to guideline-recommended care.[32] For example, screening guidelines for Aboriginal and Torres Strait Islander children recommend that weight, length or height, and head circumference be checked at age one week, four, six, 12 and 18 months of age, then at least annually to age five years. Body mass index should be plotted annually for children from two years. Recommended checks for infants and children up to 15 years generally include respiratory, ear and eye examinations, listening to the heart, oral hygiene and skin checks, with inquiries about hearing and vision concerns and other items of care.[33]

Developmental milestones are used to check a child's development, or ability to perform increasingly complex fine- and gross-motor activities, speech and language, and social interactions as they mature. Early detection of developmental problems is important for accessing interventions and maximising their positive effects. The use of standardised developmental screening tools is recommended. The Ages and Stages Questionnaire (ASQ-3) and Bayley-III tools are widely used in Australia, and a culturally adapted ASQ-Talking about Raising Aboriginal Kids (ASQ-TRAK) has been developed for monitoring the development of Australian Aboriginal children.[34] Other resources are available.[35]

Key growth and health measures

Analyses of 10,405 audit records of children collected from 132 PHC centres between 2007 and 2013 showed that many records did not include a recent record of the child's weight, or a recent record of haemoglobin monitoring. There was wide variation between PHC centres in the proportion of children with recent records. This also applied for the monitoring and recording of developmental milestones, including for vision and hearing (see below). There was wide variation between PHC centres in the recording of follow-up actions, such as a follow-up weight check, nutrition advice or action plans for children assessed with growth faltering.[36]

Developmental care and participation in CQI

Another study analysed the developmental care records of children aged from three months to five years (2,466 client records, 109 PHC centres, from 2012 to 2014), to find the following:

- All participating PHC centres (100 per cent) included the five age-specific developmental care items in their clinic's protocols (assessment of parent–child interaction, developmental milestones, vision and hearing, and advice or brief intervention about the physical and mental stimulation of the child). However, only 48 per cent of children had received the composite measure (five items) of basic developmental care in the previous 12 months: assessment of parent–child interaction, assessment of developmental milestones, assessment of vision, assessment of hearing, and advice about physical and mental stimulation of the child.

---

32   National Aboriginal Community Controlled Health Organisation and Royal Australian College 2024.
33   National Aboriginal Community Controlled Health Organisation and Royal Australian College 2024.
34   Simpson, D'Aprano et al. 2016; Strong Kids, Strong Future n.d.
35   For example, Parents' Evaluation of Developmental Status (PEDS) questionnaire.
36   R. Bailie, Matthews et al. 2014.

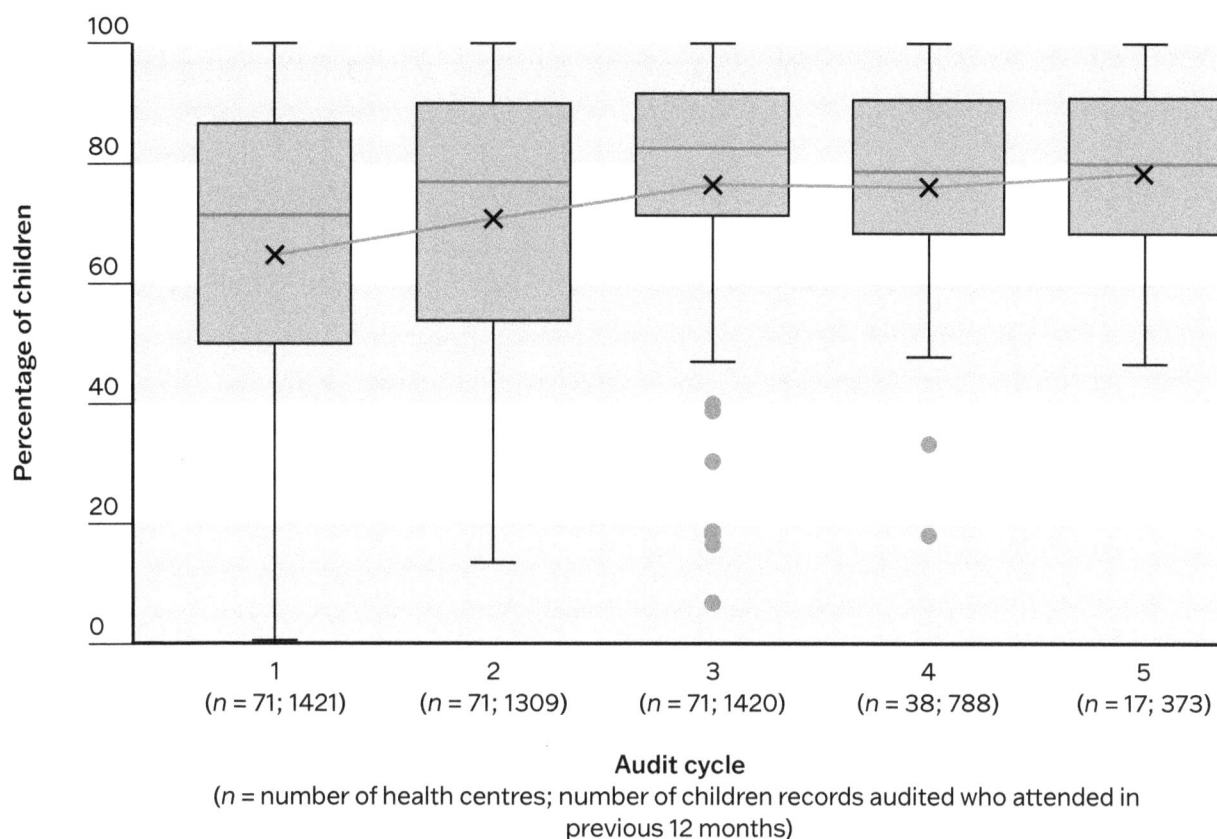

Figure 12.2 Mean percentage of children younger than four years of age attending within the previous 12 months who had a developmental milestones check, by audit cycle for health centres that have at least three years of audit data. Source: R. Bailie, Matthews et al. 2014.

- Only 4 per cent of children younger than five years were documented as having developmental problems (for example, deficits in motor, communication, play, speech and language skills, hearing, vision, learning or cognition). This percentage is far lower than global averages, indicating a need to improve practitioner skills in developmental assessment.
- Among the children who had developmental problems identified, most (93 per cent) received clinic follow-up or relevant referral or both.[37]
- Sustained participation in CQI improved access and documentation of developmental care (Figure 12.2). There was an important dose–response of improved delivery of developmental care with improved participation in CQI. Further, CQI was effective for improving developmental care in a range of PHC settings, including government-managed and community controlled PHC services, remote and non-remote locations, and small and large populations.[38]

---

37   Edmond, Tung et al. 2018.
38   Edmond, Tung et al. 2018.

- There was a need for improved resourcing of developmental care and CQI in PHC centres.[39]
- Context-specific developmental screening tools and more uniform recording methods were also needed.[40]

> Improved participation in CQI improved the delivery of developmental care.

Across CQI studies, there was a need to strengthen systems in these areas:

- recording of weight, haemoglobin and developmental milestones
- recording and follow-up action for children with growth faltering, anaemia, chronic ear infections and developmental delay
- recording and follow-up action for risks related to the domestic environment, financial situation, housing and food security
- continued participation in CQI, targeted staff training for child health and a systematic approach to delivering developmental care services for children.[41]

Immunisation

Immunisation schedules for vaccine preventable diseases (for example, diphtheria, polio, tetanus, hepatitis B, measles, mumps and rubella) vary in specific detail between countries and between jurisdictions in Australia. Child immunisation schedules are regularly and frequently updated. The table below reflects general Australian recommendations at the time of the CQI studies cited in this section.

Table 12.1 Australian vaccination recommendations.

	Vaccine
Birth	hepatitis B
2 months	HepB-DTPa_Hib_IPV (hepatitis B, diphtheria, tetanus, acellular pertussis (whooping cough), haemophilus influenza type B, polio) pneumococcal vaccine (13vPCV) rotavirus
4 months	HepB-DTPa_Hib_IPV pneumococcal vaccine (13vPCV) rotavirus

---

39 Edmond, Tung et al. 2018.
40 D'Aprano, Silburn et al. 2016.
41 R. Bailie, Matthews et al. 2014; D'Aprano, Silburn et al. 2016.

	Vaccine
6 months	HepB-DTPa_Hib_IPV influenza (annually): for those with certain medical risk factors 6 months and older, and Aboriginal and Torres Strait Islander children aged from 6 months to 5 years. pneumococcal vaccine (13vPCV): Aboriginal and Torres Strait Islander children and medically at-risk children rotavirus (3rd dose depends on brand of vaccine)
12 months	hepatitis A – 1st dose: Aboriginal and Torres Strait Islander children in high-risk areas measles, mumps and rubella (MMR) meningococcal ACWY pneumococcal vaccine (13vPCV)
18 months	DTPa haemophilus influenza type B (Hib) hepatitis A – 2nd dose: Aboriginal and Torres Strait Islander children measles, mumps, rubella, chickenpox (MMRV)
4 years	DTPa-IPV (diphtheria, tetanus, acellular pertussis (whooping cough) and polio) pneumococcal vaccine (23vPPV): medically at-risk children
10–15 years	DTPa human papilloma virus (HPV): usually 2 doses influenza – every year: Aboriginal and Torres Strait Islander peoples 15 years and older

Analysis of trend audit data (10,405 child health records, 132 PHC services, between 2007 and 2013) found that there was room for improvement in immunisation coverage in all age groups across Australian jurisdictions, and progressively lower coverage for children in older age groups. This was particularly marked for immunisations scheduled for children older than 10 years. There was some improvement in the systematic recording of immunisations and in the delivery of immunisations scheduled for delivery at two years and older, but no evidence of improvement in recording of delivery of immunisations scheduled for delivery at birth (Figure 12.3).

There is an ongoing need to strengthen attention to:

- delivery and recording of immunisations scheduled for delivery at birth[42]
- delivery and recording of immunisations scheduled at birth and at two years and older[43]

---

42   R. Bailie, Matthews et al. 2014.
43   R. Bailie, Matthews et al. 2014.

- integrating systems for the timely delivery, recording and communication between PHC centres and other providers of child health services[44]
- immunisation charts and recordings in the clinical records of children in some PHC services.[45]

Example: improving timeliness of child immunisations through CQI

An Australian PHC service, covering a large geographical area, identified problems with the timeliness of immunisation for children and with client pathways. From the infant's first visit to the child-and-family health nurse to the Aboriginal and Torres Strait Islander child health check, children and their caregivers were required to make multiple visits. This resulted in low compliance. The main clinic is in a regional town and an outreach clinic provides health care to several smaller communities. The outreach clinic has a maternity, midwife and antenatal program and a Healthy Start (newborns to 5-year-olds) program that includes immunisation, regular health checks and a children's dental team.

As part of a continuous quality improvement process, the following strategies were implemented:

- The child-and-family nurse and doctor explored clinical processes and client pathways with the service's health system support team.

- Data on completed child health checks and immunisation data were examined to establish a baseline for monitoring, and to guide discussions.

- The team reviewed client lists every morning for children who were overdue for their child health checks and immunisations. They restructured the clinic schedule to enable clients to go straight from the nurse to the doctor, ensuring that the child-and-family nurse and doctor were rostered on the same day.

- The service set up regular feedback and monitoring of results to the child health team to track improvement.

The continuous quality improvement process resulted in better team understanding of the timeliness indicator and its importance, and in monthly monitoring of timeliness data for children who have seen both a child and family health nurse and doctor in the one visit. Other outcomes of the process were increased staff interest in performance indicators and collecting and using data for CQI.[46]

---

44   R. Bailie, Si et al. 2009.
45   R. Bailie, Matthews et al. 2014.
46   Newham and Cunningham 2015.

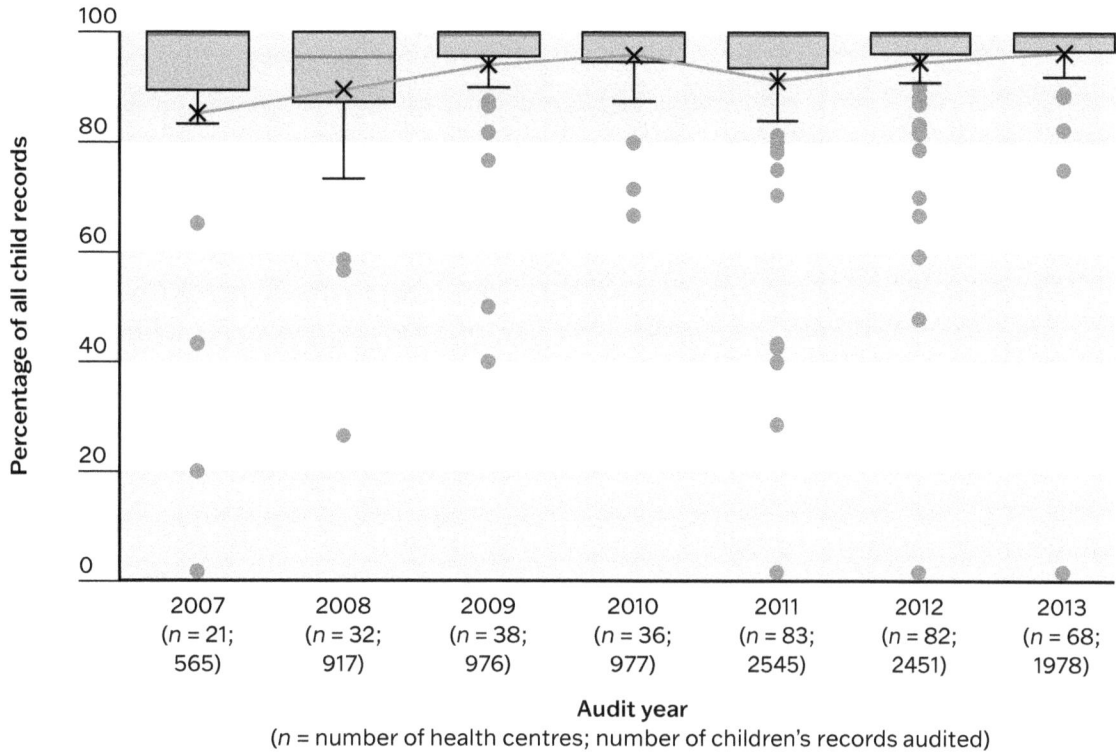

Figure 12.3a Mean percentage (by audit year for all health centres) of children with an immunisation chart present. Source: R. Bailie, Matthews et al. 2014.

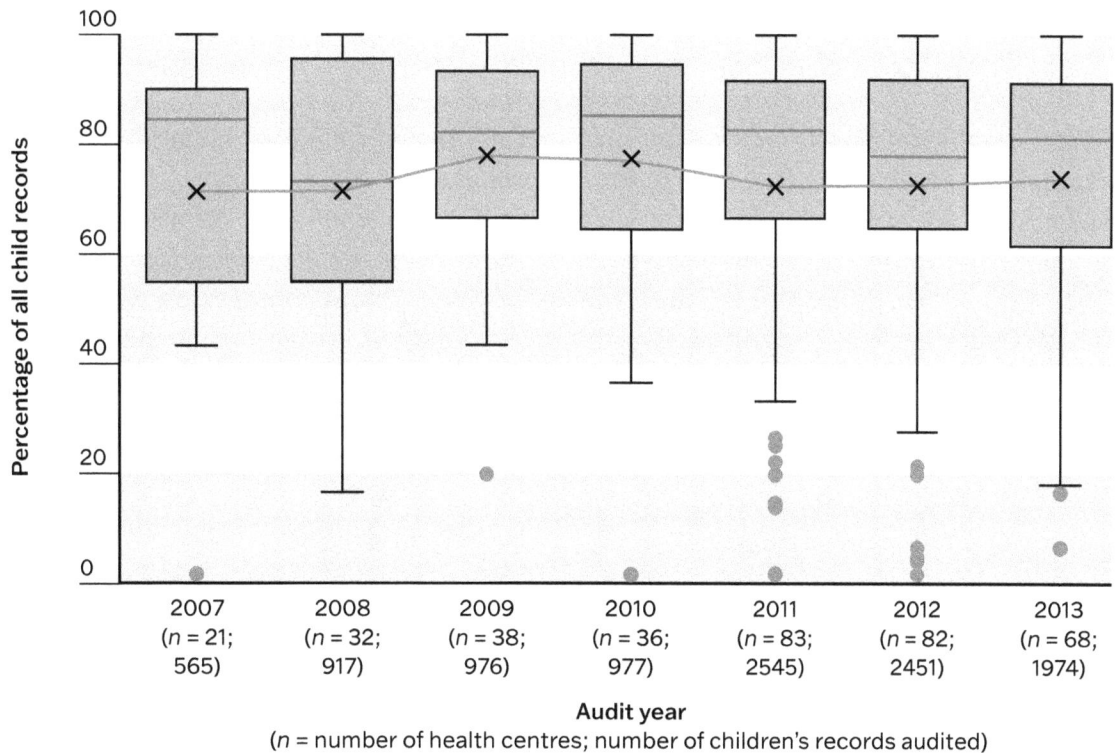

Figure 12.3b Mean percentage (by audit year for all health centres) of children with recorded hepatitis B immunisation at birth. Source: R. Bailie, Matthews et al. 2014.

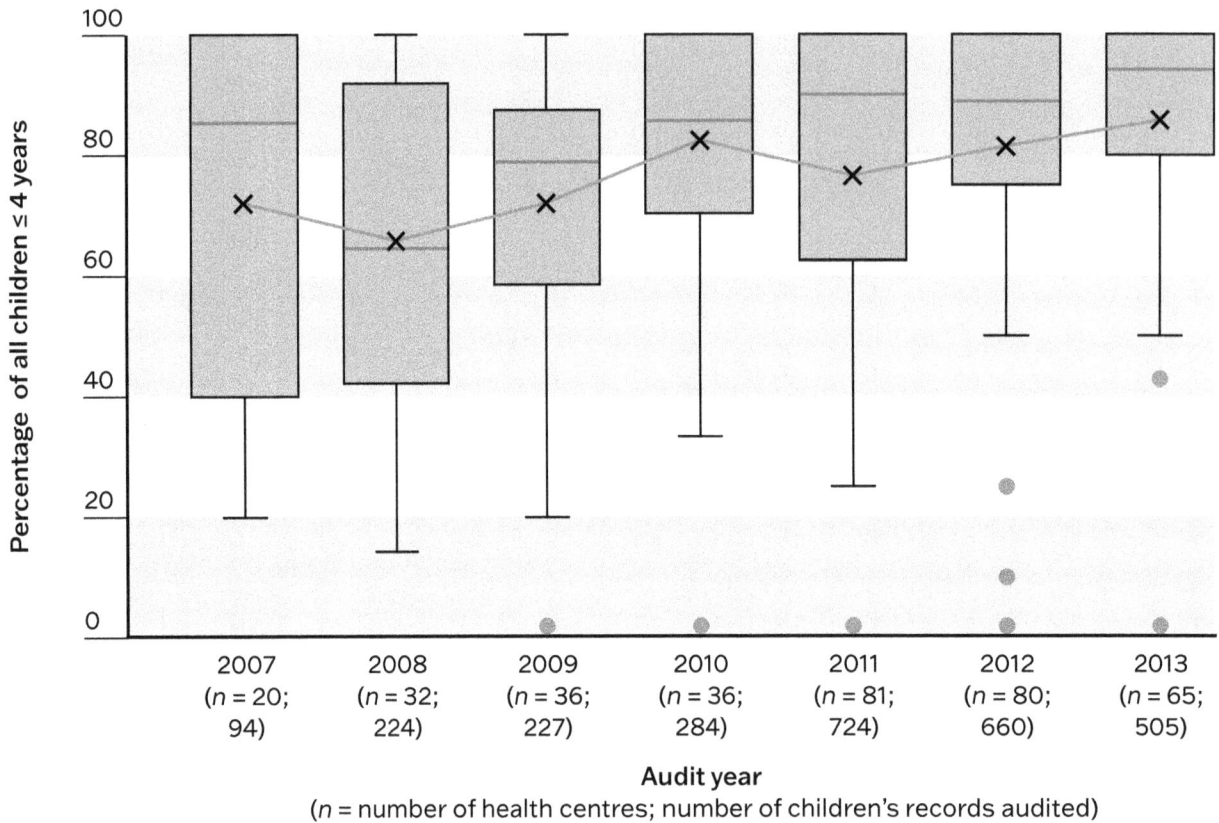

Figure 12.3c Mean percentage (by audit year for all health centres) of children with measles, mumps, rubella immunisation at four years of age. Source: R. Bailie, Matthews et al. 2014.

Childhood anaemia

A low haemoglobin reading is often a sign of iron deficiency anaemia. Anaemia is defined as a haemoglobin level less than 110 g/dl for children aged 6–59 months.[47]

In Australia, the national guide to preventive health assessments for Aboriginal and Torres Strait Islander children recommends a haemoglobin check at age 6–9 months with a repeat at 18 months, or every six months until the age of five years in conjunction with treatment if anaemia persists.[48] In geographical areas where there is a high prevalence of anaemia and parasitic infection, government policies and health service guidelines may recommend haemoglobin as a standard check, with six-monthly testing as routine to five years of age, then at 10 and 15 years. Follow-up care for abnormal findings is likely to involve nutrition advice, iron treatment, and repeat haemoglobin measurements within two months.

A study of audit records from 2007 to 2013 (10,405 children's records, 132 PHC centres) showed no clear evidence of change in the patterns of routine checking for anaemia, or in recording of anaemia, across year or audit cycles.

- A significant number of records did not include a recent record of haemoglobin monitoring and there was wide variation between PHC centres in the proportion of children with a

---

47 World Health Organization 2011.
48 National Aboriginal Community Controlled Health Organisation and Royal Australian College 2024.

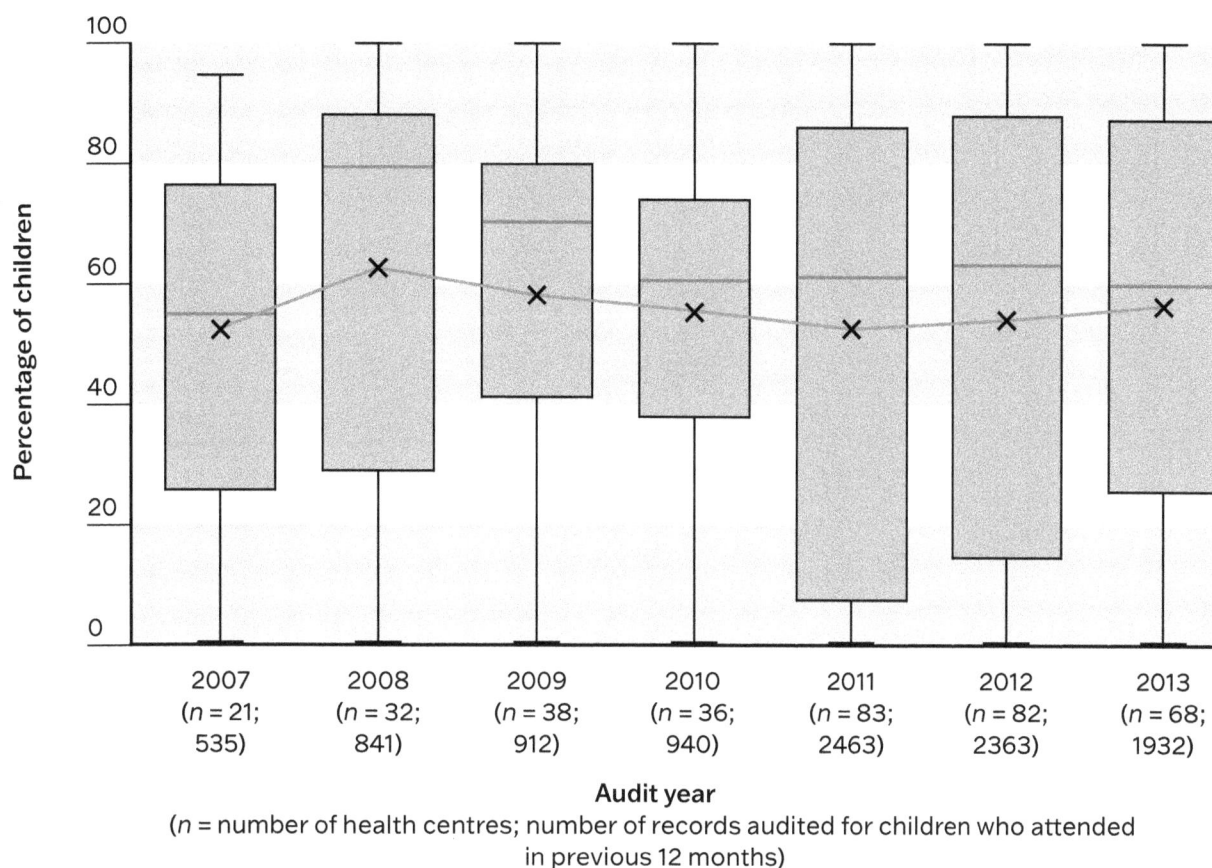

Figure 12.4 Mean percentage of children attending within the previous 12 months who had a haemoglobin check, by audit year. Source: R. Bailie, Matthews et al. 2014.

recent record – lower than expected given what we know about the population incidence of anaemia (Figure 12.4).

- There was wide variation between PHC centres in the recording of follow-up action, and generally low levels of recording of systematic actions being taken for these children – including deworming, prescription of iron supplements, nutritional advice, and follow-up monitoring of haemoglobin (Figure 12.5).[49]

A separate 2012–14 study (2,287 children's records, 109 PHC centres) had the following findings:

- both nutrition advice to carers about healthy foods and a haemoglobin measurement in the past 12 months had been completed for only 54 per cent of children
- children living in remote areas were more likely to receive both items of care than those attending PHC centres in rural and urban areas
- although abnormal haemoglobin measurements were higher in children aged 6 to 11 months, they were 71 per cent less likely to receive a haemoglobin check than children aged 1 to 5 years, and 52 per cent less likely to receive both items of care
- treatment and follow-up of children diagnosed with abnormal haemoglobin levels was low across age groups.[50]

49   R. Bailie, Matthews et al. 2014.
50   Mitchinson, Strobel et al. 2019.

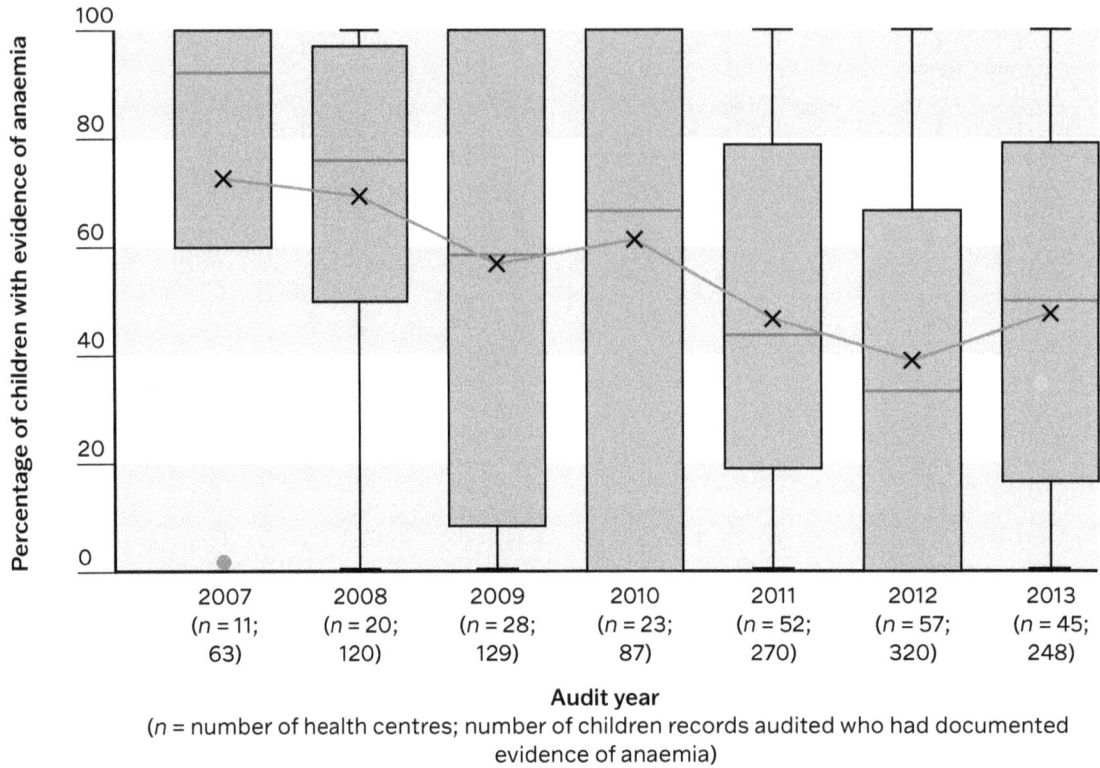

Figure 12.5a Mean percentage, by audit year, of children with anaemia who had documented evidence of deworming treatment. Source: R. Bailie, Matthews et al. 2014.

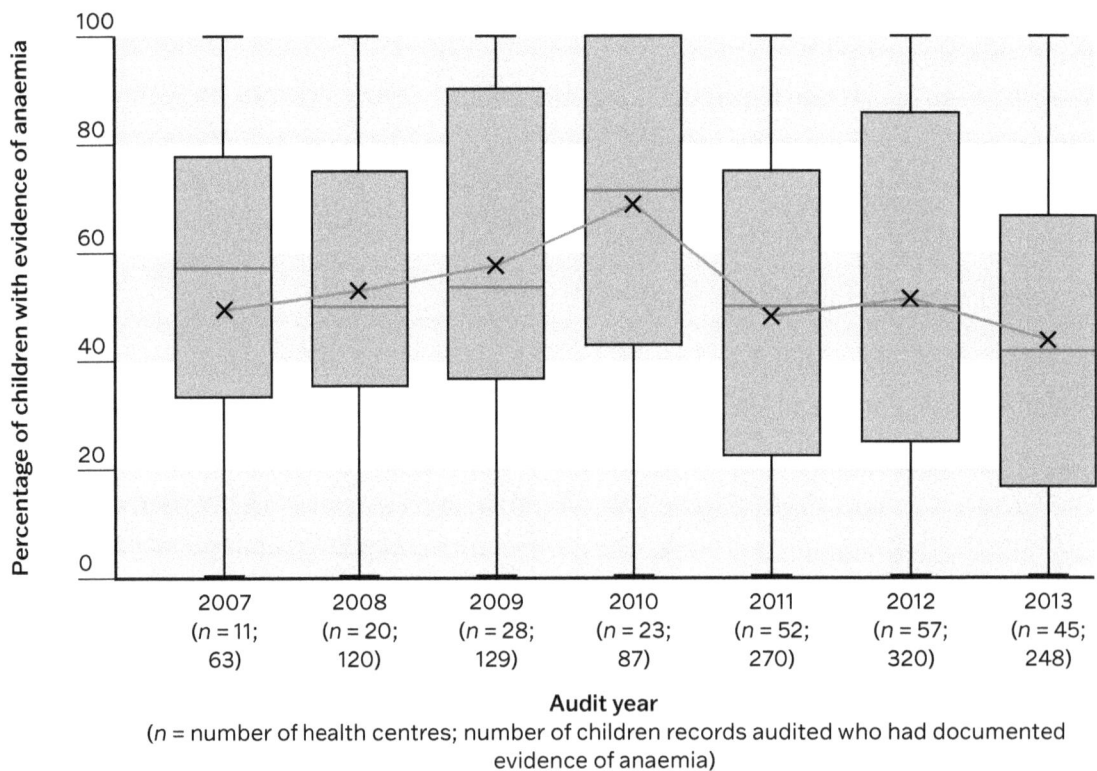

Figure 12.5b Mean percentage, by audit year, of children with anaemia who had documented evidence of a follow-up haemoglobin check. Source: R. Bailie, Matthews et al. 2014.

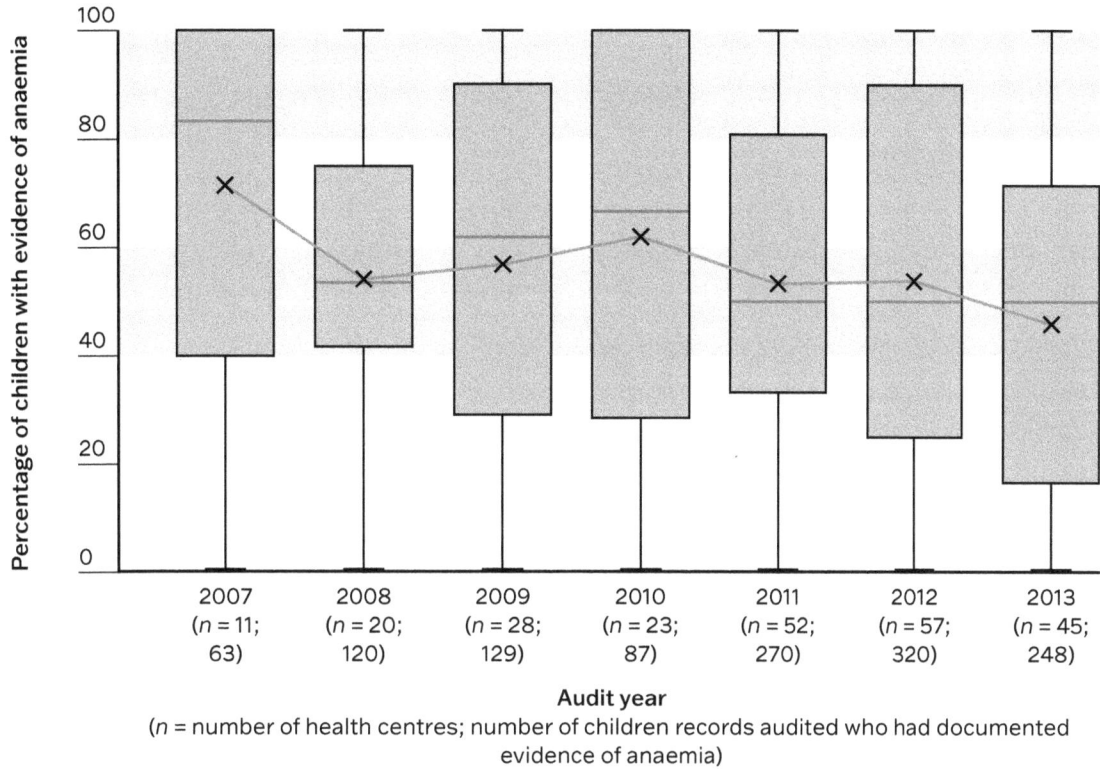

Figure 12.5c Mean percentage, by audit year, of children with anaemia who had documented evidence of an iron prescription. Source: R. Bailie, Matthews et al. 2014.

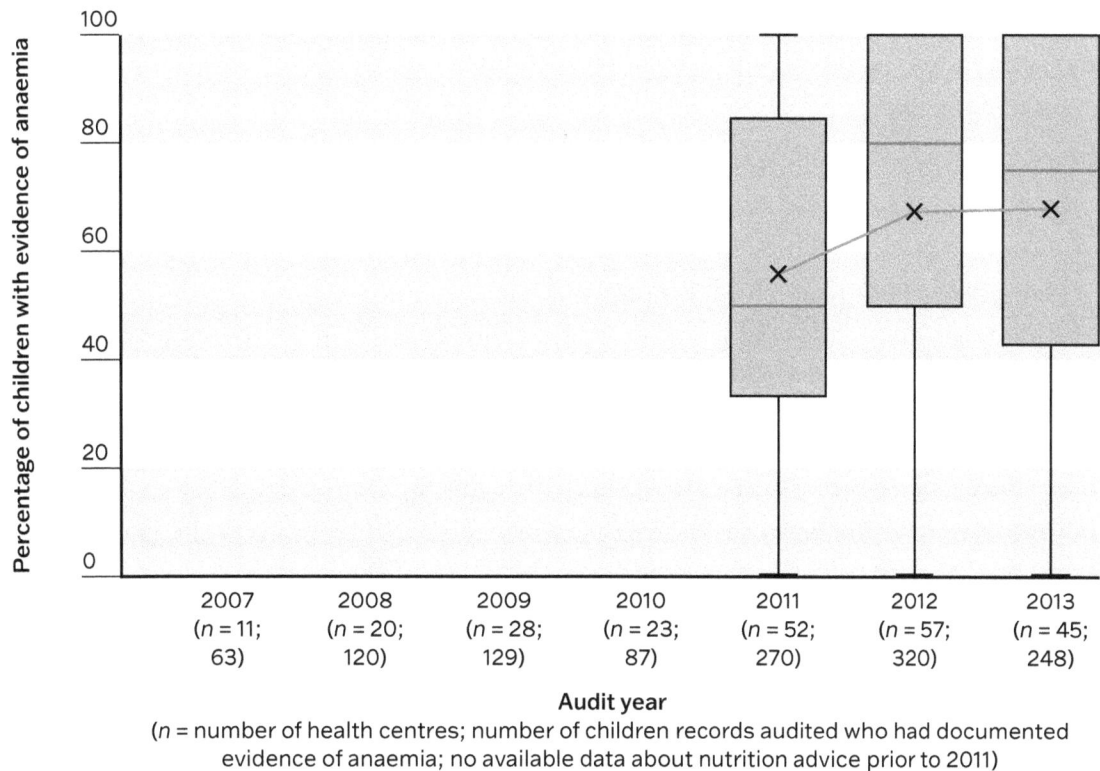

Figure 12.5d Mean percentage, by audit year, of children with anaemia who had documented evidence of nutrition advice. Source: R. Bailie, Matthews et al. 2014.

There is a need to improve monitoring and recording of haemoglobin according to best-practice guidelines, including clear processes and/or access to guidelines, and systematic approaches to screening, nutrition advice, case finding and follow-up.

Anaemia health literacy

Anaemia health literacy of community members, and health practitioner's knowledge of anaemia best-practice guidelines, was studied in a remote Indigenous community where English is not the first language. The research resulted in these findings:

- knowledge about anaemia in the community was good, but there was no evidence that this knowledge translated into improving the dietary intake of children, possibly due to food insecurity and poor knowledge about how iron-rich foods should be consumed
- community health practitioners' knowledge of follow-up procedures for anaemia ranged from fair to excellent.[51]

These findings highlight the need for holistic approaches that address the social determinants of health, such as food security and health literacy, in addition to clinical care.

Social and emotional wellbeing

PHC services have the potential to improve social and emotional wellbeing and long-term neuro-developmental outcomes in vulnerable children.[52] In Australia, there are specific guidelines for providing social and emotional wellbeing services in PHC centres. The guidelines include an assessment of the social determinants that may be affecting a child's wellbeing.

A study of the social and emotional wellbeing services delivered to families of young Indigenous children attending services (2,466 client records, 109 PHC services) found that these services were not well delivered, with little difference in services provided in remote, rural and urban areas.

- All PHC services in the study included the age-specific national best-practice guidelines for social and emotional wellbeing care in their clinic protocols.
- Delivery of service items ranged from around 11 per cent (food security) to 75 per cent (assessment of parent–child interaction).
- Families of children younger than one year old were more likely to receive these services (for example, advice about social support, child stimulation) than families of older children, but many families were not receiving these items of care.
- Almost 25 per cent of families had no follow-up or referral for concerns about domestic environment, family support and financial situation, housing or food security.
- There is a need for better resourcing, supervision and training in the skills needed to provide these services, and better documentation of the services provided.[53]

---

51   Kearns, Ward et al. 2017.
52   Engle, Fernald et al. 2011; Fremantle, Zurynski et al. 2008.
53   Edmond, McAuley et al. 2018.

Child protection

Protecting children from abuse, neglect and mistreatment is a major concern across the globe, with most Western countries confronting increasing numbers of children in need of support from child welfare services. In Australia, 174,700 children (1 in 32 children from birth to 17 years old) received child protection services in 2019–20.[54] Aboriginal and Torres Strait Islander children are over-represented in the protection and out-of-home care system.[55] Many issues affect the success of interventions: for example, cultural bias, inadequate prevention programs, cost and overburdened staff. Integration of services between different providers and continuity of engagement of parents over time can be challenging, particularly in remote areas.[56]

A review of the use of CQI in child protection systems found that strengths-based, solution-focused models of practice that were inclusive of the families engaged with child protection services consistently resulted in improved outcomes for children. Within agencies, the use of CQI had these results:

- the gathering of appropriate evidence for outcome measurement
- improvements in processes for working with children and families
- more consistent application of practice frameworks
- more positive and engaged staff.[57]

Key messages for improving the delivery of child health care

Although there are likely to be some important differences between specific settings, patterns of PHC delivery for Aboriginal and Torres Strait Islander children may reflect care delivery in many international settings. This CQI research identifies clear priorities and strategies for improving health care for children.

There are common evidence-to-practice gaps in child health care that call for system-wide and local attention:

- recording of all immunisations in children's health records, and the delivery of immunisations scheduled for delivery at birth and at two years and older

- monitoring and recording of key measures, including weight, haemoglobin and developmental milestones, and follow-up action for faltering growth, anaemia, chronic ear infections, developmental delay, and risks related to domestic environment, financial situation, housing and food security

- recording of advice or brief interventions on child nutrition, passive smoking, infection prevention and hygiene, injury prevention, domestic or social and environmental conditions, and child development

- providing follow-up or referral to other agencies for concerns about domestic environment, family support and financial situation, housing and food security

---

54   Australian Institute of Health and Welfare 2021.
55   Australian Institute of Family Studies 2018.
56   Robinson, Mares and Arney 2017.
57   Zuchowski, Miles et al. 2017.

- recording of inquiries made regarding the parents' or carers' use of alcohol, tobacco and other drugs, and discussion or advice or both provided on risks to the health of children

- developing systems for effective engagement between health centres and communities

- implementing systems that support regional health planning.

Focus on reducing barriers and strengthening enablers for providing best-practice child health care, through actions such as these:

- recruitment of PHC teams with the right mix of skills to provide child health services (for example, a child health nurse)

- staff training and development (for example, in areas of child health relevant to the evidence-practice gaps, in cultural safety)

- development of clinical information systems (for example, improve and make better use of clinical information systems including the sharing of electronic records across providers to assist follow-up, completeness of children's records and efficient use of resources for providing care)

- promotion of parenting practices that protect children's health and wellbeing (for example, encourage families to bring children to PHC services for child health checks and other scheduled services, and to seek support)

- community engagement, support and health literacy (for example, work with communities to build understanding of child health issues and priorities; involve community-based workers, community members and agencies in providing practical support for families and reducing risks to child health).

Aim for less siloed service delivery and better inter-agency coordination. Developing systems and opportunities for staff across agencies to share relevant knowledge about children and their families and carers will help to provide holistic, best-practice care.

Sustained participation in CQI activities can improve basic developmental care in PHC settings, and the overall delivery of child health care.

Sustained participation in CQI activities can improve basic developmental care in PHC settings, and the overall delivery of child health care.

Improving PHC for Aboriginal and Torres Strait Islander children

Improving the delivery of PHC for Aboriginal and Torres Strait Islander children is crucial for better health and wellbeing across the life span and for improving health equity for Aboriginal and Torres Strait Islander Australians.

Our research into the quality of care for Aboriginal and Torres Strait Islander children since 2007 highlights where significant improvements continue to be needed. Many aspects of child health care are being done well in many health centres, but common gaps and persistent wide variation in care delivery amongst health centres indicate broader system failures. Systems for delivering child health services need to be improved at local and at higher levels of the health system, including systems for coordinating service delivery across sectors (for example, child care, education, housing) and for ensuring the use of culturally appropriate resources.[58] The onset of chronic conditions at earlier ages and the prevalence of diseases that are almost eradicated in most wealthy countries, but persist for Aboriginal and Torres Strait Islander children (for example, acute rheumatic fever) are evidence of the urgency of these improvements for enabling Aboriginal and Torres Strait Islander children to thrive and fulfil their potential.

Our studies found that children younger than two years were more likely to have a recorded assessment for social and emotional wellbeing, anaemia and development than children aged from two to five years, despite older children having a greater risk of developmental problems.[59] While good care processes and organisational systems are important for improving delivery, it is imperative that parents and carers feel comfortable bringing children to PHC services. Cultural safety is essential so that PHC services can integrate high-quality clinical care with the promotion of protective factors that build children's resilience and underpin wellbeing, such as connection to Country, family, community, culture and ancestry. This has implications for the proportion of Indigenous staff employed in PHC services, staff training and mentorship (particularly in cultural safety), links with other service providers and processes for engaging communities in the design, delivery and continuous improvement of PHC services for Aboriginal and Torres Strait Islander children.

Aboriginal and Torres Strait Islander PHC services are in a strong position to lead systems-level integration of services to tackle the determinants of children's health and wellbeing by engaging community leaders and members in improving care; linking physical health and social and emotional wellbeing programs within PHC; linking with intersectoral service partners; and advocating at policy levels.[60]

> Aboriginal and Torres Strait Islander PHC services are in a strong position to lead systems-level integration of services to tackle the determinants of children's health and wellbeing.

---

58   R. Bailie, Matthews et al. 2014; D'Aprano, Silburn et al. 2016; Strobel, McAuley et al. 2018.
59   Edmond, Tung et al. 2018; Strobel, McAuley et al. 2018.
60   McCalman, R. Bailie et al. 2018.

Reporting on other indicators of quality primary health care for children

In this chapter, we have reported selected findings on the quality of child health care. The indicators were selected because they are important items of best-practice PHC for children and have been identified as priorities for improvement through our CQI research. In identifying these priorities, we drew on empirical data and the knowledge of PHC practitioners. Findings relating to other indicators are available. Table 12.2 lists all the child health indicators included in the ABCD child health audit tool, and the research papers that report results on each indicator.

Table 12.2 Child health indicators in the child health audit tool, and publications that report results for each.

Child health quality-of-care indicator	Research (full citations provided in reference list)
Record systems	
Immunisation record in child's health file Child recorded in electronic recall system	R. Bailie, Matthews et al. 2014; McAullay, McAuley et al. 2018
Record of child health check	D'Aprano, Silburn et al. 2016; McAullay, McAuley et al. 2018
Scheduled immunisations	R. Bailie, Matthews et al. 2014; R.S. Bailie, Si et al. 2009
Measurements	
Weight	R. Bailie, Matthews et al. 2014; R. Bailie, Si et al. 2008; McAullay, McAuley et al. 2018
Length or height	R. Bailie, Si et al. 2008
Head circumference	R. Bailie, Si et al. 2008
Body mass index*	
Growth chart	R. Bailie, Si et al. 2008
Haemoglobin	R. Bailie, Matthews et al. 2014; R. Bailie, Si et al. 2008; McAullay, McAuley et al. 2018; Strobel, McAuley et al. 2018
Urinalysis for proteinuria*	
Appearance	
Hip examination	R. Bailie, Si et al. 2008

Child health quality-of-care indicator	Research (full citations provided in reference list)
Gait*	
Skin check	McAullay, McAuley et al. 2018
Oral hygiene	McAullay, McAuley et al. 2018
Testes check (Male children only)	R. Bailie, Si et al. 2008
Examinations	
Cardiac auscultation	R. Bailie, Si et al. 2008
Respiratory examination*	
Ear examination	R. Bailie, Si et al. 2008; McAullay, McAuley et al. 2018
Eye examination and vision test	R. Bailie, Si et al. 2008; Burnett, Morse et al. 2016; Edmond, Tung et al. 2018
Trachoma	Burnett, Morse et al. 2016
Child development	
Developmental milestones	R. Bailie, Matthews et al. 2014; R. Bailie, Si et al. 2008; D'Aprano, Silburn et al. 2016; Edmond, Tung et al. 2018; McAullay, McAuley et al. 2018; Strobel, McAuley et al. 2018
Concerns about vision	R. Bailie, Si et al. 2008; Burnett, Morse et al. 2016; Edmond, Tung et al. 2018
Hearing	R. Bailie, Si et al. 2008; Edmond, Tung et al. 2018; McAullay, McAuley et al. 2018; Strobel, McAuley et al. 2018
Parent–child interaction	D'Aprano, Silburn et al. 2016; Edmond, McAuley et al. 2018; Edmond, Tung et al. 2018; McAullay, McAuley et al. 2018; Strobel, McAuley et al. 2018
Inquiry or brief intervention	
Breastfeeding	R. Bailie, Si et al. 2008; Gibson-Helm, J. Bailie et al. 2016; Gibson-Helm, J. Bailie et al. 2018; McAullay, McAuley et al. 2018
Nutrition	R. Bailie, Matthews et al. 2014; R. Bailie, Si et al. 2008; McAullay, McAuley et al. 2018; Strobel, McAuley et al. 2018;
SIDS (sudden infant death syndrome) or SUDI (sudden unexpected death in infancy) prevention	R. Bailie, Si et al. 2008; Gibson-Helm, J. Bailie et al. 2016, 2018

Child health quality-of-care indicator	Research (full citations provided in reference list)
Passive smoking risk	R. Bailie, Matthews et al. 2014; R. Bailie, Si et al. 2008; Gibson-Helm, J. Bailie et al. 2016, 2018
Infection prevention and hygiene	R. Bailie, Matthews et al. 2014; R. Bailie, Si et al. 2008
Oral health	R. Bailie, Si et al. 2008; McAullay, McAuley et al. 2018
Injury prevention	R. Bailie, Si et al. 2008
Domestic or social environment	R. Bailie, Matthews et al. 2014; R. Bailie, Si et al. 2008; Edmond, McAuley et al. 2018; Strobel, McAuley et al. 2018
Social or family support	R. Bailie, Si et al. 2008; Edmond, McAuley et al. 2018; Strobel, McAuley et al. 2018
Financial situation	R. Bailie, Si et al. 2008; Edmond, McAuley et al. 2018
Housing condition	R. Bailie, Si et al. 2008; Edmond, McAuley et al. 2018; Strobel, McAuley et al. 2018
Food security	R. Bailie, Si et al. 2008; Edmond, McAuley et al. 2018
Physical and mental stimulation	R. Bailie, Si et al. 2008; Edmond, McAuley et al. 2018; Edmond, Tung et al. 2018; Strobel, McAuley et al. 2018
Physical activity and rest	Edmond, Tung et al. 2018
Education progress*	
Social and emotional wellbeing	Edmond, McAuley et al. 2018; Strobel, McAuley et al. 2018
Sexual and reproductive health and safe sex advice*	
Risk factors: Smoking, alcohol use, drug or substance use	R. Bailie, Matthews et al. 2014
Follow-up of abnormal clinical findings	
Growth faltering or failure to thrive	R. Bailie, Matthews et al. 2014; R. Bailie, Si et al. 2008; McAullay, McAuley et al. 2018
Evidence of overweight or obesity*	
Recurrent or chronic ear infections	R. Bailie, Si et al. 2008; McAullay, McAuley et al. 2018

Child health quality-of-care indicator	Research (full citations provided in reference list)
Evidence of anaemia	R. Bailie, Si et al. 2008; McAullay, McAuley et al. 2018
Recurrent or chronic respiratory disease, number of respiratory infections	R. Bailie, Si et al. 2008
Infected skin sores	McAullay, McAuley et al. 2018
Scabies*	
Proteinuria*	
Developmental delay	R. Bailie, Matthews et al. 2014; R. Bailie, Si et al. 2008; D'Aprano, Silburn et al. 2016; Edmond, Tung et al. 2018
Concern and follow-up:	
Domestic environment	R. Bailie, Si et al. 2008; Edmond, McAuley et al. 2018
Social or family support and financial situation	R. Bailie, Si et al. 2008; Edmond, McAuley et al. 2018
Housing condition and food security	R. Bailie, Si et al. 2008; Edmond, McAuley et al. 2018

* Results for these indicators have not been reported in publications to date.

References

Aquino, D., D. Leonard, N. Hadgraft and J. Marley (2018). High prevalence of early onset anaemia amongst Aboriginal and Torres Strait Islander infants in remote northern Australia. *Australian Journal of Rural Health* 26(4): 245–50. DOI: 10.1111/ajr.12403.

Australian Bureau of Statistics (2019). *National Aboriginal and Torres Strait Islander health survey, 2018–19*. ABS cat. no. 4715.0. Canberra: ABS.

Australian Bureau of Statistics (2017). *National Aboriginal and Torres Strait Islander social survey, 2014–15*. ABS cat. no. 4714.0. Canberra: ABS.

Australian Institute of Family Studies (2018). The growing over-representation of Aboriginal and Torres Strait Islander children in care. *AIFS*. https://aifs.gov.au/cfca/2018/05/07/growing-over-representation-aboriginal-and-torres-strait-islander-children-care.

Australian Institute of Health and Welfare (2023). *Aboriginal and Torres Strait Islander Health Performance Framework summary report 2023*. Canberra: AIHW.

Australian Institute of Health and Welfare (2021). Child protection Australia 2019–20. Canberra: Australian Government. https://www.aihw.gov.au/reports/child-protection/child-protection-australia-2019-20/summary.

Bailie R., V. Matthews, J. Bailie and A. Laycock (2014). *Primary health care for Aboriginal and Torres Strait Islander children: priority evidence–practice gaps and stakeholder views on barriers and strategies for improvement. Final report.* Brisbane: Menzies School of Health Research.

Bailie R., D. Si, M. Dowden, C. Connors, L. O'Donoghue, H. Liddle et al. (2008). Delivery of child health services in Indigenous communities: implications for the federal government's emergency intervention in the Northern Territory. *Medical Journal of Australia* 188(10): 615–18. DOI: 10.5694/j.1326-5377.2008.tb01806.x

Bailie R., D. Si, M. Dowden, C. Selvey, C. Kennedy, R. Cox et al. (2009). A systems approach to improving timeliness of immunisation. *Vaccine* 27: 3669–74. DOI: 10.1016/j.vaccine.2009.02.068.

Barker, D., J. Eriksson, T. Forsén and C. Osmond (2002). Fetal origins of adult disease: strength of effects and biological basis. *International Journal of Epidemiology* 31(6): 1235–39. DOI: 10.1093/ije/31.6.1235.

Blair, M., and D. Hall (2006). From health surveillance to health promotion: the changing focus in preventive children's services. *Archives of Disease in Childhood* 91(9): 730–5. DOI: 10.1136/adc.2004.065003.

Burnett, A., A. Morse, T. Naduvilath, A. Boudville, H. Taylor and R. Bailie (2016). Delivery of eye and vision services in Aboriginal and Torres Strait Islander primary health care centers. *Frontiers in Public Health* 4: 276. DOI: 10.3389/fpubh.2016.00276.

Chando, S., J. Craig, L. Burgess, S. Sherriff, A. Purcell, H. Gunasekera et al. (2020). Developmental risk among Aboriginal children living in urban areas in Australia: the study of environment on Aboriginal resilience and child health (SEARCH). *BMC Pediatrics* 20(1): 13. DOI: 10.1186/s12887-019-1902-z.

Closing the Gap (n.d.). https://www.closingthegap.gov.au/.

D'Aprano, A., S. Silburn, V. Johnston, R. Bailie, F. Mensah, F. Oberklaid et al. (2016). Challenges in monitoring the development of young children in remote Aboriginal health services: clinical audit findings and recommendations for improving practice. *Rural and Remote Health* 16(3852): 1–10. DOI: 10.22605/RRH3852.

Department of Health (2019). *National immunisation strategy for Australia 2019 to 2024*. Canberra: Australian Government.

Department of Health and Aged Care (2022). *Annual health checks for Aboriginal and Torres Strait Islander people*. https://www.health.gov.au/health-topics/aboriginal-and-torres-strait-islander-health/primary-care/annual-health-checks.

Edmond, K., K. McAuley, D. McAullay, V. Matthews, N. Strobel, R. Marriott et al. (2018). Quality of social and emotional wellbeing services for families of young Indigenous children attending primary care centers: a cross sectional analysis. *BMC Health Services Research* 18(1). DOI: 10.1186/s12913-018-2883-6.

Edmond, K., S. Tung, K. McAuley, N. Strobel and D. McAullay (2018). Improving developmental care in primary practice for disadvantaged children. *Archives of Disease in Childhood* 104: 372–80. DOI: 10.1136/archdischild-2018-315164.

Engle, P., L. Fernald, H. Alderman, J. Behrman, C. O'Gara, A. Yousafzai et al. (2011). Strategies for reducing inequalities and improving developmental outcomes for young children in low-income and middle-income countries. *Lancet* 378(9799): 1339–53. DOI: 10.1016/S0140-6736(11)60889-1.

Fremantle, E., Y. Zurynski, D. Mahajan, H. D'Antoine and E. Elliott (2008). Indigenous child health: urgent need for improved data to underpin better health outcomes. *Medical Journal of Australia* 188(10): 588–91. DOI: 10.5694/j.1326-5377.2008.tb01797.x.

Gibson-Helm, M., J. Bailie, V. Matthews, A. Laycock, J. Boyle and R. Bailie (2018). Identifying evidence–practice gaps and strategies for improvement in Aboriginal and Torres Strait Islander maternal health care. *PLOS One* 13(2): e0192262. DOI: 10.1371/journal.pone.0192262.

Gibson-Helm, M., J. Bailie, V. Matthews, A. Laycock, J. Boyle and R. Bailie (2016). *Priority evidence-practice gaps in Aboriginal and Torres Strait Islander maternal health care final report: engaging stakeholders in identifying priority evidence–practice gaps and strategies for improvement in primary health care (ESP project)*. Brisbane: Menzies School of Health Research.

Grantham-McGregor, S. and C. Ani (2001). A review of studies on the effect of iron deficiency on cognitive development in children. *Journal of Nutrition* 131(2S-2): 649S–68S. DOI: 10.1093/jn/131.2.649S.

Grantham-McGregor, S., Y. Cheung, S. Cueto, P. Glewwe, L. Richter and B. Strupp (2007). Developmental potential in the first 5 years for children in developing countries. *Lancet (British edition)* 369(9555): 60–70. DOI: 10.1016/S0140-6736(07)60032-4.

Hertzman, C. and C. Power (2004). Child development as a determinant of health across the life course. *Current Paediatrics* 14(5): 438–43. DOI: 10.1016/j.cupe.2004.05.008.

Kearns, T., F. Ward, S. Puszka, R. Gundjirryirr, B. Moss and R. Bailie (2017). Anaemia health literacy of community members and health practitioners knowledge of best practice guidelines in a remote Australian Aboriginal community. *Universal Journal of Public Health* 5(1): 32–9. DOI: 10.13189/ujph.2017.050105.

McAullay, D., K. McAuley, R. Bailie, V. Mathews, P. Jacoby, K. Gardner et al. (2018). Sustained participation in annual continuous quality improvement activities improves quality of care for Aboriginal and Torres Strait Islander children. *Journal of Paediatrics and Child Health* 54(2): 132–40. DOI: 10.1111/jpc.13673.

McCalman, J., R. Bailie, R. Bainbridge, K. McPhail-Bell, N. Percival, D. Askew et al. (2018). Continuous quality improvement and comprehensive primary health care: a systems framework to improve service quality and health outcomes. *Frontiers in Public Health* 6: 76. DOI: 10.3389/fpubh.2018.00076.

McDonald, E., R. Bailie, A. Rumbold, P. Morris and B. Paterson (2008). Preventing growth faltering among Australian Indigenous children: implications for policy and practice. *Medical Journal of Australia* 188(8 Suppl): S84–6. DOI: 10.5694/j.1326-5377.2008.tb01753.x.

Menzies School of Health Research and One21seventy (2015). *Child health clinical audit tool*. Brisbane: Menzies School of Health Research.

Mitchinson, C., N. Strobel, D. McAullay, K. McAuley, R. Bailie and K. Edmond (2019). Anemia in disadvantaged children aged under five years; quality of care in primary practice. *BMC Pediatrics* 19(1): 178. DOI: 10.1186/s12887-019-1543-2.

National Aboriginal Community Controlled Health Organisation and Royal Australian College of General Practitioners (2024). *National guide to a preventative health assessment for Aboriginal and Torres Strait Islander people*, 4th edn. Melbourne: RACGP.

Newham, J. and F. Cunningham (2015). *Continuous quality improvement success stories: identifying effective strategies for CQI in Aboriginal and Torres Strait Islander primary health care – study report*. ABCD National Research Partnership. Brisbane: ABCD National Research Partnership, Menzies School of Health Research.

Priest, N., T. Mackean, E. Waters, E. Davis and E. Riggs (2009). Indigenous child health research: a critical analysis of Australian studies. *Australian and New Zealand Journal of Public Health* 33(1): 55–63. DOI: 10.1111/j.1753-6405.2009.00339.x.

Productivity Commission (2023). *Closing the Gap: annual data compilation report July 2023*. Canberra: Australian Government.

Productivity Commission (2020). Overcoming Indigenous disadvantage: key indicators 2020. Canberra: Australian Government. https://www.pc.gov.au/research/ongoing/overcoming-indigenous-disadvantage/2020.

Robinson, G., S. Mares and F. Arney (2017). Continuity, engagement and integration: early intervention in remote Australian Aboriginal communities. *Australian Social Work* 70(1): 116–24. DOI: 10.1080/0312407X.2016.1146315.

Sabanathan, S., B. Wills and M. Gladstone (2015). Child development assessment tools in low-income and middle-income countries: how can we use them more appropriately? *Archives of Disease in Childhood* 100(5): 482–8. DOI: 10.1136/archdischild-2014-308114.

Siddiqi, K. and J. Newell (2005). Putting evidence into practice in low-resource settings. *Bulletin of the World Health Organization* 83(12): 882.

Simpson, S., A. D'Aprano, C. Tayler, S. Toon Khoo and R. Highfold (2016). Validation of a culturally adapted developmental screening tool for Australian Aboriginal children: early findings and next steps. *Early Human Development* 103: 91–5. DOI: 10.1016/j.earlhumdev.2016.08.005.

Strobel, N., K. McAuley, V. Matthews, A. Richardson, J. Agostino, R. Bailie et al. (2018). Understanding the structure and processes of primary health care for young indigenous children. *Journal of Primary Health Care* 10(3): 267–78. DOI: 10.1071/HC18006.

Strong Kids, Strong Future (n.d.). ASQ-TRAK. https://www.strongkidsstrongfuture.com.au/asqtrak/.

Walker, S., T. Wachs, S. Grantham-McGregor, M. Black, C. Nelson, S. Huffman et al. (2011). Inequality in early childhood: risk and protective factors for early child development. *Lancet* 378(9799): 1325–38. DOI: 10.1016/S0140-6736(11)60555-2.

Williamson, A., C. D'Este, K. Clapham, S. Redman, T. Manton, S. Eades et al. (2016). What are the factors associated with good mental health among Aboriginal children in urban New South Wales, Australia? Phase I findings from the study of environment on Aboriginal resilience and child health (SEARCH). *BMJ Open* 6(7): e011182–e82. DOI: 10.1136/bmjopen-2016-011182.

World Health Organization (2020). *Children: improving survival and well being.* Fact sheets. https://www.who.int/en/news-room/fact-sheets/detail/children-reducing-mortality.

World Health Organization (2011). *Haemoglobin concentrations for the diagnosis of anaemia and assessment of severity.* Vitamin and Mineral Nutrition Information System, WHO/NMH/NHD/MNM/11.1. Geneva: World Health Organization.

Zuchowski, I., D. Miles, C. Woods and K. Tsey (2017). Continuous quality improvement processes in child protection: a systematic literature review. *Research on Social Work Practice* 19(4): 1–12. DOI: 10.1177/1049731517743337.

Improving maternal health care

Maternal care in PHC

Primary healthcare (PHC) services have a vital role in providing integrated pre-conception, pregnancy and postnatal care, and in many places, care during childbirth. High-quality maternal care lays foundations for babies to have the best possible start in life and includes these key elements:

- identifying risks to health
- preventing and managing pregnancy-related complications, illnesses, or concurrent diseases
- supporting the transition to birthing and motherhood
- health education and health promotion.

There have been significant gains in maternal outcomes in recent decades. Between 2000 and 2017, the number of maternal deaths per 100,000 live births dropped by about 38 per cent worldwide. The infant mortality rate more than halved from an estimated 65 deaths per 1,000 live births in 1990, to 29 deaths per 1,000 live births in 2017. However, inequalities persist. Low-income countries reported 462 maternal deaths per 100,000 live births compared with 11 per 100,000 live births in high-income countries, and risk of infant mortality was highest in the World Health Organization African Region.[1] These statistics reflect poor access to good-quality health services (for example, lack of skilled health workers or local birthing facilities) and other underlying determinants of health and health care. Poverty, lack of information, and poor integration of cultural practices into health services may also prevent women from seeking or receiving care from health professionals during pregnancy and childbirth.[2] Parental capacity to provide nurturing care is linked to social determinants of health and to experiences of health inequity and poverty.[3]

Global improvement in maternal outcomes has shifted the focus from survival to maximising maternal health and wellbeing through best-practice women-centred care. Good antenatal care aims for a positive pregnancy experience and supports women to make informed choices about their care and childbirth. It includes effective communication, emotional support, respect and

1   World Health Organization 2020.
2   World Health Organization 2019.
3   Marmot, M., P. Goldblatt, J. Allen, et al. 2010.

dignity, medical care, and relevant and timely information.[4] Access to appropriate care and counselling for diseases (for example, tuberculosis, HIV, malaria), and chronic conditions such as diabetes, kidney disease and heart disease are important components of antenatal care.

> Good antenatal care aims for a positive pregnancy experience and supports women to make informed choices about their care and childbirth.

Postnatal care (usually provided for 6–8 weeks after birth) should be a continuation of the care provided through pregnancy, labour and childbirth. It focuses on clinical care needs (for example, preventing and treating postpartum complications), rest and nutrition, baby feeding, parent–baby attachment, social and emotional support, contraception and, often, cervical screening. The complexity of providing holistic woman-centred care is one of the reasons that CQI has such positive potential in maternal health care.

Health of Aboriginal and Torres Strait Islander mothers and their babies

Aboriginal and Torres Strait Islander mothers account for around 5 per cent of women who give birth in Australia. In recent years, improvements in outcomes have included an increase in the percentage of Aboriginal and Torres Strait Islander mothers who seek early and regular antenatal care. In 2021, 72 per cent of Aboriginal and Torres Strait Islander mothers attended an antenatal visit in the first trimester compared with 50 per cent in 2012, and 88 per cent of those who sought antenatal care attended five or more pregnancy care visits. Over a similar period, the proportion of women who smoked during pregnancy and the proportion of babies with a low birth weight born to Aboriginal and Torres Strait Islander mothers decreased.[5] These improvements have been achieved despite system barriers such as variability in culturally safe care, some expectations that women in rural areas transfer to bigger cities for birthing, and staff shortages (particularly in rural and remote areas). The proportion of babies with a healthy birth weight still needs to increase to reach the Closing the Gap target of 91 per cent by 2031,[6] and the significant reduction in sudden unexpected death in infancy in Australia since the early 1990s has not been experienced among Aboriginal and Torres Strait Islander communities.[7]

Many Aboriginal and Torres Strait Islander women experience medical, behavioural, environmental, economic, and social and emotional wellbeing risk.[8] For example the incidence of diabetes, including gestational diabetes, is higher among Aboriginal and Torres Strait Islander peoples, and people living in lower socio-economic areas and remote areas.[9] Gestational diabetes is a strong predictor of future type 2 diabetes[10] and children exposed to hyperglycaemia

---

4   White Ribbon Alliance 2011; World Health Organization 2016.
5   Australian Institute of Health and Welfare 2023.
6   Australian Institute of Health and Welfare 2021.
7   Freemantle and Ellis 2018; Heazell 2020.
8   Marmot, M., P. Goldblatt, J. Allen, et al. 2010.
9   Australian Institute of Health and Welfare 2024.
10   Chamberlain, Oldenburg et al. 2016.

(high blood glucose) in utero are at risk of developing diabetes at an early age.[11] Low birth weight also increases the risk of children developing chronic illnesses in later life.[12] Risk factors for chronic illnesses are relatively common among young Indigenous women,[13] and many of the risk factors (for example, infections, smoking, high-risk alcohol use, being obese or underweight) are associated with poor pregnancy outcomes.[14] High levels of psychological distress and stressors during pregnancy may also be associated with low birth weight and preterm birth.[15]

The relatively high levels of risk are a legacy of government policies that ruptured family and cultural connections and removed many Aboriginal and Torres Strait Islander children from their families. The positive counter effects of extended kinship and community care for parents, spiritual connection to Country and active cultural practices are vitally important for protecting the health and wellbeing of many Aboriginal and Torres Strait Islander mothers and their families. These protective factors need to be supported through culturally safe PHC that builds on community and cultural strengths.

High-quality preventive and pre-conception care, and best-practice care during and after pregnancy and birthing, is crucial for closing the gap in maternal health outcomes between Aboriginal and Torres Strait Islander and non-Indigenous women in Australia.

Recommended maternal care

High-quality maternal care includes emotional support and advice, clinical care, and relevant and timely information.

The World Health Organization recommends that all pregnant women have a minimum of eight contacts with a health provider. Antenatal care should include nutrition interventions (for example, advice about healthy eating and exercise, iron supplements); maternal and foetal assessment (for early detection of pregnancy complications, and identification of women at risk of complications during birthing); interventions for smoking, alcohol and other drug use; disease testing and care (for example, for gestational diabetes); preventive health measures (for example, tetanus vaccination); and interventions for common physiological symptoms (for example, nausea). Women-held case notes, midwife-led continuity of care, and sharing of care across a range of providers are also recommended.[16] National guidelines outline context- and population-specific interventions, and routine and targeted maternal health tests during different stages of pregnancy.

Recommended postnatal care includes at least four postnatal assessments in the 6 weeks following delivery (and delivery-related care for the mother and newborn). These visits should include clinical assessment and care, breastfeeding support, emotional wellbeing and other risk assessment (for example, food security, safety, housing, smoking, alcohol and other drug use), contraception advice and psychosocial support.[17]

---

11   Dabelea 2007; MacKay, Kirkham et al. 2020.
12   McMillen and Robinson 2005; Saigal and Doyle 2008.
13   Crinall, Boyle et al. 2017.
14   Abell, Nankervis et al. 2016; Lee, Hiscock et al. 2007.
15   Cunningham and Paradies 2012; Ding, Wu et al. 2014.
16   World Health Organization 2016.
17   World Health Organization 2015.

Findings: quality of maternal health care

The data presented below on the quality of maternal care come mainly from nine research papers and key reports published by the Audit and Best Practice for Chronic Disease Continuous Quality Improvement Research research program between 2010 and 2018. Studies analysed more than 4,402 records of Aboriginal and Torres Strait Islander mothers with infants aged between 2 and 14 months, and 242 systems assessments completed by PHC teams. Audit data were collected from 91 health centres serving Aboriginal and Torres Strait Islander populations between 2007 and 2014; these are the most recent audit data available for analysis. Stakeholders participated in data interpretation to identify priority evidence–practice gaps and factors influencing improvement.

Comprehensive maternal primary health care

The maternal health clinical audit tool and protocol[18] were used to collect data about the delivery of pregnancy and postnatal services. The data were analysed to assess how well the services reflected best-practice guidelines for maternal care. In general, pregnancy care was delivered at higher levels than postnatal care and there was also less variation between health centres in the delivery of antenatal care compared with postnatal care, indicating a need for increased emphasis on improving postnatal care as part of our efforts to improve maternal PHC in general.

Overall pregnancy care

The results for delivery of antenatal care brought together audit data for the recording of pregnancy risk factors, routine antenatal checks, laboratory investigations and brief interventions and counselling. (The audit tool contained these 26 best-practice indicators: seven or more antenatal visits; estimated gestational age is 13 weeks or less at the first antenatal visit; blood pressure recorded (in the first, second and third trimesters); urinalysis undertaken (in the first and second trimesters); body mass index recorded (in the first trimester); fundal height recorded (second and third trimesters); foetal movements recorded (third trimester); blood glucose level recorded (second trimester); blood group recorded; antibody, rubella and hepatitis B status recorded; mid-stream urine test; full blood examination; syphilis serology; PCR test for HIV; smoking and drinking (alcohol) status recorded (first and third trimesters); social risk and emotional wellbeing assessments conducted; plans for care and birthing discussed; nutrition discussed; domestic, social environment and cultural considerations discussed.)

These were the observations for PHC centres that completed maternal health audit cycles between 2007 and 2014:

- the average level of overall delivery of pregnancy care ranged between 60 and 80 per cent. This means that, on average, 60–80 per cent of mothers received all 26 best-practice indicators (items of antenatal care) during their pregnancy
- the average level of overall service delivery improved
- variation in the quality of antenatal care between health centres persisted (Figure 13.1).[19]

18   Menzies School of Health Research and One21seventy 2014.
19   Gibson-Helm, J. Bailie et al. 2016.

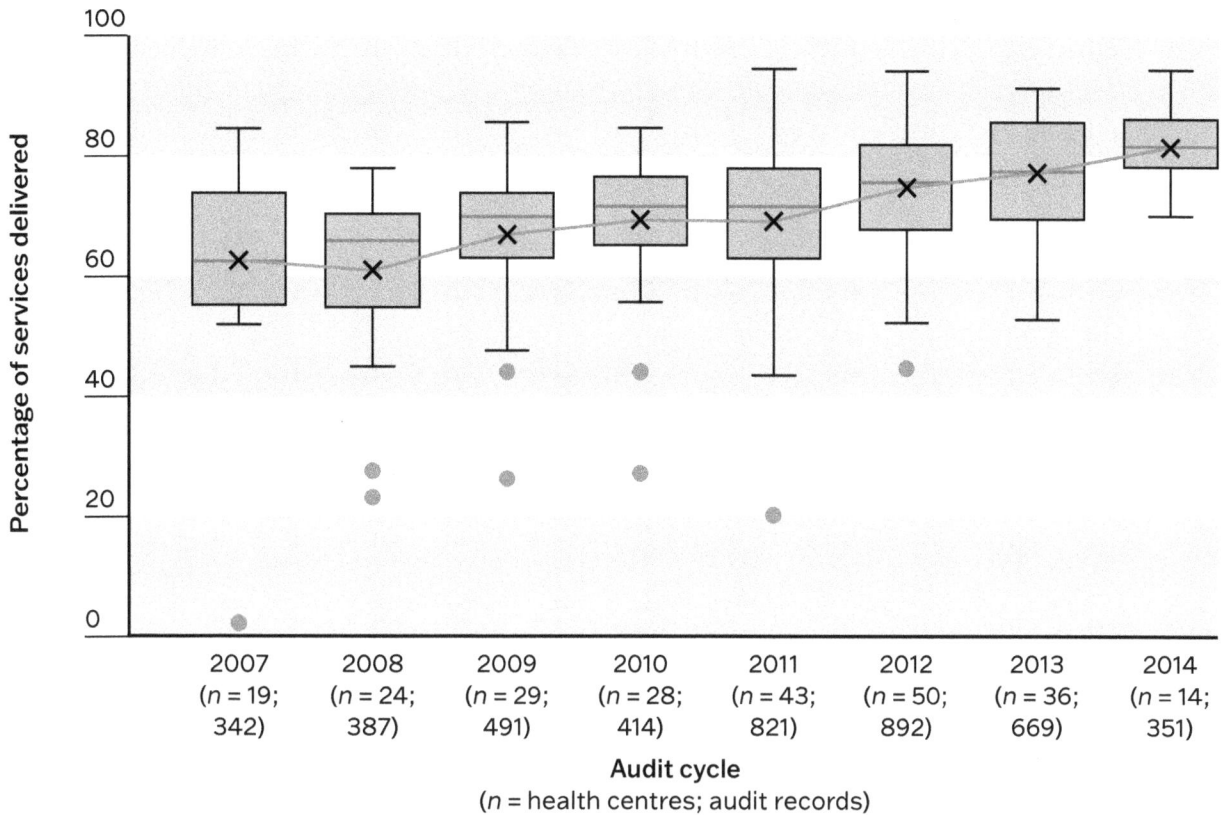

Figure 13.1 Trends in overall pregnancy care. Source: Gibson-Helm, J. Bailie et al. 2016.

Postnatal brief interventions and counselling

The results for delivery of postnatal care focused on the recording of brief interventions and counselling for a range of health risk factors: smoking; nutrition; breastfeeding; infection prevention; injury prevention; sudden infant death syndrome (SIDS) prevention; alcohol and other substance abuse; physical activity; mood (depression); contraception; domestic and social environment; social and family support; financial support; housing condition; and food security.

These were the observations for PHC centres that completed maternal health audit cycles between 2007 and 2014:

- the average level of overall delivery of postnatal care for brief interventions and counselling ranged between 20 and 45 per cent (this means that, on average, 20–45 per cent of mothers received all 15 best-practice indicators for brief interventions and counselling in postnatal care)
- the average level of overall delivery of brief interventions and counselling improved
- wide variation between health centres in the delivery of brief interventions and counselling did not reduce across audit cycles (Figure 13.2).[20]

---

20   Gibson-Helm, J. Bailie et al. 2016.

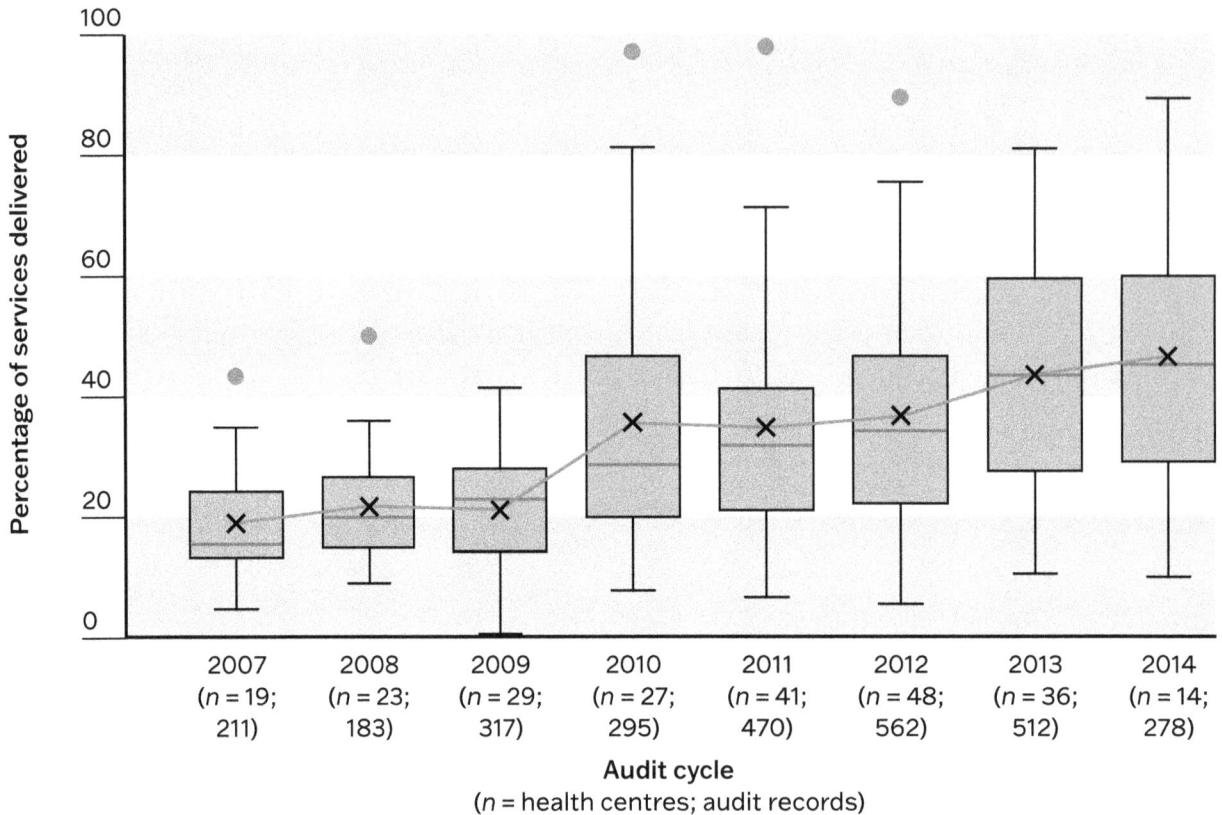

Figure 13.2 Trends in overall postnatal care. Source: Gibson-Helm, J. Bailie et al 2016.

The average level of overall service delivery improved over audit cycles for antenatal and postnatal care.

Routine pregnancy care

Audit data from 65 PHC centres (1,091 patient records, from 2012 to 2014) were analysed in four areas: antenatal visits and care plans; risk factors and brief interventions; laboratory investigations; and routine antenatal checks and abnormal findings.

The findings for antenatal visits and care plans indicated a need to improve care leading up to and during the first months of pregnancy, and to improve communication between hospitals and PHC centres:

- most records (average of 90 per cent, range of 77–100 per cent) contained a pregnancy care plan and a delivery summary from the hospital where the mother gave birth; delivery summaries were less likely to be complete than pregnancy care plans (average of 80 per cent, range of 35–100 per cent)
- there was wide variation in quality of care between health centres for first trimester visits (average of 60 per cent, range of 15–85 per cent), with less variation in quality of care for second and third trimester visits

- recording of folate prescription before pregnancy was low at all health centres (average of 6 per cent, range of 0–25 per cent), suggesting a need to raise community and staff awareness of pre-conception health and pre-conception care.[21]

For risk factors and brief interventions, the data showed considerable scope for improvement in follow-up for social risk factors and social and physical wellbeing. The findings suggest a need to train and support the workforce to have sensitive conversations with women about social and emotional wellbeing, and to increase options for referral to appropriate local services:

- smoking status, alcohol use, and social and medical risk factors were generally recorded
- follow-up, brief interventions or counselling for physical and social wellbeing were often not provided
- brief interventions for smoking were documented for most women who reported smoking tobacco (almost 85 per cent on average), with lower rates of brief interventions for alcohol use or illicit drug use
- despite very high levels of social and medical risk factor assessments, and follow-up for medical risk factors, follow-up for social risk factors varied greatly. Brief interventions or counselling about maternal wellbeing during pregnancy was not provided in many cases (for example, financial situation, food security, housing environment, cultural considerations). [22]

The analysis of data for laboratory investigations had mixed outcomes, with some very good results and some highlighting of areas where improvements can be made:

- levels of laboratory investigations were very high (nearly all over 80 per cent average)
- across PHC centres fewer than 60 per cent of women were offered foetal anomaly screening. This may relate to local availability and accessibility of screening, staff time constraints, communication difficulties caused by language differences (for example, difficulty explaining the concept of risk of foetal abnormalities and testing).[23]
- the average level of delivery of glucose challenge tests and glucose tolerance tests was high (70–80 per cent), although there was wide variation between health centres (0–100 per cent)[24]
- follow-up actions for anaemia and abnormal glucose challenge and tolerance tests were generally well done
- follow-up for anti-D injections, during pregnancy and post-birth, and post-birth rubella immunisations was generally not well done.[25]

As with the other categories of data, the changes here revealed some areas where care provision was widely of a high quality, and other items where quality of care can be substantially improved.

- Most women who attended during the first trimester were weighed (average of 90 per cent; range of 60–100 per cent) (Figure 13.3).

---

21   Gibson-Helm, J. Bailie et al. 2016, data supplement.
22   Gibson-Helm, J. Bailie et al. 2016, Gibson-Helm, Teede et al. 2015.
23   Gibson-Helm, J. Bailie et al. 2016, data supplement; Rumbold, Wild et al. 2015.
24   Note that screening for diabetes has changed since these data were collected.
25   Gibson-Helm, J. Bailie et al. 2016, data supplement.

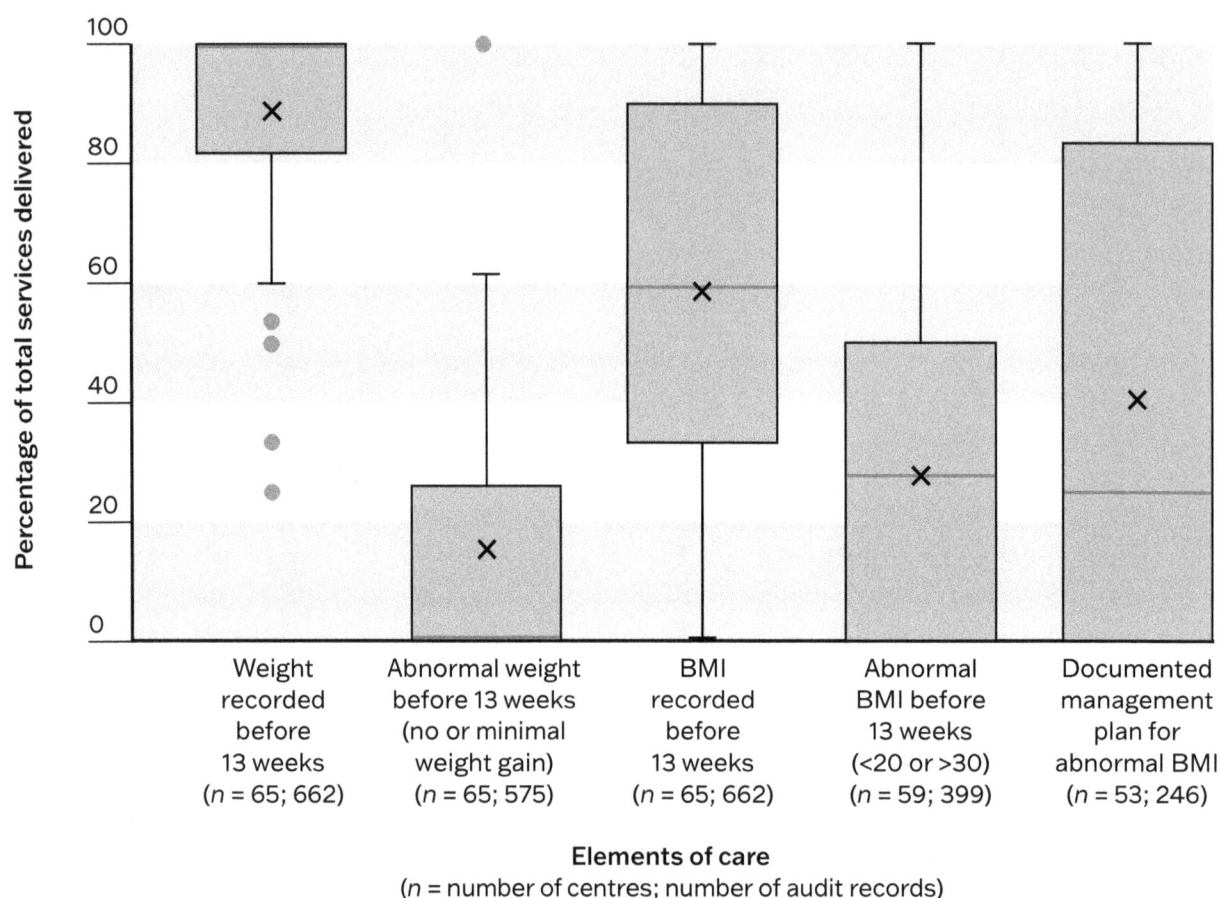

Figure 13.3 Record of scheduled maternal care services received by Indigenous women at Indigenous primary health care centres, 2012–2014. Source: J. Bailie, Boyle and R. Bailie 2018.

- The recording of body mass index (BMI) varied. On average, it was approximately 60 per cent with a range of 0–100 per cent (Figure 13.3). Many women with an abnormal BMI (average of 30 per cent; range 0–100 per cent), did not have a BMI management plan in their client record (average of 40 per cent; range of 0–100 per cent). The recording of both BMI and BMI management plans varied between PHC centres (Figure 13.3).[26]
- Most women had their blood pressure measured during antenatal visits at all stages of pregnancy, with a record of follow-up testing if blood pressure was abnormal.[27]
- Urine sample analysis was provided at relatively high levels at all stages, but there was wide variation in subsequent mid-stream urine tests following abnormal urinalysis results and this is important for the prevention of preterm labour.[28]
- Nearly all women received fundal height, foetal heart rate and foetal movement checks, but women with a record of abnormal foetal movement had little or no record of follow-up use of kick charts. Cardiotocograph monitoring or referral to a specialist service varied widely, possibly due to lack of access to equipment or specialist.[29]

---

26   J. Bailie, Boyle and R. Bailie 2018.
27   Gibson-Helm, J. Bailie et al. 2016.
28   Gibson-Helm, J.Bailie et al. 2016.
29   Gibson-Helm, J. Bailie et al. 2016.

Routine postnatal care

Analysis of audit data from 65 PHC centres (1,091 patient records, 2012–14) revealed a need to improve discussion and brief interventions for social and physical risk factors as part of routine postnatal care:

- the majority of women had a recorded postnatal visit
- breastfeeding and contraception were usually discussed and recorded in the client's file
- there was wide variation in discussing and providing brief intervention for nutrition, infection prevention, mood, domestic and social environment, and social and family support
- smoking, injury prevention for the infant, prevention of sudden unexpected death in infancy, the woman's financial situation, housing and food security were infrequently raised and discussed by PHC staff.[30]

Social and emotional wellbeing of pregnant women and mothers

The CQI research identified the need to improve social and emotional wellbeing care for pregnant women and mothers, as part of antenatal and postnatal care. This improvement priority was identified from the analysis of maternal health audit data from 65 PHC centres (1,091 audit records; 58 systems assessments; 2012–14) and input from people providing PHC services. The quality of social and emotional wellbeing care was then tracked from 2010 to 2014 to assess trends in care quality.

- Risk of social and emotional distress was associated with factors such as use of alcohol and other drugs.[31]
- Women attending urban and regional health centres were more likely to be at risk of distress than those attending remote health centres.[32]
- From 2010 to 2014, the delivery of screening for emotional wellbeing using standard screening tools (for example, PHQ and aPHQ-9) improved steadily.[33] Records showed an average of 15 per cent in 2010, when the audit item was introduced, which increased to 60 per cent in 2014 (Figure 13.4a).[34]
- There was wide and persistent variation between PHC centres in the delivery of screening for emotional wellbeing, ranging from 0 to 100 per cent (Figure 13.4a).[35]
- Follow-up for women identified as "at risk", based on assessment of emotional wellbeing during pregnancy, improved. In 2014, follow-up ranged from around 75 to 100 per cent (average of 90 per cent) across PHC centres (Figure 13.4b).[36]

30   Gibson-Helm, J. Bailie et al. 2016.
31   Gausia, Thompson et al. 2015.
32   Gausia, Thompson et al. 2015.
33   For culture-specific screening tools, see Chapters 11 and 15.
34   Gibson-Helm, J. Bailie et al. 2016, 2018.
35   Gibson-Helm, J. Bailie et al. 2016, 2018.
36   Gibson-Helm, J. Bailie et al. 2016, 2018.

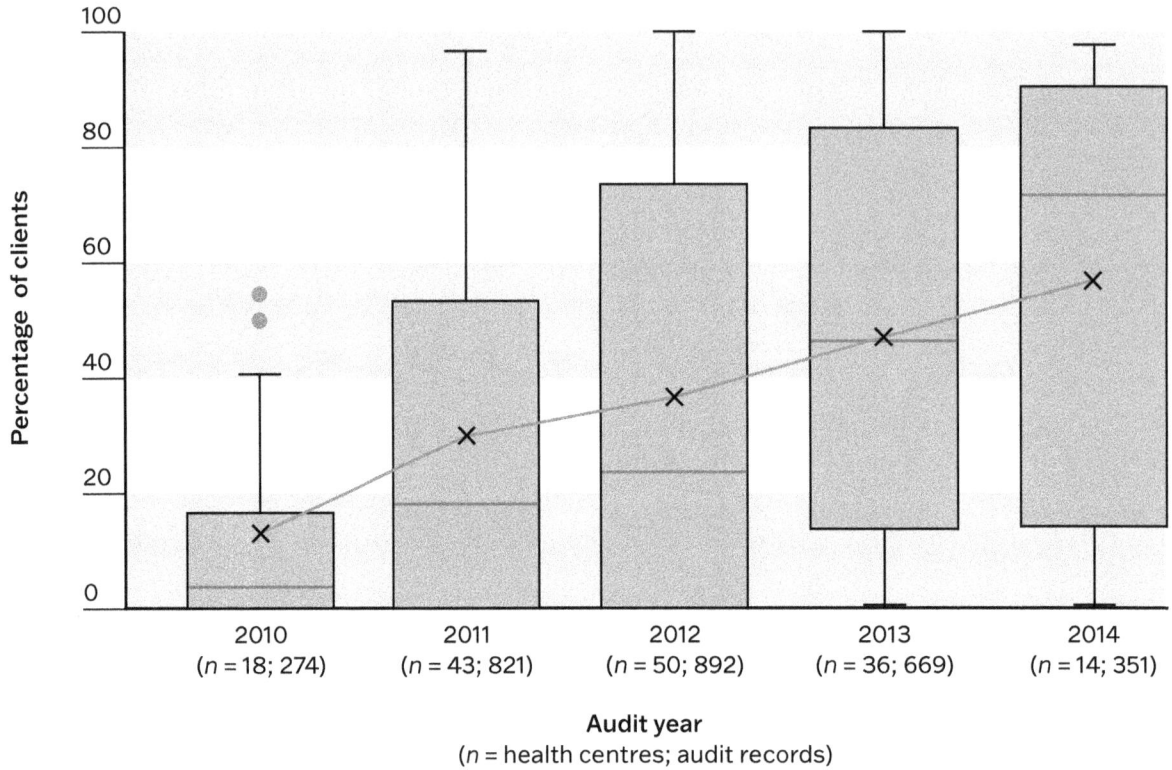

Figure 13.4a Screening for maternal social and emotional wellbeing.
Source: Gibson-Helm, J. Bailie et al. 2018.

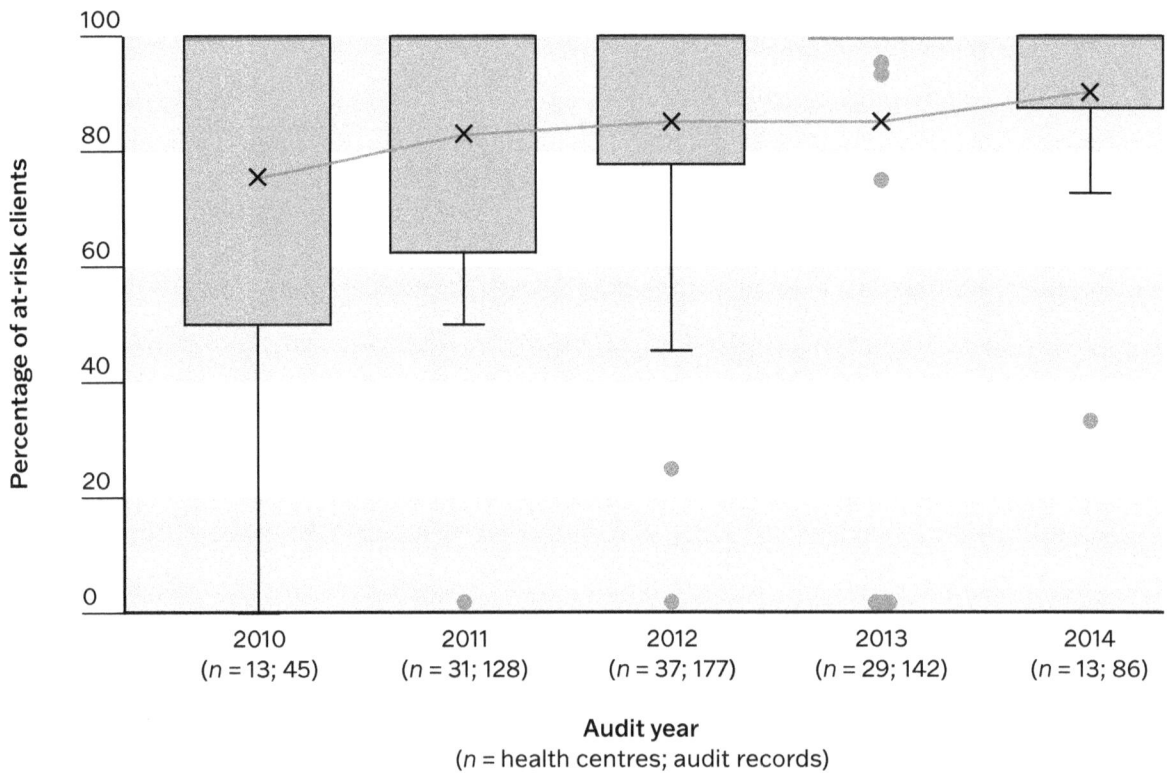

Figure 13.4b Follow-up action for clients identified at risk for social and emotional wellbeing. Source: Gibson-Helm, J. Bailie et al. 2018.

Did using CQI improve maternal care?

Our research found that women who attended a PHC centre that conducted audits for maternal care were more likely to receive recommended screening and brief interventions for lifestyle-related risk factors than women attending centres that did not use CQI.[37] Even one cycle of CQI improved screening for BMI, blood pressure and diabetes.[38]

PHC teams that completed three or more systems assessments for maternal health noted improvements over time in how systems worked to deliver maternal care.[39] (For information about the ABCD systems assessment tool, see Chapter 5.)

> Women who attended a PHC centre that conducted audits for maternal care were more likely to receive recommended screening and brief interventions for lifestyle-related risk factors than women attending centres that did not use CQI.

Key messages for improving maternal health care in PHC

Common evidence-to-practice gaps in maternal care affect the health of both women and babies. This CQI research identifies clear priorities and strategies for improving maternal health care and includes stakeholder interpretation of CQI data. Patterns of PHC delivery for Aboriginal and Torres Strait Islander maternal care are likely to reflect, at least to some extent, care delivery in international settings.

PHC teams should focus on improving aspects of pregnancy and postnatal care in which there are system-wide evidence-to-practice gaps in delivery. This means improving systems to support best-practice care before, during and after pregnancy:

- Before pregnancy, these activities should be undertaken:
  - raising community and staff awareness of pre-conception health and pre-conception care
  - offering health promotion and prevention activities (for example, to stop smoking, to support social and emotional wellbeing).
- In pregnancy, as part of routine maternal care, these items of care should be included:
  - asking women about smoking and drinking alcohol and providing brief counselling
  - assessing social risk factors and emotional wellbeing and taking the appropriate follow-up action.

37   J. Bailie, Boyle and R. Bailie 2018; Gibson-Helm, Rumbold et al. 2016; Gibson-Helm, J. Bailie et al. 2018.
38   Gibson-Helm, Teede et al. 2015.
39   Gibson-Helm, Teede et al. 2015.

- At the postnatal visit, these areas should be discussed:
  - how a smoking environment increases the risk of sudden unexpected death in infancy
  - how to protect babies from harm
  - how diet and nutrition are important for the mother and baby.

In addition, follow-up or referral to programs and services as needed should be provided at the postnatal visit.

Encourage women to share decision-making and have an active role in their health care (for example, to make choices about foetal anomaly screening), and develop community-based programs that increase health literacy and raise community expectations of receiving best-practice woman-centred maternal health care.

Health systems should ensure that all PHC providers are empowered and equipped with the necessary skills and resources to deliver continuity of maternal care, including the following:

- systems to coordinate team care (wraparound care) before, during and after pregnancy
- systems to recruit, train and support adequate staff to provide maternal care through a mix of roles (for example, midwives, doctors, medical specialists, community and mental health workers)
- systems and training to support culturally safe care
- training and support for staff to confidently provide best-practice care relating to sensitive issues (for example, conversations about family violence, social and emotional wellbeing)
- clear pathways for referral to local and appropriate services
- appropriate awareness-raising and education resources, and partnering with communities on health promotion and prevention projects and resource development
- partnership with participatory women's groups and other community groups that connect and support women and their families.

Participate in CQI. Sustained commitment to CQI can improve the quality of maternal health care.

Improving maternal care for Aboriginal and Torres Strait Islander women

Research into the quality of maternal care since 2010 highlights many aspects of care that are being done well by PHC centres serving Aboriginal and Torres Strait Islander communities. It also highlights a need to enhance the delivery of recommended services.[40] Despite generally high levels of attendance for antenatal care, an early study across multiple PHC centres found that only one in five Aboriginal and Torres Strait Islander women was screened for depression in pregnancy using a standard screening tool.[41] Delivery of this service item has improved, but not sufficiently and not consistently across PHC centres. The development and uptake of place-based screening tools (for example, Kimberley Mum's Mood Scale[42]) could help to improve delivery.

There are many examples of variation in service delivery for routine items of maternal care. These common and persistent gaps in care indicate broader system weaknesses and a need to focus on the functioning of organisational systems and the root causes of gaps in care (rather than on isolated issues or staff roles). Establishing systems to train and support PHC staff to use standard screening tools and provide brief interventions and referrals, for example, can improve care for a range of health risk factors and client groups, as long as appropriate referral options are available.

> Sustained commitment to CQI can improve the quality of maternal health care.

Australian governments are investing in culturally responsive maternity care, but limited availability of birthing services outside urban centres means that many women who live in remote communities are still separated from family, community and PHC services during the final weeks of their pregnancies and while giving birth. The separation can be a significant stress. The connectedness of Aboriginal and Torres Strait Islander families and communities is a strength and a source of learning and support for mothers. Community-based maternal care, including family-focused programs that enable women to pass on cultural birthing and parenting practices, have potential for improving outcomes. Studies highlight the importance of the relationships established between healthcare teams and mothers, access to Aboriginal and Torres Strait Islander practitioners and other community-based workers, and culturally safe care.[43] An evaluation of the Strong Women, Strong Babies, Strong Culture program in the Northern Territory identified several features required for program success, with transferrable lessons for other maternal care initiatives:

- respect for Aboriginal knowledge and practice as a vital component of health care
- organisational commitment for a high level of community participation and control
- competence in intercultural collaborative practice of staff.[44]

---

40 Gibson-Helm, Rumbold et al. 2016; Gibson-Helm, Teede et al. 2015; Rumbold, R. Bailie et al. 2011.
41 Gausia, Thompson et al. 2013.
42 Marley, Kotz et al. 2017.
43 Gibson-Helm, J. Bailie et al. 2016, 2018; Kildea, Hickey et al. 2018; Kildea, Stapleton et al. 2012; McCalman 2014.
44 Lowell, Kildea et al. 2015.

Continuity of care and carer are highly valued by Aboriginal and Torres Strait Islander mothers and present many opportunities for reducing health risks.[45] PHC services need to connect well with young women to provide culturally safe preventive care, and to deliver best-practice, woman-centred maternal care before, during and after pregnancy. Good documentation and coordination between hospital and PHC teams is important for reducing health risks for mothers and babies following delivery,[46] while continuity of care through an infant's early years provides further opportunities to improve outcomes.[47] In summary, collaboration between health professionals is needed in all phases and women should expect to be provided with information to make informed choices about their care.[48]

> Collaboration between health professionals is needed in all phases and women should expect to be provided with information to make informed choices about their care.

The translation of evidence into policy and clinical practice is a common challenge. Mechanisms and funding support provided through the Closing the Gap and other government programs can increase workforce investment and strengthen systems for effective, culturally appropriate maternal care at higher levels of the system. CQI initiatives within PHC services are key to strengthening systems for high-quality maternal care at the community level, as part of comprehensive, holistic and culturally safe PHC.[49]

References

Abell, S., A. Nankervis, K. Khan and H. Teede (2016). Type 1 and type 2 diabetes preconception and in pregnancy: health impacts, influence of obesity and lifestyle, and principles of management. *Seminars in Reproductive Medicine* 34(2): 110–20. DOI: 10.1055/s-0035-1571196.

Australian Institute of Health and Welfare (2024). *Diabetes: Australian facts – gestational diabetes.* Canberra: Australian Government.

Australian Institute of Health and Welfare (2023). Australia's mothers and babies. *First Nations mothers and babies.* Canberra: AIHW.

Australian Institute of Health and Welfare (2021). *Australia's mothers and babies.* Canberra: AIHW. https://www.aihw.gov.au/reports/mothers-babies/australias-mothers-babies/contents/about.

Bailie, J., J. Boyle and R. Bailie (2018). Population attributable fractions of perinatal outcomes for nulliparous women associated with overweight and obesity, 1990–2014. *Medical Journal of Australia* 208(11): 505–6. DOI: 10.5694/mja18.00263.

Bar-Zeev, S., L. Barclay, C. Farrington and S. Kildea (2012). From hospital to home: the quality and safety of a postnatal discharge system used for remote dwelling Aboriginal mothers and infants in the top end of Australia. *Midwifery* 28(3): 366–73. DOI: 10.1016/j.midw.2011.04.010.

Chamberlain, C., B. Oldenburg, A. Wilson, S. Eades, K. O'Dea, J. Oats et al. (2016). Type 2 diabetes after gestational diabetes: greater than fourfold risk among Indigenous compared with non-Indigenous Australian women. *Diabetes/Metabolism Research and Reviews* 32(2): 217–27. DOI: 10.1002/dmrr.2715.

---

45   Sivertsen, Anikeeva et al. 2020.
46   Bar-Zeev, Barclay et al. 2012.
47   Sivertsen, Anikeeva et al. 2020.
48   Royal Australian and New Zealand College of Obstetricians and Gynaecologists 2017.
49   Harfield, Davy et al. 2018.

Crinall, B., J. Boyle, M. Gibson-Helm, D. Esler, S. Larkins and R. Bailie (2017). Cardiovascular disease risk in young Indigenous Australians: a snapshot of current preventive health care. *Australian and New Zealand Journal of Public Health* 41(5): 460–6. DOI: 10.1111/1753-6405.12547.

Cunningham, J. and Y. Paradies (2012). Socio-demographic factors and psychological distress in Indigenous and non-Indigenous Australian adults aged 18–64 years: analysis of national survey data. *BMC Public Health* 12(1 Feb 2012): 95. DOI: 10.1186/1471-2458-12-95.

Dabelea, D. (2007). The predisposition to obesity and diabetes in offspring of diabetic mothers. *Diabetes Care* 30(Supplement_2): S169–S74. DOI: 10.2337/dc07-s211.

Ding, X., Y. Wu, S. Xu, R. Zhu, X. Jia, S. Zhang et al. (2014). Maternal anxiety during pregnancy and adverse birth outcomes: a systematic review and meta-analysis of prospective cohort studies. *Journal of Affective Disorders* 159: 103–10. DOI: 10.1016/j.jad.2014.02.027.

Freemantle, J. and L. Ellis (2018). An Australian perspective. In J.R. Duncan and R.W. Byard (eds), *SIDS sudden infant and early childhood death: the past, the present and the future*. Adelaide: University of Adelaide Press. https://www.ncbi.nlm.nih.gov/books/NBK513382/.

Gausia, K., S. Thompson, T. Nagel, A. Rumbold, C. Connors, V. Matthews et al. (2013). Antenatal emotional wellbeing screening in Aboriginal and Torres Strait Islander primary health care services in Australia. *Contemporary Nurse: A Journal for the Australian Nursing Profession* 46(1): 73–82. DOI: 10.5172/conu.2013.46.1.73.

Gausia, K., S.C. Thompson, T. Nagel, G. Schierhout, V. Matthews and R. Bailie (2015). Risk of antenatal psychosocial distress in indigenous women and its management at primary health care centres in Australia. *General Hospital Psychiatry* 37(4): 335–9. DOI: 10.1016/j.genhosppsych.2015.04.005.

Gibson-Helm, M., J. Bailie, V. Matthews, A. Laycock, J. Boyle and R. Bailie (2018). Identifying evidence–practice gaps and strategies for improvement in Aboriginal and Torres Strait Islander maternal health care. *PLOS One* 13(2): e0192262. DOI: 10.1371/journal.pone.0192262.

Gibson-Helm, M., J. Bailie, V. Matthews, A. Laycock, J. Boyle and R. Bailie (2016). *Priority evidence–practice gaps in Aboriginal and Torres Strait Islander maternal health care final report: engaging stakeholders in identifying priority evidence–practice gaps and strategies for improvement in primary health care (ESP project)*. Brisbane: Menzies School of Health Research.

Gibson-Helm, M., A. Rumbold, H. Teede, S. Ranasinha, R. Bailie and J. Boyle (2016). Improving the provision of pregnancy care for Aboriginal and Torres Strait Islander women: a continuous quality improvement initiative. *BMC Pregnancy and Childbirth* 16(118). DOI: 10.1186/s12884-016-0892-1.

Gibson-Helm, M., H. Teede, A. Rumbold, S. Ranasinha, R. Bailie and J. Boyle (2015). Continuous quality improvement and metabolic screening during pregnancy at primary health centres attended by Aboriginal and Torres Strait Islander women. *Medical Journal of Australia* 203(9): 369.e1–69.e7. DOI: 10.5694/mja14.01660.

Harfield, S., C. Davy, A. McArthur, Z. Munn, A. Brown and N. Brown (2018). Characteristics of Indigenous primary health care service delivery models: a systematic scoping review. *Globalization Health* 14(1): 12. DOI: 10.1186/s12992-018-0332-2.

Heazell, A. (2020). Need to ensure that improvements in stillbirth rates are also achieved in high-risk groups. *Paediatric and Perinatal Epidemiology* 34(1): 1–2. DOI: https://doi.org/10.1111/ppe.12609.

Kildea, S., S. Hickey, C. Nelson, J. Currie, A. Carson, M. Reynolds et al. (2018). Birthing on Country (in our community): a case study of engaging stakeholders and developing a best-practice Indigenous maternity service in an urban setting. *Australian Health Review* 42(2): 230–8. DOI: 10.1071/AH16218.

Kildea, S., H. Stapleton, R. Murphy, N.B. Low and K. Gibbons (2012). The Murri clinic: a comparative retrospective study of an antenatal clinic developed for Aboriginal and Torres Strait Islander women. *BMC Pregnancy and Childbirth* 12(1): 159. DOI: 10.1186/1471-2393-12-159.

Lee, A., R. Hiscock, P. Wein, S. Walker and M. Permezel (2007). Gestational diabetes mellitus: clinical predictors and long-term risk of developing type 2 diabetes: a retrospective cohort study using survival analysis. *Diabetes Care* 30(4): 878–83. DOI: 10.2337/dc06-1816.

Lowell, A., S. Kildea, M. Liddle, B. Cox and B. Paterson (2015). Supporting Aboriginal knowledge and practice in health care: lessons from a qualitative evaluation of the Strong Women, Strong Babies, Strong Culture program. *BMC Pregnancy and Childbirth* 15(1): 19. DOI: 10.1186/s12884-015-0433-3.

MacKay, D., R. Kirkham, N. Freeman, K. Murtha, P. Van Dokkum, J. Boyle et al. (2020). Improving systems of care during and after a pregnancy complicated by hyperglycaemia: a protocol for a complex health systems intervention. *BMC Health Services Research* 20(1): 814. DOI: 10.1186/ s12913-020-05680-x.

Marley, J., J. Kotz, C. Engelke, M. Williams, D. Stephen, S. Coutinho et al. (2017). Validity and acceptability of Kimberley Mum's Mood Scale to screen for perinatal anxiety and depression in remote Aboriginal health care settings. *PLOS One* 12(1): e0168969. DOI: 10.1371/journal.pone.0168969.

Marmot, M., P. Goldblatt, J. Allen, et al. *Fair society, healthy lives (The Marmot Review)*. London: Institute of Health Equity.

McCalman, J. (2014). Evaluating the Baby Basket program in north Queensland. *Lowitja Institute*. https://www.lowitja.org.au/projects/baby-basket/.

McMillen, I. and J. Robinson (2005). Developmental origins of the metabolic syndrome: prediction, plasticity, and programming. *Physiological Reviews* 85(2): 571–633. DOI: 10.1152/physrev.00053.2003.

Menzies School of Health Research and One21seventy (2014). *Maternal health clinical audit tool*. One21seventy. Brisbane: Menzies School of Health Research.

Royal Australian and New Zealand College of Obstetricians and Gynaecologists (2017). *Maternity care in Australia: a framework for a healthy new generation of Australians*. https://ranzcog.edu. au/wp-content/uploads/2022/01/Maternity-Care-in-Australia-Web.pdf

Rumbold, A., R. Bailie, D. Si, M. Dowden, C. Kennedy, R. Cox et al. (2011). Delivery of maternal health care in Indigenous primary care services: baseline data for an ongoing quality improvement initiative. *BMC Pregnancy and Childbirth* 11(1): 16. DOI: 10.1186/1471-2393-11-16.

Rumbold, A., K. Wild, E. Maypilama, S. Kildea, L. Barclay, E. Wallace et al. (2015). Challenges to providing fetal anomaly testing in a cross-cultural environment: experiences of practitioners caring for Aboriginal women. *Birth (Berkeley, Calif.)* 42(4): 362–8. DOI: 10.1111/birt.12182.

Saigal, S. and L. Doyle (2008). An overview of mortality and sequelae of preterm birth from infancy to adulthood. *Lancet* 371(9608): 261–9. DOI: 10.1016/S0140-6736(08)60136-1.

Sivertsen, N., O. Anikeeva, J. Deverix and J. Grant (2020). Aboriginal and Torres Strait Islander family access to continuity of health care services in the first 1000 days of life: a systematic review of the literature. *BMC Health Services Research* 20(1): 829. DOI: 10.1186/s12913-020-05673-w.

White Ribbon Alliance (2011*). The respectful maternity care charter: the universal rights of childbearing women*. Washington: White Ribbon Alliance. http://www.healthpolicyproject.com/index. cfm?ID=publications&get=pubID&pubID=46.

World Health Organization (2020). Global Health Observatory (GHO) data. Infant mortality: situations and trends. Geneva, Switzerland: WHO.

World Health Organization (2019). *Maternal mortality*. Fact sheets. https://www.who.int/news-room/ fact-sheets/detail/maternal-mortality.

World Health Organization (2016). *WHO recommendations on antenatal care for a positive pregnancy experience*. https://www.who.int/reproductivehealth/publications/maternal_perinatal_health/ anc-positive-pregnancy-experience/en/.

World Health Organization (2015). *Postnatal care for mothers and newborns: highlights from the World Health Organization 2013 guidelines*. Geneva, Switzerland: WHO.

Developing an audit tool to improve youth health care – a case study

This chapter differs from the other chapters in Part III. It describes how a youth health audit tool was developed and applied in primary health care (PHC). The chapter offers guidance for those developing an audit tool in any area of PHC with less developed clinical guidelines and a less well-established evidence base.

Youth health

Youth is a critical period of development and transition in a person's life. Young people who are in good health between the ages of 12 and 24 are more likely to achieve better educational outcomes, transition successfully into work, develop healthy adult lifestyles, and experience fewer challenges when establishing families and parenting than young people who experience poor health and wellbeing.[1]

How the transition from childhood to adulthood is defined differs between cultures and over time, nevertheless adolescence is a time of intense physical, neurological, social and emotional change. We build our sense of self, grow more concerned about peers' opinions, learn to manage emotions and relationships, and seek independence from parents and other adults in our lives as we develop more ability to reason and to think logically, critically and morally.[2] This occurs within a complex system of family, peer, school, community, media and broader cultural influences.[3]

Youth is a time when behaviours and habits can be formed, experimentation and taking risks may occur and mental health problems are likely to emerge.[4] Accidental injuries and violence, poor mental health, substance misuse, and problems related to nutrition, infectious diseases and sexual reproductive health are among the health issues commonly experienced by young people in many countries.[5] These occur regardless of wealth, with mental health problems being the most common health issues facing young people worldwide.[6] Furthermore, in many low-income countries, more than 50 per cent of the population is younger than

---

1   Australian Institute of Health and Welfare 2011.
2   World Health Organization 2014.
3   Viner, Ozer et al. 2012.
4   Puszka, Nagel et al. 2015.
5   Moya 2002.
6   Institute for Health Metrics and Evaluation 2018.

20 years.[7] Seventy-five per cent of global mental illness starts by age 24;[8] globally, almost one in seven young people meets diagnostic criteria for a mental health disorder[9] but fewer than two-thirds of young people with mental health problems and their families are likely to access professional help.[10] Focusing on the prevention of mental health problems early in life is important for improving population health and lives.

As the first point of contact with the health system for many young people and their families, it is critical that PHC professionals have the expertise and resources to engage with young people and to provide high-quality PHC for this group, including mental health care and trauma-informed care. From the perspective of PHC services, this life phase presents an opportunity for supporting healthy lifestyles, identifying and reducing risk factors for future ill health and promoting social and emotional wellbeing.[11] It also presents an opportunity to make up for any developmental deficits and health threats caused by a child's living environment (for example, food shortages, lack of access to school, conflict and displacement, violence and abuse).[12] Yet many barriers prevent access to health services for this group, including availability, acceptability and equity.[13] Some PHC professionals say they lack skills and confidence relating to young people.[14]

The need to make health services more adolescent- and youth-friendly has been identified as a priority,[15] and international standards of health care for youth have been developed.[16] Improving PHC for young people is an important investment in creating healthy futures for individuals and for public health and prevention more generally.

What we know about improving youth health through PHC

The international literature offers general strategies for improving youth health.

Targeted strategies and information

Adolescents and young adults, like other specific population groups, need targeted primary healthcare strategies and information. PHC services should aim to achieve these outcomes:

- provide youth-specific health facilities, or facilities that are appealing, that acknowledge the diversity of young people and are appropriately equipped and easily accessible
- use strategies that make PHC services more acceptable and accessible for young people, such as opening hours that allow young people to come outside school hours, staff who relate well to them, and assurance that confidentiality will be respected
- provide accurate health information and age-appropriate programs and resources

---

7   WorldData.info 2020.
8   McGorry, Purcell et al. 2011.
9   Polanczyk, Salum et al. 2015.
10 Sadler, Vizard et al. 2018.
11 Puszka, Nagel et al. 2015.
12 World Health Organization 2010.
13 World Health Organization 2012a.
14 O'Brien, Harvey et al. 2016.
15 James, Pisa et al. 2018.
16 World Health Organization 2012a.

- use the internet when appropriate or possible to deliver information and evidence-based programs, including via mobile phone apps and social media
- regularly update and share information about age-appropriate health, education, social, cultural and recreational resources available to young people in the local community
- use marketing strategies that encourage young people to access preventive services.[17]

Mental health care

A strong focus on youth mental health care is essential – now more than ever. Youth mental health care needs were well documented prior to 2020. The Covid-19 pandemic further inequitably affected the mental health of young people, putting them at higher risk of mental illness. Extended time away from education, friendships and relationships, sport, social life, cultural and community events had a particular effect on young people, for whom peer relationships are especially significant. Many have felt lonely. Many young people worldwide have suffered loss and grief from losing important people in their lives to the virus. The Covid-19 experience highlights these needs:

- focusing on developing young people's resilience and preventing mental health problems early
- providing mental health training for PHC practitioners tailored to youth needs, including locally available referral options and skills to identify and support young people in distress[18]
- strengthening links between PHC services, schools and community resources for young people, such as social services, mental health and counselling services, alcohol and other drugs programs, suicide prevention programs and crisis response services
- overcoming known barriers to young people seeking and accessing mental health care
  - barriers for young people include stigma, embarrassment, concerns about confidentiality and trust in a person they don't know, cost, difficulties with recognising problems and a desire to deal with difficulties themselves[19]
  - barriers for families include cost, wait times, trust and confidence in health professionals, and knowing where to get help[20]
  - barriers for communities are having little or no access to affordable or appropriate mental health services.

Sexual and reproductive health

Often sexual and reproductive health, an important aspect of youth health, is the entry point to health services for adolescents. Primary healthcare services should prepare in these ways to help young people:

- train practitioners to share information with young people about sexual and reproductive health, in ways that promote understanding[21]

---

17   James, Pisa et al. 2018; Leung, Brennan et al. 2022; World Health Organization 2012a.
18   Dudgeon, Darwin et al. 2018; O'Brien, Harvey et al. 2016.
19   Gulliver, Griffiths and Christensen 2010; Reardon, Harvey et al. 2017.
20   Reardon, Harvey et al. 2017.
21   World Health Organization 2012a, b.

- ensure that sexual and reproductive health services can be accessed confidentiality and without judgement
- include sexual and reproductive health services discreetly as part a wider range of services (rather than a specialised clinic).

Community- and systems-based approaches

Comprehensive PHC for young people integrates clinical care with other wellbeing programs and services. These services may offer points of contact between youth and health service staff. In this area of practice, primary healthcare services should have these aims:

- working with schools and other agencies to provide holistic care, such as homelessness, counselling, disability and employment services
- connecting with young people in the places where they spend time – through school programs, sports and social clubs, entertainment venues and social media[22]
- where possible, engaging young people through peer educators and influencers.

Community- and systems-based approaches to PHC are described in Part IV. Chapter 15 includes an example of a school-based program to strengthen the resilience of teenagers in boarding schools.

Young Aboriginal and Torres Strait Islander peoples

In Australia, Aboriginal and Torres Strait Islander peoples aged 10–24 represent 5 per cent of the total Australian youth population. Many are connected to their culture, and participation in sporting, social or community events is high. Of those living in remote areas, more than 80 per cent surveyed recognised their traditional homelands, and participated in cultural activities. More than 75 per cent of those aged 15 to 24 years reported being happy all or most of the time.[23] Another positive wellbeing indicator for young Aboriginal and Torres Strait Islander people is the proportion completing secondary education (Year 12 or equivalent), which has increased from 47 per cent in 2006 to 68 per cent in 2021.[24] Around 74 per cent of young Aboriginal and Torres Strait Islander people aged 15–19 consider family relationships extremely or very important, and most aged 15–24 reported they had family or friends to confide in. The proportion of this age group who smoke decreased from 45 per cent in 2002 to 31 per cent in 2014–15.[25]

Building on these strengths is crucial, because young Aboriginal and Torres Strait Islander people have poorer health, as a population group, than other Australian young people. This is largely due to higher rates of mental illness, substance use and injuries[26] – a legacy of colonisation that resulted in dispossession of land, disruption of family structures and social and cultural practices, and exclusion from societal opportunities. In 2014–15, for example, racial discrimination was experienced by young Aboriginal and Torres Strait Islander people

---

22   World Health Organization 2012a.
23   Australian Institute of Health and Welfare 2018.
24   Productivity Commission 2023.
25   Australian Institute of Health and Welfare 2018.
26   Australian Institute of Health and Welfare 2019.

aged 15–24 in most types of settings (for example, educational, health, work, public places);[27] in 2022, two in five (40 per cent) young Aboriginal and Torres Strait Islander people reported that they had been treated unfairly or discriminated against in the past year.[28] Young people exposed to racism are much more likely than others to have anxiety, depression, be at suicide risk, and have poor overall mental health.[29] Compared with their non-Indigenous peers, young Aboriginal and Torres Strait Islander people also experience higher rates of chronic conditions, including diabetes, hearing loss, rheumatic heart disease and other health challenges.[30] Aboriginal and Torres Strait Islander adolescents living in remote areas have the poorest adolescent health outcomes in Australia.[31] Reducing these inequities for a healthier future requires systemic and social change and high-quality health care.

> Reducing inequities for a healthier future for Aboriginal and Torres Strait Islander young people requires systemic and social change and high-quality health care.

Aboriginal and Torres Strait Islander youth underuse health services and engage with health care at more advanced stages of illness and for shorter periods in comparison to non-Indigenous youth.[32] For example, in 2014–15, only 23 per cent of the young Aboriginal and Torres Strait Islander people reporting high or very high levels of distress in the previous 12 months had been seen by a health professional.[33] The quality, capacity and cultural appropriateness of health services are key factors in whether or not young people engage with services and in their health outcomes.[34] Understanding the effect of intergenerational trauma, racism and socio-economic inequality is important for understanding the experiences of young Aboriginal and Torres Strait Islander people, the challenges they face in the transition to adulthood and their interactions with healthcare providers.[35] The experiences of particular groups (for example, young people in out-of-home care, boarding school students), the context and language in which interactions take place (for example, clinic or community venue, first language), and the relationship between a young person and a health professional (for example, kinship links, cultural understandings or differences) are also likely to influence their engagement with health care.

The *National guide to a preventative health assessment for Aboriginal and Torres Strait Islander people*[36] includes guidelines for youth health checks, and recommendations for reducing risks of unplanned pregnancy, sexually transmissible infections and illicit drug use. Useful tools, as recommended by National Aboriginal Community Controlled Health Organisation and the Royal Australian College of General Practitioners, include the HEEADSSS assessment tool and

---

27   Australian Institute of Health and Welfare 2018.
28   Leung, Brennan et al. 2022.
29   Priest, Paradies et al. 2011.
30   Australian Institute of Health and Welfare 2011.
31   Australian Institute of Health and Welfare 2018.
32   Price and Dalgleish 2013; Westerman 2010.
33   Australian Bureau of Statistics 2017.
34   Australian Institute of Health and Welfare 2011.
35   Australian Institute of Health and Welfare 2018.
36   National Aboriginal Community Controlled Health Organisation and Royal Australian College 2024.

the Aboriginal and Torres Strait Islander youth social and emotional wellbeing assessment and question guide. The HEEADSSS assessment tool includes items relating to home and environment, education and employment, eating and exercise, activities and peer relationships, drug use/tobacco/alcohols, sexuality, suicide and depression, and safety.

Social and emotional wellbeing assessments for young people (as for other age groups) can be done opportunistically or as part of an annual youth health check to obtain a holistic assessment of health and to determine risk factors affecting wellbeing. Assessment should take a strengths-based approach that focuses on the capabilities of the young person and the community, advocates for a positive sense of cultural identity, and acknowledges potential for change, growth and success. When referrals are needed, the services and programs need to be culturally appropriate.

These health and care needs reinforce the need for PHC services to build the Aboriginal and Torres Strait Islander workforce and to connect positively with young people to provide culturally safe, affirming and holistic care. Strategies may include the following:

- increasing the number of Aboriginal and Torres Strait Islander staff, including Elders and young workers
- supporting community-led and youth-guided PHC solutions based on Aboriginal and Torres Strait Islander ways of knowing, being and doing
- connecting with young people and their families in the places they come together (for example, sports and cultural events)
- engaging young people to develop and spread health messages using preferred media and communication tools (for example, social media, digital technologies)
- using or co-designing age-appropriate resources[37] and health promotion activities
- integrating care with the work of other youth and family services (for example, schools, training providers, child and youth protection, housing and youth justice) (see also Chapter 15).

The ongoing development and use of CQI approaches are important for monitoring progress and improving young people's access to high-quality PHC. Good documentation of care processes in health records is essential for effective CQI. Community stories about what works well and not so well to improve services and outcomes for young people should also be documented and should reflect the voices of young people and their families. This aspect of CQI remains under-documented, and such stories are an important source of data for improving health promotion activities as part of comprehensive PHC.

Developing a clinical audit tool to measure the quality of care for youth – an implementation case study

Recognising that systems for monitoring and improving the performance of youth health services were limited, our research group developed and piloted a clinical audit tool for assessing the quality of PHC for young Aboriginal and Torres Strait Islander people aged 12–24, including mental health services provided within primary care. Few published pilot and validation studies of audit tools contain explicit information about the methodology used

---

37   For examples: https://cbpatsisp.com.au/ and https://wellmob.org.au/

to develop indicators or the assessment criteria used to evaluate them.[38] Here we explain the systematic approach taken to develop the audit tool, and how challenges that emerged during the development process were overcome.

Approach and methods

Traditionally, the development of quality indicators follows Donabedian's theoretical approach to measuring quality of health care based on structures, processes and outcomes of care (see Chapter 4), and involves a combination of evidence-based guidelines and expert consensus. Where standards of care have not been defined, evidence-based guideline recommendations are identified and audit items developed using a systematic expert consensus approach and explicit selection criteria.[39] This was the approach the group took in the absence of agreed standards of care for Aboriginal and Torres Strait Islander youth health.

As part of the project design, opportunities were provided for developing the capacity of Aboriginal and Torres Strait Islander researchers and stakeholders at all levels of the project, including two chief investigators. The development process, as detailed in a paper by Puszka and colleagues,[40] is summarised here:

- *Establishment of expert reference group* (to determine content validity of the tool). Members from primary healthcare services and research organisations had collective expertise in Aboriginal and Torres Strait Islander youth health. They represented diverse PHC settings and services, and had knowledge of factors relevant to the health system and youth population (for example, appropriateness of services, priority health conditions and risk factors) and to PHC services (for example, client information systems, feasibility to complete audit). The group met monthly for 18 months.
- *Development of audit items.* Relevant guidelines for Aboriginal and Torres Strait Islander youth health were identified (16 in total) and used as a basis for development of initial audit items. Six criteria for including or excluding an audit item were developed (see Box 14.1). Group facilitation techniques were used to achieve consensus amongst members about audit items. Where members disagreed on the inclusion of a specific item in the audit, disagreements were generally resolved with reference to the inclusion criteria.
- *Pilot tested.* Four health centres ranging in size and governance arrangements piloted the tool in urban, regional and remote communities. Pilot testing aimed to assess the recording in client records of specific items of care and the ease of use of the audit tool. Testing was done using both paper-based and electronic patient information systems. At each pilot site, 30 client records were audited by trained auditors and health service staff.
- *User feedback.* Notes and feedback from auditors were used to assess performance and, at one site, a focus group discussion explored user experiences of the tool. Analysed data were fed back to the expert reference group for consideration.
- *Refinement.* The audit tool and protocol underwent four further phases of development as the expert reference group considered an initial draft and results from pilot testing and user feedback at the pilot sites. Each phase enabled revision and further refinement,

---

38   Hearnshaw, Harker et al. 2002.
39   Kötter, Blozik and Scherer 2012.
40   Puszka, Nagel et al. 2015.

taking account of user feedback, the gaps and conflicts in relevant guidelines for Aboriginal and Torres Strait Islander youth health, a lack of agreed standards of care, and the state of development of client information systems.[41]

Box 14.1 Criteria for determining audit items for the delivery of primary health care to Aboriginal and Torres Strait Islander youth

1. Every audit item needs to have a specific justification for inclusion.

2. Every item related to a clinical or other service, or a health condition, must be relevant to an important health problem for the target youth population.

3. For every item related to a clinical or other service, the item should be backed by good justification in terms of its value in assessment of health or social conditions, or its effectiveness as an intervention, or in terms of appropriate follow-up care.

4. For every item there needs to be a reasonable expectation that the relevant information would be documented in the clinical records of a busy health centre, and that this information is "auditable" (we can reasonably expect the information to be documented in a way that can be found in the clinical record by a person with some training in the audit process).

5. Together, the audit items should reflect best-practice service delivery for the prevention, screening or treatment for risk factors and conditions identified as priority issues for the health and wellbeing of Aboriginal and Torres Strait Islander youth.

6. For every item related to a clinical or other service, there needs to be a reasonable expectation that the service would be routinely provided if indicated.[42]

Youth audit tool content

The audit tool[43] includes items under five main headings:

- client information recorded in attendance records
- health checks
- scheduled immunisations
- protective factors, risk factors and brief interventions and referrals
- scheduled services including preventive health care.

A key component of the tool is its assessment of protective factors, risk factors, brief interventions and referrals. Audit items in this section are based on the internationally accepted youth psychosocial assessment known as HEEADSSS (see above in "Young Aboriginal and Torres Strait Islander people").

---

41   Puszka, Nagel et al. 2015.
42   Puszka, Nagel et al. 2015.
43   Menzies School of Health Research and One21seventy 2014. Download tool and protocol: https://www.menzies.edu.au/page/Resources/Youth_health_clinical_audit_tool/.

Results of testing

The testing process[44] showed that a few audit items had lower reliability. These items were refined and reviewed. While the tool was found to be user friendly, the time taken to complete the audit and feedback on the length of the tool provided impetus to prioritise audit items. The availability of information in client records led to further refinement.

The variable quality of documentation in client records presented challenges. Some audit items were not well documented and were difficult to audit. For example, there were inconsistencies in the recording of non-clinical items such as referrals and reports received from referral services, and in the terminology used in client records (for example, relating to psychosocial wellbeing). In response, clear definitions of terms were included in the audit protocol.

The documentation of screening for the psychosocial wellbeing of young people was found to vary greatly between psychosocial domains and between testing sites. There were also differences in the provision of treatment or referral in response to different psychosocial concerns. For example, there were gaps in service delivery for tobacco use. A decision was made to group some psychosocial items into a "lifestyle discussion".

Brief interventions were the most common form of treatment provided, with the exceptions of mental health, where referral was more common, and sexual behaviour risks where "other treatment" was commonly provided (usually recorded as testing for sexually transmitted infections). An unexpected finding during the pilot study was that no prescription or discussion of contraception was documented in response to concerns about sexual behaviour risks across all sites.

The testing process demonstrated how the audit could help educate staff about best practice for youth health and encourage reflective practice. It reinforced the role of a clear, user-friendly audit protocol for collecting consistent data for measuring the quality of care for youth and tracking improvements over successive audit cycles. The practitioners who tested the tool questioned whether there should be scope to note why care standards were not met (for example, clients refusing treatment and their reasons), and whether the audit should include communication with referral services.[45] While out of scope of the audit tool, this feedback highlighted the need to combine clinical audit results with other assessments of how well PHC systems are functioning to engage young people and respond to their healthcare needs. The One21seventy Youth Health Clinical Audit Tool was published in 2014.[46]

Wider implications of the tool for improving the quality of care for young people

The potential health benefits and savings of health systems with a focus on prevention and early intervention are well documented.[47] A greater emphasis on prevention and early intervention, particularly for psychosocial issues, caring staff who relate well to young people and the sustained use of measurement and monitoring frameworks for youth health may help reduce

---

44   Puszka, Nagel et al. 2014.
45   Puszka, Nagel et al. 2014.
46   Menzies School of Health Research 2014. Download: https://www.menzies.edu.au/page/ Resources/Youth_health_clinical_audit_tool/.
47   Australian Institute of Health and Welfare 2020.

the gap in health outcomes between young Aboriginal and Torres Strait Islander people and young non-Indigenous Australians. In this PHC context, frameworks need to incorporate Aboriginal and Torres Strait Islander perspectives on health and wellbeing.

Audits can only capture care processes and indicators that are documented in clients' health records. When care processes are well documented, there is more likelihood that audit findings will be accurate and that improvement strategies based on the data will be effective. Well-functioning client information systems are also crucial for the follow-up and management of young people's health needs. Use of the Youth Health Clinical Audit Tool provides new evidence for improving PHC for young people. The participation of Aboriginal and Torres Strait Islander PHC team members (particularly young team members) in interpreting CQI data and guiding improvement strategies helps to ensure the evidence is put into practice in ways that build on youth and community strengths to improve care quality.

> When care processes are well documented, there is more likelihood that audit findings will be accurate and that improvement strategies based on the data will be effective.

Lessons learnt

The researchers identified several generalisable lessons[48] from their experience of developing a youth health clinical audit tool for use in PHC.

- In the context of no articulated standards of care, it is possible to develop an audit process premised on relevant available evidence.

- The justification for each audit item must be explicit and realistic.

- Engagement with stakeholders and experts is essential for determining key measures of quality.

- Consider the feasibility of the audit process and whether you can reasonably expect a service item to be delivered and documented, given the resources available in your PHC context.

- Allow for further refinement of the audit tool and audit tool protocol post-implementation.

- Use a clinical audit tool in combination with other CQI tools and processes to assess and improve the way a PHC service provides comprehensive PHC.

---

48   Puszka, Nagel et al. 2015.

Conclusion

Developing the youth health audit tool required the developers to determine key measures of evidence-based care. This involved a systematic approach, drawing on existing evidence and expert consensus in combination with a more pragmatic process of determining the key items of care that could reasonably be expected to be provided and documented in the PHC context.

Audits and audit tools need to reflect the state of development of healthcare systems, client record systems and clinical guidelines or standards of care. They also need to reflect reasonable expectations about what care is feasible, even in relatively well-resourced health systems like those in Australia. Particularly in low-resource settings, but also more generally, policymakers and clinicians developing audit processes would need to ensure that audits are not used to assess practitioners and health services against unreasonable expectations. When audits are used in combination with systems assessments and with sensitivity to context, the findings are particularly useful for informing achievable goals and strategies for improving systems of care. The aim of introducing and using any CQI tools is to support teams and services to continuously learn and improve healthcare quality.

References

Australian Bureau of Statistics (2017). *National Aboriginal and Torres Strait Islander social survey, 2014–15*. ABS cat. no. 4714.0. Canberra: ABS.

Australian Institute of Health and Welfare (2020). *Australia's health 2020*. No. 17. Cat. no. AUS 232. Canberra: AIHW.

Australian Institute of Health and Welfare (2019). *Australian Burden of Disease study: impact and causes of illness and death in Australia, 2015*. Australian Burden of Disease series no. 19. Cat. no. BOD 22. Canberra: AIHW.

Australian Institute of Health and Welfare (2018). *Aboriginal and Torres Strait Islander adolescent and youth health and wellbeing 2018*. Cat. no. IHW 202. Canberra: AIHW.

Australian Institute of Health and Welfare (2011). *Young Australians: their health and wellbeing 2011*. Cat. no. PHE 140. Canberra: AIHW.

Dudgeon, P., L. Darwin, R. McPhee, C. Holland, S. von Helle and L. Halliday (2018). *Implementing integrated suicide prevention in Aboriginal and Torres Strait Islander communities: a guide for primary health networks*. Perth: University of Western Australia and Black Dog Institute.

Gulliver, A., K. Griffiths and H. Christensen (2010). Perceived barriers and facilitators to mental health help-seeking in young people: a systematic review. *BMC Psychiatry* 10(1): 113. DOI: 10.1186/1471-244X-10-113.

Hearnshaw, H., R. Harker, F. Cheater, R. Bake and G. Grimshaw (2002). A study of the methods used to select review criteria for clinical audit. *Health Technology Assessment* 6(1): 1–78. DOI: 10.3310/hta6010.

Institute for Health Metrics and Evaluation (2018). *Findings from the Global Burden of Disease Study 2017*. Seattle, WA: IHME.

James, S., P.T. Pisa, J. Imrie, M. Beery, C. Martin, C. Skosana et al. (2018). Assessment of adolescent and youth friendly services in primary health care facilities in two provinces in South Africa. *BMC Health Services Research* 18(1): 809. DOI: 10.1186/s12913-018-3623-7.

Kötter, T., E. Blozik and M. Scherer (2012). Methods for the guideline-based development of quality indicators – a systematic review. *Implementation Science* 7(1): 21. DOI: 10.1186/1748-5908-7-21.

Leung, S., N. Brennan, T. Freeburn, W. Waugh and R. Christie (2022). *Youth Survey report 2022*. Sydney: Mission Australia.

McGorry, P., R. Purcell, S. Goldstone and G. Amminger (2011). Age of onset and timing of treatment for mental and substance use disorders: implications for preventive intervention strategies and models of care. *Current Opinion in Psychiatry* 24(4): 301–6. DOI: 10.1097/YCO.0b013e3283477a09.

Menzies School of Health Research and One21Seventy (2014). Youth health clinical audit tool. Darwin: Menzies School of Health Research. https://www.menzies.edu.au/page/Resources/Youth_health_clinical_audit_tool/

Moya, C. (2002). Creating youth-friendly sexual health services in sub-Saharan Africa. Washington, DC: Advocates for Youth.

National Aboriginal Community Controlled Health Organisation and Royal Australian College of General Practitioners (2024). *National guide to a preventative health assessment for Aboriginal and Torres Strait Islander people*, 4th edn. Melbourne: RACGP.

O'Brien, D., K. Harvey, J. Howse, T. Reardon and C. Creswell (2016). Barriers to managing child and adolescent mental health problems: a systematic review of primary care practitioners' perceptions. *British Journal of General Practice* 66(651): e693. DOI: 10.3399/bjgp16X687061.

Polanczyk, G., G. Salum, L. Sugaya, A. Caye and L. Rohde (2015). Annual research review: a meta-analysis of the worldwide prevalence of mental disorders in children and adolescents. *Journal of Child Psychology and Psychiatry* 56(3): 345–65. DOI: 10.1111/jcpp.12381.

Price, M. and J. Dalgleish (2013). Help-seeking behaviour among Indigenous Australian adolescents: exploring attitudes, behaviours and barriers. *Youth Studies Australia* 32(1): 10–18.

Priest, N., Y. Paradies, W. Gunthorpe, S. Cairney and S. Sayers (2011). Racism as a determinant of social and emotional wellbeing for Aboriginal Australian youth. *Medical Journal of Australia* 194(10): 546–50.

Productivity Commission (2023). *Closing the Gap: annual data compilation report July 2023*. Canberra: Australian Government.

Puszka, S., T. Nagel, V. Matthews, D. Mosca, R. Piovesan, A. Nori et al. (2015). Monitoring and assessing the quality of care for youth: developing an audit tool using an expert consensus approach. *International Journal of Mental Health Systems* 9(28): 1–12. DOI: 10.1186/s13033-015-0019-5.

Puszka, S., T. Nagel, A. Nori, V. Daniel, E. Williams and V. Matthews (2014). *Development of the One21seventy youth health audit tool: final report*. Darwin: Menzies School of Health Research.

Reardon, T., K. Harvey, M. Baranowska, D. O'Brien, L. Smith and C. Creswell (2017). What do parents perceive are the barriers and facilitators to accessing psychological treatment for mental health problems in children and adolescents? A systematic review of qualitative and quantitative studies. *European Child and Adolescent Psychiatry* 26(6): 623–47. DOI: 10.1007/s00787-016-0930-6.

Sadler, K., T. Vizard, T. Ford, F. Marcheselli, N. Pearce, D. Mandalia et al. (2018). *Mental health of children and young people in England, 2017*. Leeds, UK: Health and Social Care Information Centre.

Viner, R., E. Ozer, S. Denny, M. Marmot, M. Resnick, A. Fatusi et al. (2012). Adolescence and the social determinants of health. *Lancet* 379(9826): 1641–52. DOI: 10.1016/S0140-6736(12)60149-4.

Westerman, T. (2010). Engaging Australian Aboriginal youth in mental health services. *Australian Psychologist* 45(3): 212–22. DOI: 10.1080/00050060903451790.

World Health Organization (2014). *Health for the world's adolescents: a second chance in the second decade*. Geneva, Switzerland: WHO.

World Health Organization (2012a). *Making health services adolescent friendly: developing national quality standards for adolescent-friendly health services*. Geneva, Switzerland: WHO.

World Health Organization (2012b). *WHO strategy on health policy and systems research: changing mindsets*. Geneva, Switzerland: WHO.

World Health Organization (2010). *Strengthening the health sector response to adolescent health and development*. Geneva, Switzerland: WHO.

WorldData.info (2020, updated 2024). Median and average age in global comparison. https://www.worlddata.info/average-age.php.

Improving mental health and wellbeing care

Mental health and wellbeing

Mental health is "an integral and essential component of health . . . a state of wellbeing in which an individual realises his or her own abilities, can cope with the normal stresses of life, can work productively and is able to make a contribution to his or her community".[1] The diminishment of mental health can affect people of almost any age, and mental health disorders affect hundreds of millions of people globally. In 2019, mental health disorders caused approximately 5 per cent of the global burden of disease and 16 per cent of all years lived with disability.[2] In Australia, mental health and substance use disorders accounted for 13 per cent of the total disease burden in 2018, the fourth-highest cause after cancer, cardiovascular diseases and musculoskeletal conditions, and almost half of all Australians will experience a mental health disorder at some stage in their lives.[3] Youth is a particularly important life stage for prevention and early intervention, since 75 per cent of global mental illness starts by age 24.[4] By 2030, depression is likely to be the second-highest cause of the global disease burden (second to HIV-AIDS) and the highest single contributor in high-income countries.[5] People are more likely to have depression when they have physical illnesses (for example, diabetes, cancer)[6] and may be more vulnerable to depression at particular life phases. A recent review found that 21 per cent of women worldwide experienced depression during pregnancy.[7]

Around the world, health systems are slow to respond effectively to the increasing burden of mental health disorders. In low- and middle-income countries, between 76 and 85 per cent of people with mental health disorders receive no treatment.[8] In wealthy countries, insensitivity to client preferences, context and culture when treating mental disorders has led to waste and harm. The United States mental health system, for example, fails to reach more than half of people with the most serious mental health disorders.[9]

---

1   World Health Organization 2018, 1.
2   Rehm and Shield 2019.
3   Australian Institute of Health and Welfare 2022b.
4   McGorry, Purcell et al. 2007.
5   Mathers and Loncar 2006.
6   Ngo, Rubinstein et al. 2013.
7   Yin, Sun et al. 2021.
8   Wang, Aguilar-Gaxiola et al. 2007; World Health Organization 2019.
9   Drake, Binagwaho et al. 2014.

Integrating mental health services into PHC across the life course is a viable way of closing the treatment gap and increasing access to appropriate support.[10] PHC has been found to deliver better care and clinical outcomes than psychiatric hospitals for common mental health disorders, such as depression, anxiety and substance disorders, and for less acute or severe mental illness.[11] There are several likely reasons. For example, PHC staff with mental health training can provide a holistic and coordinated approach to care for people who experience mental illness in combination with physical health problems. Stigma for clients with mental illness may be reduced when seeking care at a PHC service (compared with using a stand-alone mental health service), making care more acceptable. Family life and employment, and client recovery, are less disrupted when treatment can occur closer to home.[12] PHC also provides more scope for non-medicalised approaches, family and community involvement in mental health care, and care models that take account of social, political and cultural environments.[13]

Best-practice PHC for mental health includes prevention strategies, and screening, diagnosis and treatment for people with mental health disorders and mental health issues that affect wellbeing and physical health.[14] Evidence has shown that with adequate training and support, PHC workers can screen clients for mental health and wellbeing issues, recognise psychological distress and mental health disorders, treat common problems such as anxiety and depression, and provide brief interventions for the management of hazardous substance use.[15] But, traditionally, attempts to integrate mental health in PHC have been fraught with systems, resource and organisational challenges.[16]

The integration of mental health services into PHC requires multidisciplinary and collaborative care models supported by effective policy and systems.[17] Complementary services are needed, particularly secondary care facilities and specialist mental health professionals to whom PHC practitioners can turn for referrals, support and supervision. Care tasks should be limited and doable by staff, and clients must have access to essential psychotropic medications. Good service coordination, and collaboration with non-health sectors such as education, social and spiritual welfare, justice or employment are required to support recovery and social and emotional wellbeing.[18]

Mental health and social and emotional wellbeing of Aboriginal and Torres Strait Islander peoples

Social and emotional wellbeing (SEWB) is a term preferred by many First Nations people because it includes, but extends beyond, conventional understandings of mental health and mental disorder.[19] For Aboriginal and Torres Strait Islander Australians, SEWB is based on a holistic concept of health and culturally informed practices, "shaped by connections to body,

---

10   Ngo, Asarnow et al. 2009; World Health Organization 2019.
11   Kwan and Nease 2013; WHO and Wonca 2008.
12   WHO and Wonca 2008.
13   Drake, Binagwaho et al. 2014; Ngo, Rubinstein et al. 2013.
14   WHO and Wonca 2008.
15   Funk, Wutzke et al. 2005; Patel, Araya et al. 2007.
16   Haswell-Elkins, Hunter et al. 2005; Nguyen, Tran et al. 2021.
17   Ngo, Rubinstein et al. 2013.
18   WHO and Wonca 2008.
19   Gee, Dudgeon et al. 2014.

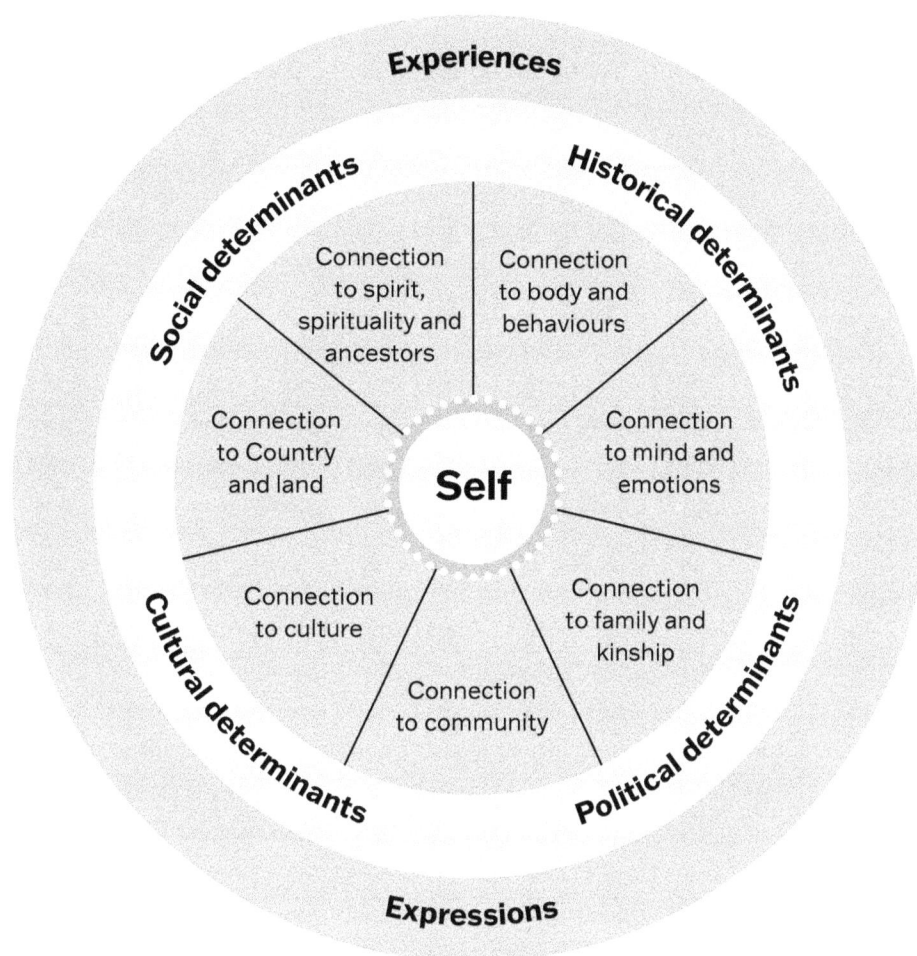

Figure 15.1 Social and emotional wellbeing (SEWB) from an Aboriginal and Torres Strait Islander perspective. Source: Adapted from Gee, Dudgeon et al. 2014.

mind and emotions, family and kinship, community, culture, land and spirituality"[20] and by a range of social, historical, political and cultural influences (see Figure 15.1). People's understanding of social and emotional wellbeing varies between different cultural groups and individuals, and may change across the life course (for example, factors important to a child's SEWB compared with factors important to Elders).[21]

The domains of SEWB, as illustrated in Figure 15.1, can be seen as protective factors for Aboriginal and Torres Strait Islander mental health across the life course. For many people, good mental health comes through a collective sense of self and belonging, strong cultural identity, positive relationships and understanding of social roles, and connection to other aspects of life that are a source of strength and resilience. Conversely, poor mental health can be influenced by stressors such as grief and trauma, forced removal from family and Country, racism and discrimination, incarceration, displacement from culture, intergenerational trauma and economic exclusion[22] – ongoing legacies of colonisation. Exposure to adverse experiences

---

20   Gee, Dudgeon et al. 2014, 58.
21   Gee, Dudgeon et al. 2014.
22   Dudgeon, Milroy and Walker 2014; Gee, Dudgeon et al. 2014.

or stressful life events are risk factors for mental health disorders[23] and "Western" mental health approaches that do not incorporate Aboriginal and Torres Strait Islander knowledge systems have contributed to poor access and treatment outcomes for many Aboriginal and Torres Strait Islander people.[24]

Mental health and substance use disorders are a leading contributor (19 per cent) to the illness experienced by Aboriginal and Torres Strait Islander people.[25] In 2018–19, an estimated 24 per cent (187,500) of those surveyed reported a mental health or behavioural condition, with a higher rate among men than women. Anxiety was most reported (17 per cent), followed by depression (13 per cent). Sixty-six per cent of adults reported "low or moderate" levels of psychological distress and 31 per cent reported "high or very high" levels.[26] Lower access to primary mental health care according to need has resulted in over-representation of First Nations clients in other parts of the health and mental health system. Hospitalisation rates for mental health, behavioural disorders and alcohol-related conditions are disproportionally high and suicide rates are especially concerning.[27]

As discussed in Chapter 14, Aboriginal and Torres Strait Islander young people are deeply concerned about mental health. The Mission Australia 2022[28] youth survey found that, while 28 per cent of Aboriginal and Torres Strait Islander young people (aged 15–19) rated their mental health as excellent or very good, over one third (34 per cent) reported feeling high psychological distress. Forty per cent didn't know where to go for help and only 62 per cent of those who sought help consulted a health professional. Accessible culturally safe treatment pathways that can cater for the complex sociocultural factors faced by Aboriginal and Torres Strait Islander children and young people are essential for healthy futures.

Improving the mental health and wellbeing of Aboriginal and Torres Strait Islander families and communities requires systemic and transformative change,[29] deep respect for Indigenous perspectives on wellbeing, Indigenous-led responses and a workforce skilled in trauma-informed care. Current policies refer to the importance of strengthening the cultural – as well as social and biomedical – determinants of health through languages, relationships, customs and community networks.[30] Across Australia, Aboriginal and Torres Strait Islander communities have developed programs to strengthen Indigenous identity, resilience, wellbeing and empowerment. These programs, like the Family Wellbeing Program (see Box 15.1), focus on strengths while also reducing social and emotional wellbeing stressors (risks) and improving the capacity of communities and services to cope with these.[31] They are an important part of comprehensive primary health care for Aboriginal and Torres Strait Islander people.

23   Commonwealth of Australia 2017; Dudgeon, Milroy and Walker 2014; Paradies, Ben et al. 2015.
24   Dudgeon, Bray et al. 2020.
25   Australian Institute of Health and Welfare 2016.
26   Australian Bureau of Statistics 2019.
27   Australian Institute of Health and Welfare 2022b; Commonwealth of Australia 2017; Dudgeon, Milroy and Walker 2014.
28   Leung, Brennan et al. 2022.
29   McGorry, Bates and Birchwood 2013.
30   Department of Health 2017.
31   Dudgeon, Bray et al. 2017.

> **Box 15.1 The Family Wellbeing Program**
>
> The Family Wellbeing Program is a learning and empowerment program based on Aboriginal and Torres Strait Islander cultural knowledge and frameworks, while incorporating Western knowledge. Completion of all five stages of the program provides participants with a nationally accredited qualification in counselling.[32]
>
> > "The Family Wellbeing Program involves teaching participants about social and emotional needs in a way that allows them to go on and share this learning with others … It teaches problem-solving skills that help us to build resilience and deal with managing relationships, conflicts, addiction and violence. We then use this empowerment to … bring community members together to take action on larger social issues that matter to us."
>
> – Leslie Baird, National Centre for Family Wellbeing.
>
> Since the Family Wellbeing Program was developed in 1993, by and for Aboriginal people, the program has been adapted and delivered in at least 60 locations. It has helped Aboriginal and Torres Strait Islander participants to take control over the conditions affecting their lives and target critical issues like suicide using community-based solutions. Quality improvement processes have been used to adapt the program to local communities.[33]
>
> There is further potential to use CQI to systematically strengthen links between program activities and clinical PHC, and to capture and build on community wellbeing stories.

Recommended mental health and social and emotional wellbeing care in clinical PHC

Stresses on social and emotional wellbeing exist for all populations and all age groups. Therefore, screening and care for social and emotional wellbeing is relevant across the life course and as part of the management of many health conditions. It can prevent mental health and wellbeing issues from developing into more serious disorders and supports early intervention. High-quality PHC supports children and adults living with mental illness – and those who care for and support them – with effective clinical and non-clinical services.

These are among the essential clinical services in PHC:

- mental health and social and emotional wellbeing promotion and prevention services
- screening for social and emotional wellbeing
- brief interventions or referral when people are assessed as at risk for social and emotional wellbeing challenges
- screening, brief interventions and referral for substance misuse
- early identification and treatment of mental health disorders

---

32   Prince, Jeffrey et al. 2018.
33   McCalman, Bainbridge et al. 2018.

- management of stable psychiatric clients
- counselling for common mental health disorders
- referral to other services when required.

PHC practitioners should provide client-centred care within their expertise and capabilities, and coordinate clients' access to other care providers (for example, psychologists, social workers, occupational therapists) and appropriate agencies. These might be government, private or community-based services, cultural healers, community Elders or religious leaders, community or family members.

Some clients experience multiple social and emotional wellbeing and mental health issues in addition to the negative effects of social determinants such as poverty, racism and housing issues. In these circumstances, it may be appropriate to begin with case management and problem-solving approaches to tackle these issues, and to support clients to establish safety, security and stability before focusing on other healing processes.[34] Individualised mental health care plans can provide a framework for coordination and continuity of care. A well-designed care plan, reviewed on a regular basis, promotes communication across disciplines and client engagement.

Clinical practice guidelines are available for the prevention and management of mental health disorders. They include guidelines for managing specific conditions, such as depression, complex trauma and post-traumatic stress, and guidelines for working with specific groups, such as refugees or First Nations people. We recommend searching reliable online sources for guidelines and resources that are relevant for your PHC context and clients' needs.

Findings: quality of mental health care

The data presented below come mainly from six research papers and a key report published by the ABCD CQI research program between 2011 and 2019. A mental health audit tool[35] and the systems assessment tool[36] were used to collect data about the delivery of mental health care from 21 PHC centres between 2009 and 2014. These are the most recent audit data available. Analysis was conducted on 975 records for Aboriginal and Torres Strait Islander clients with a diagnosed mental health disorder to assess how well care reflected best-practice guidelines for mental health and wellbeing care. Stakeholders participated in data interpretation to identify priority evidence–practice gaps and factors influencing improvement.

---

34   Gee, Dudgeon et al. 2014.
35   Menzies School of Health Research 2014.
36   Menzies School of Health Research and One21seventy 2012.

Routine items of mental health care

Risk factors and brief interventions

Analysis of 314 client records in 17 services (2012–2014) found that, in the 12 months before the audit, the recording of risk factors and brief interventions varied between PHC centres and risk factors:

- 80 per cent of mental health clients had their alcohol use recorded; 70 per cent of high-risk alcohol users received brief interventions or counselling for alcohol use
- 85 per cent had their tobacco use recorded; 55 per cent of smokers received brief interventions or counselling for smoking
- 75 per cent (range 30–100 per cent) of clients who had drug misuse noted received brief intervention or counselling for drug misuse
- 33 per cent (range 0–80 per cent) of clients with a body mass index of more than 25 had a record of brief intervention or counselling for overweight or obesity
- the recording of mental health risk factors and interventions varied widely across PHC centres.[37]

Follow-up if mental health deteriorated

The research also examined whether follow-up action was recorded for clients who experienced worsening or deteriorating symptoms and behaviours related to a mental health disorder. These concerns included sleep patterns and mood, hallucinations, psychotic symptoms, medication side effects, aggressive behaviour, social withdrawal or deterioration in self-care. When worsening symptoms were recorded in client records:

- an average of 70 per cent of clients (range 30–100 per cent) were referred to another health professional, and 75 per cent received psychosocial or culturally appropriate interventions
- 70 per cent of clients had their medication reviewed; 40 per cent of these clients had their medication adjusted.[38]

Mental health care plans and shared care arrangements

- On average, only 50 per cent of mental health clients had a mental health care plan.
- Where care plans were recorded, most included both clinical goals and self-management or recovery goals (average of 90 per cent and 83 per cent respectively). There was more variation in the recording of self-management or recovery goals than clinical goals.
- Review of goals in the three months before the audit varied widely across PHC centres (average of 65 per cent; range 0–100 per cent) (see Figure 15.2).[39]
- Shared care arrangements and referrals were not well documented (median 55 per cent, range 0–100 per cent).[40]

---

37   Matthews, J. Bailie et al. 2016.
38   Matthews, J. Bailie et al. 2016.
39   Matthews, J. Bailie et al. 2016.
40   Matthews, J. Bailie et al. 2016.

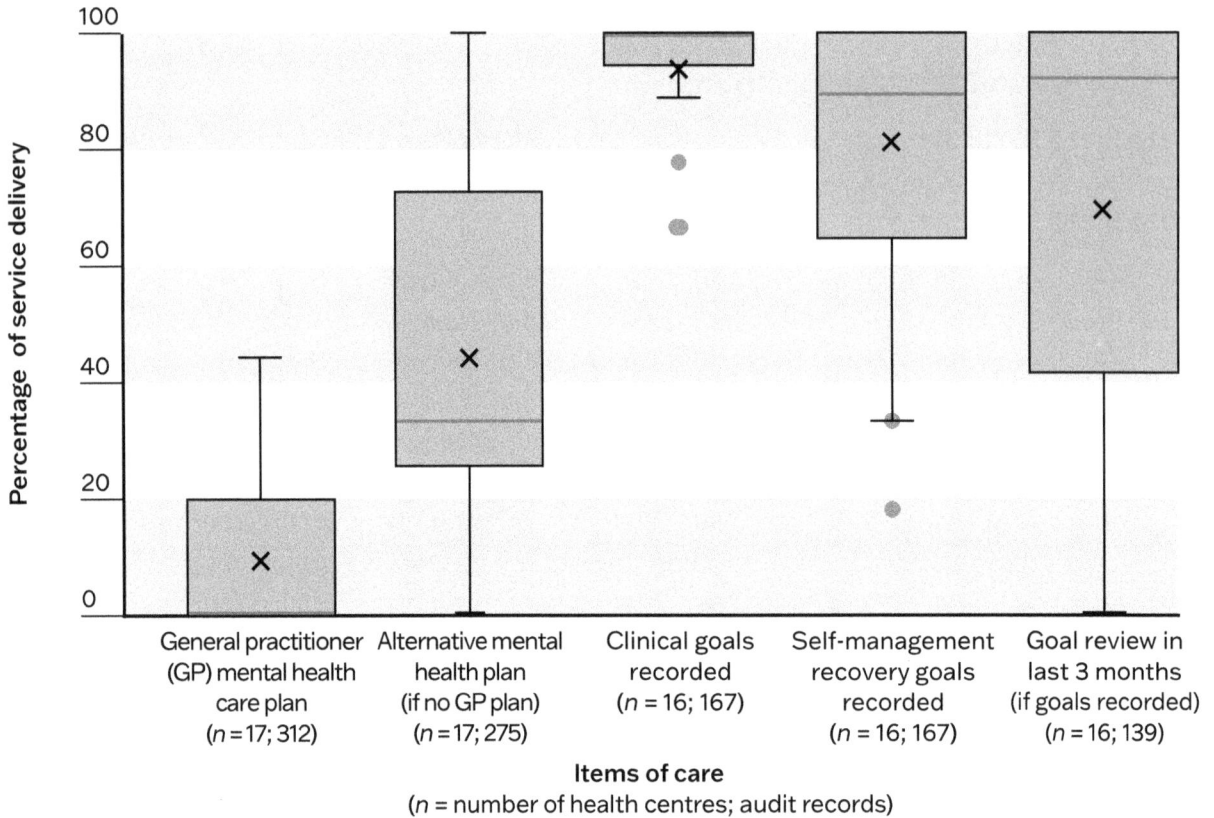

Figure 15.2 Mean percentage of health centre clients with a care plan and associated goals in their medical records. Source: Matthews, J. Bailie et al. 2016.

Overall mental health care

We analysed mental health audit data from PHC centres over three years (2011–2013). While overall levels of service delivery for mental health care were steady, lower performing health centres had improved care for clients diagnosed with mental health conditions.

- There was no clear improvement in the overall service delivery of mental health and wellbeing care. The mean and median level of care delivery was about 60 per cent over the three years (see Figure 15.3).
- There was less variation in quality of care between PHC centres, mainly because lower performing PHC centres improved their delivery of mental health services.
- Based on 12 best-practice indicators for mental health care, the lower performing PHC centres improved their overall delivery of mental health care, from 30 per cent in 2011 to around 50 per cent in 2012 and 2013[41] (see Figure 15.3).

The 12 best-practice indicators were recording of alchohol, tobacco and drug use; brief interventions for alcohol and drug misuse; health check withing the last 12 months; blood pressure check within the last 6 months; mental health assessment, if client had attended within the last 3 months; provision of social issues and family or individual counselling, if client had attended within the last 3 months; joint discussion regarding culturally apppropiate interventions, if client had attended within the last 3 months; liver function test; serum

---

41   Matthews, J. Bailie et al. 2016.

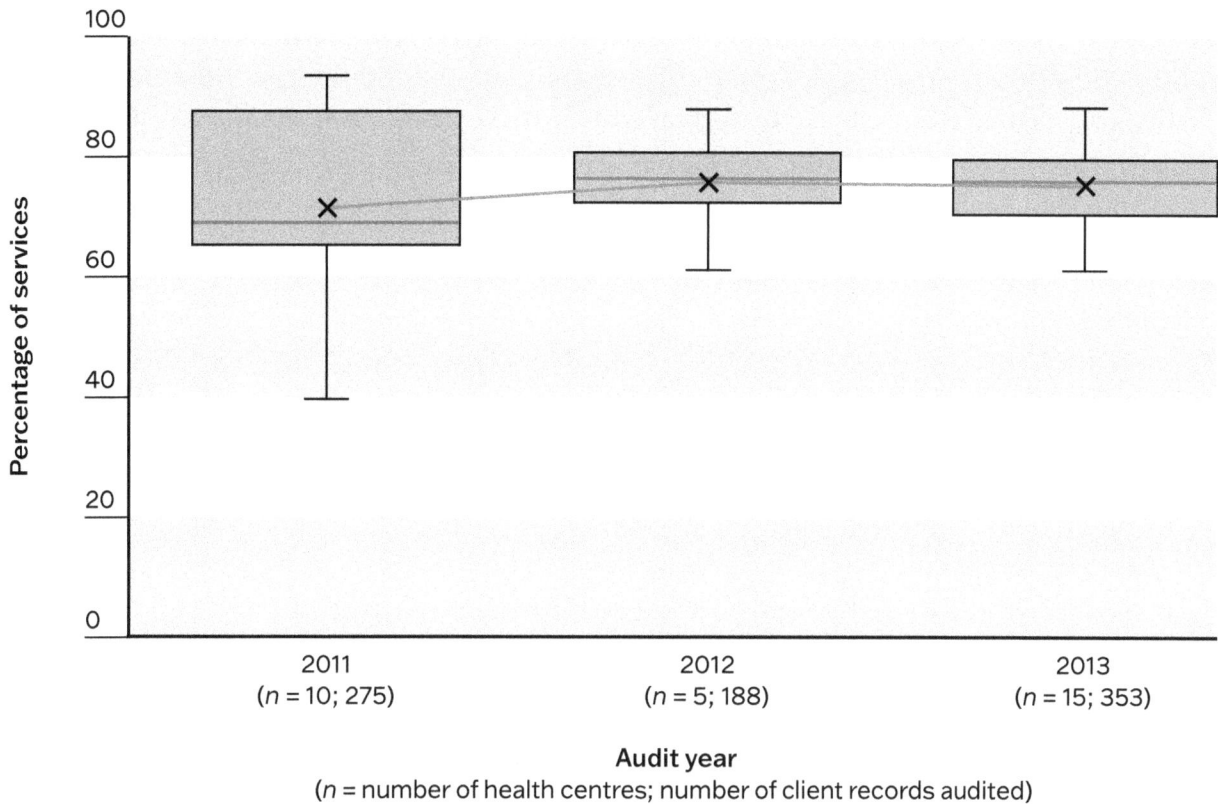

Figure 15.3 Trends in overall mental health care for 12 best-practice indicators. Source: Matthews, J. Bailie et al. 2016.

creatinine; thyroid function test; full blood count; and follow-up action, including medication review and adjustment, referral or psychosocial or culturally appropriate intervention if deteroriation in symptoms.

Systems supporting mental health care

Twenty-nine assessments of the PHC systems supporting mental health care were also analysed by researchers and PHC stakeholders. Systems assessments evaluate delivery system design, information systems and decision support, client self-management support, links with community, other health services and resources, and organisational influence and system integration.[42] There were two key findings for informing system improvement:

- 100 per cent of surveyed stakeholders viewed organisational commitment to structures and processes for safe, high-quality mental health care as a priority for improvement
- 90 per cent viewed community involvement in planning mental health and wellbeing services as a priority.[43]

---

42   Menzies School of Health Research and One21seventy 2012.
43   Matthews, J. Bailie et al. 2016.

Findings: quality of screening and care for social and emotional wellbeing

The findings about the quality of screening and care for social and emotional wellbeing come from the use of four ABCD audit tools: adult preventive care, type 2 diabetes care, maternal care and child health. Altogether, more than 9,400 health records were analysed. Across the audit data, patterns emerged about the quality of social and emotional wellbeing care.

Preventive care

Preventive health records for 3,407 adults in 100 PHC centres (2012–2014) were analysed. According to health records:

- social and emotional wellbeing screening was not undertaken for 73 per cent of clients
- no further action was taken for 25 per cent of screened clients for whom a concern was recorded
- when a treatment plan was documented, follow-up was poor.

As Figure 15.4 illustrates, this represents a combined management gap of 75 per cent.

The analysis also found there was more screening of younger adults (younger than 30 years) and people older than 55 years compared with other age groups. Lower rates of screening were associated with larger service populations (more than 1,000) and health service participation in fewer CQI cycles.[44]

It is a similar story across care for health conditions, not just for preventive care.

Diabetes care

Comorbidity of mental health disorders with chronic conditions is common. Given the increased likelihood of poor levels of SEWB for those with diabetes, screening and follow-up action is an important aspect of clinical care. A study of 1,174 records of people with diabetes from 44 PHC centres (2009) also found low screening rates for social and emotional wellbeing.

- Only 5 per cent of clients with diabetes had been screened, with only four of the 44 PHC centres using a standard depression or distress screening tool in the past year.
- 37 to 67 per cent of people with diabetes were screened in those health centres where screening had been done. A record of screening was much less likely for people with severe diabetes-related disease compared to people with less severe disease.
- Documented depression ranged from 0 to 33 per cent between health centres. Regardless of whether they had been screened, 6 per cent of clients across 24 health centres had a documented diagnosis of depression, while 5 per cent had a diagnosis of another mental illness.
- 39 per cent of clients with a current prescription for antidepressant medication did not have a documented diagnosis of depression or other mental illness in their health records.[45]

---

44   Langham, McCalman et al. 2017.
45   Schierhout, Nagel et al. 2013.

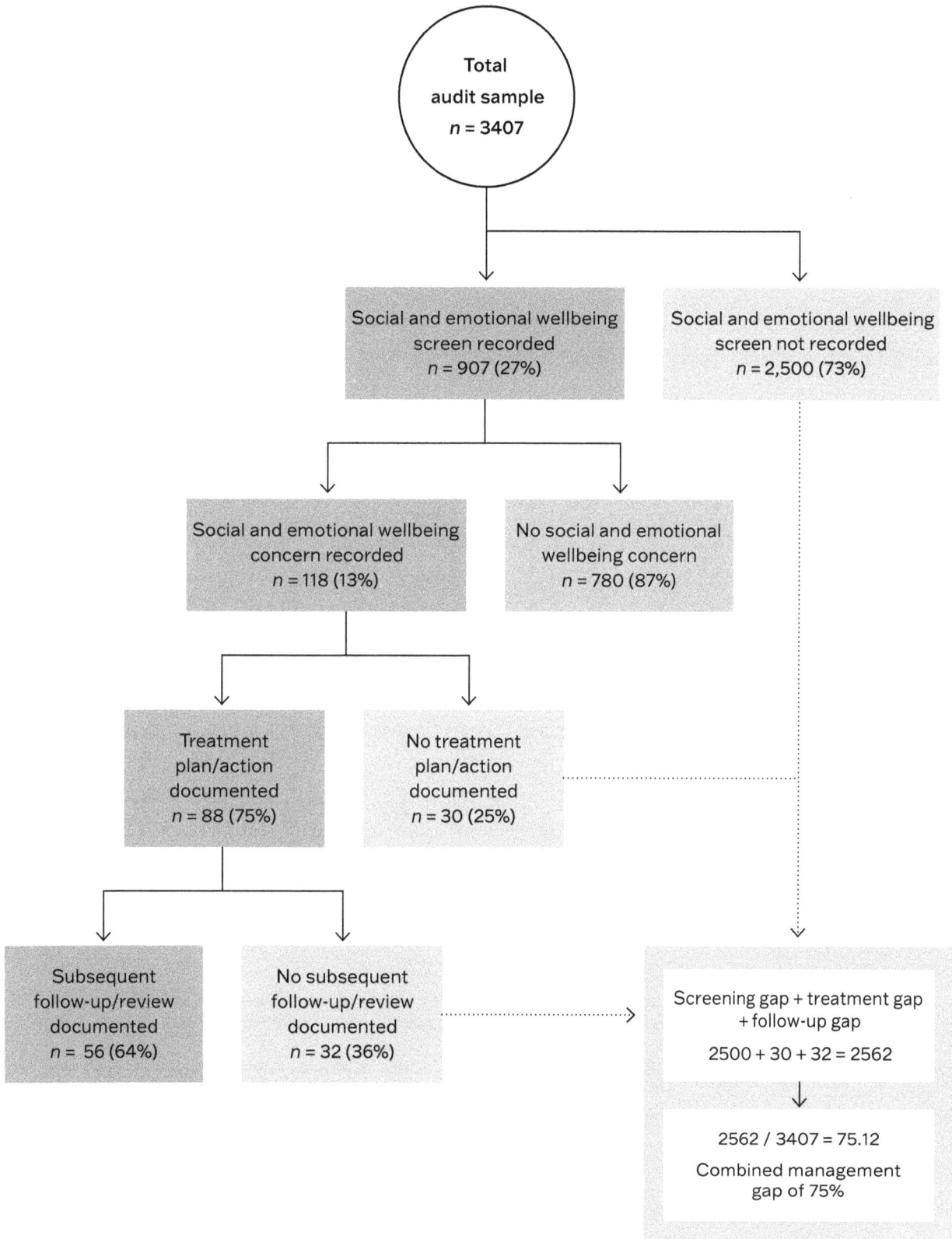

Figure 15.4 Social and emotional wellbeing screening and management: gaps in screening, treatment and follow-up. Source: Langham, McCalman et al. 2017.

An earlier study of 1,592 records of people with diabetes from 62 PHC settings had also found inconsistencies in the recording of diagnoses for depression and prescribed medications:

- 62 out of the 140 clients with a recorded diagnosis of depression had no record of antidepressant medication being prescribed
- 45 clients with diabetes had a prescription for selective serotonin reuptake inhibitors (SSRIs) recorded, without a recorded diagnosis of depression.[46]

The study raised questions about whether health professionals working in Indigenous settings chose not to use screening tools based in Western medical models (see "Improving mental health and wellbeing care in Aboriginal and Torres Strait Islander PHC" section below), whether they resisted making a diagnosis of depression, or whether other mental disorders were being treated with antidepressant medications.

Pregnancy care

Analysis of 797 maternal health records from 36 PHC settings (2010–2012) found scope for improvement, particularly for emotional wellbeing screening.

- Only 17 per cent of all women had a record of emotional wellbeing screening during pregnancy, despite 86 per cent of women having at least four antenatal visits.
- Most women had records of assessment for social (79 per cent) and medical (86 per cent) risk factors, and risk factors such as use of cigarettes (78 per cent), alcohol (57 per cent) and illicit drugs (53 per cent) in pregnancy.
- Emotional wellbeing screening was more likely when social risk factors were noted, and when health professionals noted plans for care and birthing, antenatal education and breastfeeding.[47]
- 16 per cent of women identified at risk of depression were prescribed antidepressant drugs during their pregnancy.[48]
- Non-pharmaceutical interventions for pregnant women assessed as being at risk of having their SEWB affected included brief intervention (61 per cent), counselling (57 per cent) and cognitive behaviour therapy (5 per cent).
- About 39 per cent of women at risk of having their SEWB affected were referred to external services.[49]

Care for families of young children

Analysis of 2,466 health records of Indigenous children from 109 PHC centres (2012–14) found scope for improvement in service provision and in follow-up or referral when concerns were noted.

- PHC centres used the national best-practice guidelines for social and emotional wellbeing care and included important services (for example, advice about child stimulation and behaviour, and parent–child interaction).

---

46   Si, Dowden et al. 2011.
47   Gausia, Thompson et al. 2013.
48   Gausia, Thompson et al. 2015.
49   Gausia, Thompson et al. 2015.

- The proportion of families receiving social and emotional wellbeing services ranged from 11 per cent (advice about nutrition and food security) to 75 per cent (assessment of parent–child interaction).
- Almost 25 per cent of families had no clinical follow-up or referral for concerns about domestic environment, family support and financial situation, housing condition and food security.
- Families of children aged 3–11 months (40 per cent) were more likely to receive social and emotional wellbeing services than families of children aged 12–59 months (30 per cent).
- Families living in remote areas received similar services to rural and urban families.[50]

Emerging patterns and recent developments

Our research found that some aspects of social and emotional wellbeing care were being done well (for example, assessment of risk factors for pregnant women). However, data collected using four different audit tools (adult preventive care, type 2 diabetes care, maternal care and child health) showed many opportunities for improvement. There was considerable variation in quality of care between health centres. This is not surprising. Until recently, social and emotional wellbeing care received relatively less attention than care for physical conditions in PHC. Since we analysed these CQI data, there have been important developments in mental health, social and emotional wellbeing care and in suicide prevention for Aboriginal and Torres Strait Islander communities. Culturally sensitive screening tools (for example, aPHQ-9), [51] clinical guidelines and social and emotional wellbeing services have become more widely available. We would expect these developments to be reflected in more recently collected CQI data. Services that start from a low baseline have greater potential for large and rapid improvements in care quality.

> Services that start from a low baseline have greater potential for large and rapid improvements in care quality.

Australia has adopted a stepped care model of primary mental health care. Stepped care aims to deliver the most effective yet least resource-intensive treatment to clients first, only "stepping up" to intensive and specialist services as clinically required.[52] CQI has an important role in advancing the system changes needed to strengthen stepped care and to implement further evidence-based developments. CQI processes can be used to improve systems at each of the five steps:

- health promotion and preventive care for well populations
- early intervention for at-risk groups
- access to low-intensity services for those with mild mental illness
- provision of services and interventions for people with moderate illness
- adequate levels of intervention to maximise recovery, prevent escalation and provide wraparound coordinated care for people with severe mental illness.

---

50   Edmond, McAuley et al. 2018.
51   Getting it Right Collaborative Group, Hackett et al. 2019.
52   Commonwealth of Australia 2017.

Key messages for improving mental health and wellbeing care in PHC

Although there are important differences between settings, the patterns of delivery for mental health and wellbeing care in Aboriginal and Torres Strait Islander PHC are likely to reflect care delivery in many international settings. In addition, the issues experienced and the solutions suggested by Aboriginal and Torres Strait Islander communities may be relevant to other populations that experience a high burden of grief and trauma.

The CQI research (2005–14) supports long-standing key messages from international PHC[53] about how to improve mental health and wellbeing care across the life span, as part of PHC. There is a need for these features to be acted on:

- organisational commitment to a culture, structures and processes that promote high-quality mental health and wellbeing care across the life span

- integrated care strategies that are tailored to PHC and community settings

- teamwork that creates collaborative healthcare teams with the right mix of skills and clear allocation of roles and responsibilities

- training, supervision and support of PHC staff by mental health professionals

- strong links between PHC services, communities, schools and support groups for mental health promotion and prevention, service planning and resource development

- connection by PHC services with other agencies and sectors that address social, economic and environmental determinants of health (for example, safety, social support, housing, education, employment, food security)

- embedding of CQI processes into mental health and wellbeing services and programs.

Common gaps

To improve care for people diagnosed with a mental health disorder, systems need to be strengthened in these ways:

- increase staff understanding of mental health and disorders, and ability to recognise and respond to psychosocial distress and depression

- record mental health plans, shared care arrangements and referrals

- record risk factors and brief interventions, particularly for alcohol and drug misuse

- follow up clients with mental disorders whose symptoms are getting worse.

To improve social and emotional wellbeing care for all clients, systems need to be strengthened in these ways:

---

53   WHO and Wonca 2008; Davis, Balasubramanian et al. 2013.

- educate staff to understand the many influences on social and emotional wellbeing, including risk factors and protective factors specific to population groups served (for example, LGBTQI+ people, refugees, Indigenous people)

- train PHC staff in social and emotional wellbeing assessment, brief interventions, counselling and management

- provide social and emotional wellbeing screening across client groups of all ages as part of holistic care

- document wellbeing assessments, actions taken and follow-up care in client health records[54]

- integrate community-based, youth-guided and children- and family-centred care into social and emotional wellbeing services[55] (see also Chapter 14).

All of these strategies require ongoing policy commitment to improve PHC systems and resources for providing high-quality mental health and wellbeing care.

Improving mental health and wellbeing care in Aboriginal and Torres Strait Islander PHC

Our CQI research findings support calls for strategies that integrate mental health and social and emotional wellbeing care into PHC; engage communities in social and emotional wellbeing programs; and strengthen cross-sector action to address mental health risks and protect wellbeing. Community-controlled health services are well positioned to lead the way in developing such strategies, because they have developed from models of comprehensive PHC based on a holistic concept of health with the cultural, social and emotional wellbeing of families at their centre.[56]

Whatever governance arrangements are in place, responding to high demands for acute and chronic illness care amongst service populations can constrain the capacity of PHC services to provide social and emotional wellbeing services. In addition, practitioners working in Aboriginal and Torres Strait Islander communities are often confronted with complex client presentations for mental health care. For example, community members may be simultaneously experiencing mental health issues, loss and cultural disconnection, financial hardship and child removal.[57] Aboriginal and Torres Strait Islander staff may themselves experience significant wellbeing stressors, including stressors that come from identifying with the trauma experienced by their clients. Supporting the social and emotional wellbeing of the Aboriginal and Torres Strait Islander workforce is critical.

Our CQI research identified enablers for improving mental health and wellbeing care for Aboriginal and Torres Strait Islander clients and communities, including these features:

---

54   Edmond, McAuley et al. 2018; Gausia, Thompson et al. 2015; Langham, McCalman et al. 2017; Schierhout, Nagel et al. 2013.

55   McCalman, Bainbridge et al. 2020.

56   Anaf, Baum et al. 2014; Edmond, McAuley et al. 2018.

57   Gee, Dudgeon et al. 2014.

- good systems for recruiting, supporting and retaining PHC staff, particularly Aboriginal and Torres Strait Islander staff
- strong systems for providing PHC teams with training and support from mental health professionals
- effective strategies for building and sharing staff understanding and skills in culturally appropriate mental health and wellbeing care
- strong links between health services, communities and other agencies providing mental health and SEWB care, focusing on holistic and strengths-based approaches.[58]

The research findings showed that, at the time of data collection, many opportunities for social and emotional wellbeing screening and care were not taken up. One suggested reason was practitioners' concern about the cultural suitability of screening tools based on Western medical models. This concern is being tackled through the development or adaptation of assessment tools such as the Here and Now Aboriginal Assessment tool,[59] the Aboriginal and Torres Strait Islander Perinatal Mental Health guide for PHC professionals[60] and the adapted Patient Health Questionnaire 9, which has phrasing culturally adapted for five Australian Aboriginal language groups.[61] The Centre of Best Practice in Aboriginal and Torres Strait Islander Suicide Prevention Clearing House has links to a range of validated tools and checklists. The *National guide to a preventive health assessment for Aboriginal and Torres Strait Islander people* includes guidance for the prevention of depression and suicide.[62] The uptake of screening tools should continue to improve as more culturally based tools and guidelines are developed.

Screening alone provides minimal benefit and has the potential to cause harm.[63] To be beneficial at an individual client or population level, screening needs to be part of a broader, culturally competent assessment process entailing these aspects:

- formal training in culturally appropriate assessment
- a comprehensive client interview to explain and determine the appropriate assessment processes and any required screening
- reflective documentation of the process
- interpretation and reporting of results using cultural explanations and avoidance of labelling.[64]

As with all clinical assessments, there must be systems in place to ensure that a diagnosis of abnormal findings is followed by guideline-based treatment and follow-up care.[65]

Screening tools focus on identifying deficits and risk factors. While these are useful, identifying strengths and protective factors is integral to a comprehensive assessment[66] and can support a social and emotional wellbeing care plan that helps to empower the person.

---

58   Matthews, J. Bailie et al. 2016.
59   Janca, Lyons et al. 2015.
60   Beyondblue 2013.
61   Getting it Right Collaborative Group, Hackett et al. 2019.
62   National Aboriginal Community Controlled Health Organisation and Royal Australian College 2024.
63   Martin, Potter et al. 2016; Woolf and Harris 2012.
64   Langham, McCalman et al. 2017.
65   Dobrow, Sullivan et al. 2018.
66   Haswell-Elkins, Hunter et al. 2009.

Such a plan builds on individual, family and community strengths (for example, education, loving family, support networks, cultural involvement). Resources for frontline health and wellbeing workers, made by and for Aboriginal and Torres Strait Islander people, are brought together on the Wellmob website.[67] Other resources are available.[68]

Aboriginal and Torres Strait Islander leadership and policy support for social and emotional wellbeing, mental health and suicide prevention are well established.[69] In communities, culturally capable and responsive PHC services, shaped by community-led health initiatives, have a key role in protecting social and emotional wellbeing, improving mental health and wellbeing care and supporting the self-determination of individuals and communities. PHC teams need to be supported by respected community leaders and organisations, using best-practice guidelines that identify appropriate strategies for developing care plans, including protocols for treatment, referral pathways and follow-up with PHC staff.[70]

The use of CQI supports PHC teams and communities to improve mental health and social and emotional wellbeing care. Coordination between health and other service providers, such as education, employment, housing and justice, will help to support a holistic approach to promoting social and emotional wellbeing (see Box 15.2).[71]

Box 15.2 Improving social and emotional wellbeing services for boarding school students

In recent years, Australian government policies have promoted access to secondary education through boarding schools for Aboriginal and Torres Strait Islander students from remote communities. These students experience the poorest health of any Australian adolescent group. Adjusting to being away from family and community, changes in culture and language, school and academic expectations can further challenge wellbeing. While these students have high levels of risk and distress, they report themselves as having good health: this raises the possibility that they are normalising stress. This in turn creates the potential that boarding schools may fail to identify students' needs and refer the students appropriately.[72]

Boarding school health staff support student-centred health care and wellbeing by weaving a relational network with students, families, school staff and external healthcare providers, but as one Aboriginal and Torres Strait Islander healthcare practitioner commented: "It can't just be left to individuals to know everybody. It's gotta be in the system and we've got to work out ways to make sure that none of our students drop through holes."[73]

---

67   WellMob. n.d. https://wellmob.org.au/.
68   Australian Indigenous Health*InfoNet*. n.d. https://healthinfonet.ecu.edu.au/.
69   Gayaa Dhuwi (Proud Spirit) Australia. n.d. https://www.gayaadhuwi.org.au/.
70   Langham, McCalman et al. 2017.
71   Carson, Dunbar et al. 2007; McCalman, Langham et al. 2020.
72   McCalman, Bainbridge and Benveniste 2019.
73   McCalman, Langham et al. 2020, 11.

Providing and integrating care to meet the needs of remote-dwelling Indigenous students is complex and needs an integrated, systems approach. Communication and feedback linkages between students, parents and kin, healthcare services and schools are key.[74] A CQI approach can help to identify and take opportunities to strengthen systems for student care.

See also Chapter 14.

References

Anaf, J., F. Baum, T. Freeman, R. Labonte, S. Javanparast, G. Jolley et al. (2014). Factors shaping intersectoral action in primary health care services. *Australian and New Zealand Journal of Public Health* 38(6): 553–9. DOI: 10.1111/1753-6405.12284.

Australian Bureau of Statistics (2019). *National Aboriginal and Torres Strait Islander health survey, 2018–19*. Cat. no. 4715.0. Canberra: ABS.

Australian Indigenous Health*InfoNet*. n.d. Edith Cowan University. https://healthinfonet.ecu.edu.au/.

Australian Institute of Health and Welfare (2022a). *Australia's health 2022: First Nations People – Indigenous health and wellbeing*. Canberra: Australian Government.

Australian Institute of Health and Welfare (2022b). *Mental health services in Australia: mental health: prevalence and impact*. Canberra: Australian Government.

Australian Institute of Health and Welfare (2016). *Australian Burden of Disease study: impact and causes of illness and death in Aboriginal and Torres Strait Islander people 2011*. Australian Burden of Disease Study. Canberra: AIHW.

Beyondblue (2013). *Aboriginal and Torres Strait Islander perinatal mental health: a guide for primary care health professionals*. Melbourne: beyondblue.

Carson, B., T. Dunbar, R. Chenhall and R. Bailie, eds (2007). *Social determinants of Indigenous health*. Sydney: Allen & Unwin.

Commonwealth of Australia (2017). *National Strategic Framework for Aboriginal and Torres Strait Islander Peoples' mental health and social and emotional wellbeing 2017–2023*. Canberra: Department of the Prime Minister and Cabinet.

Davis, M., B. Balasubramanian, E. Waller, B. Miller, L. Green and D. Cohen (2013). Integrating behavioral and physical health care in the real world: early lessons from Advancing Care Together. *Journal of the American Board of Family Medicine* 26(5): 588–602. DOI: 10.3122/jabfm.2013.05.130028.

Department of Health (2017). *My life my lead – opportunities for strengthening approaches to the social determinants and cultural determinants of Indigenous health: report on the national consultations December 2017*. Canberra: Commonwealth of Australia.

Dobrow, M., T. Sullivan, L. Rabeneck, V. Hagens and R. Chafe (2018). Consolidated principles for screening based on a systematic review and consensus process. *Canadian Medical Association Journal* 190(14): E422–E29. DOI: 10.1503/cmaj.171154.

Drake R., A. Binagwaho, H. Martell and A. Mulley. (2014). Mental health care in low and middle income countries. *BMJ* 349(g7086). DOI: 10.1136/bmj.g7086.

Dudgeon, P., A. Bray, D. Darlaston-Jones and R. Walker (2020). *Aboriginal participatory action research: an Indigenous research methodology strengthening decolonisation and social and emotional wellbeing*. Discussion Paper. Melbourne: Lowitja Institute.

Dudgeon, P., A. Bray, B. D'Costa and R. Walker (2017). Decolonising psychology: validating social and emotional wellbeing. *Australian Psychologist* 52(4): 316–25. DOI: 10.1111/ap.12294.

Dudgeon, P., H. Milroy and R. Walker, eds (2014). *Working together: Aboriginal and Torres Strait Islander mental health and wellbeing principles and practice*, 2nd edn. Canberra: Australian Council

---

74   McCalman, Bainbridge et al. 2020.

for Education Research and Telethon Institute for Child Health Research, Office for Aboriginal and Torres Strait Islander Health, Department of Health and Ageing.

Edmond, K., K. McAuley, D. McAullay, V. Matthews, N. Strobel, R. Marriott et al. (2018). Quality of social and emotional wellbeing services for families of young Indigenous children attending primary care centers; a cross sectional analysis. *BMC Health Services Research* 18(1). DOI: 10.1186/s12913-018-2883-6.

Funk, M., S. Wutzke, E. Kaner, P. Anderson, L. Pas, R. McCormick et al. (2005). A multicountry controlled trial of strategies to promote dissemination and implementation of brief alcohol intervention in primary health care: findings of a World Health Organization collaborative study. *Journal of Studies on Alcohol and Drugs* 66(3): 379–88. DOI: 10.15288/jsa.2005.66.379.

Gausia, K., S. Thompson, T. Nagel, A. Rumbold, C. Connors, V. Matthews et al. (2013). Antenatal emotional wellbeing screening in Aboriginal and Torres Strait Islander primary health care services in Australia. *Contemporary Nurse: A Journal for the Australian Nursing Profession* 46(1): 73–82. DOI: 10.5172/conu.2013.46.1.73.

Gausia, K., S. Thompson, T. Nagel, G. Schierhout, V. Matthews and R. Bailie (2015). Risk of antenatal psychosocial distress in Indigenous women and its management at primary health care centres in Australia. *General Hospital Psychiatry* 37(4): 335–9. DOI: 10.1016/j.genhosppsych.2015.04.005.

Gayaa Dhuwi (Proud Spirit) Australia (n.d.). *Aboriginal and Torres Strait Islander Leadership in social and emotional wellbeing, mental health and suicide prevention.* https://www.gayaadhuwi.org.au/.

Gee, G., P. Dudgeon, C. Schultz, A. Hart and K. Kelly (2014). Aboriginal and Torres Strait Islander social and emotional wellbeing. In P. Dudgeon, H. Milroy and R. Walker, eds. *Working together: Aboriginal and Torres Strait Islander health and wellbeing principles and practice*, 2nd edn, 55–68. Canberra: Australian Council for Education Research and Telethon Institute for Child Health Research, Office for Aboriginal and Torres Strait Islander Health, Department of Health and Ageing.

Getting it Right Collaborative Group, M. Hackett, A. Teixeira-Pinto, S. Farnbach, N. Glozier, T. Skinner et al. (2019). Getting it right: validating a culturally specific screening tool for depression (aPHQ- 9) in Aboriginal and Torres Strait Islander Australians. *Medical Journal of Australia* 211(1): 24–30. DOI: 10.5694/mja2.50212.

Haswell-Elkins, M., E. Hunter, T. Nagel, C. Thompson, B. Hall, R. Mills et al. (2005). Reflections on integrating mental health into primary health care services in remote Indigenous communities in Far North Queensland and the Northern Territory. *Australian Journal of Primary Health* 11(2): 62–9. DOI: 10.1071/PY05023.

Haswell-Elkins, M., E. Hunter, R. Wargent, B. Hall, C. O'Higgins and R. West (2009). *Protocols for the delivery of social and emotional well being and mental health services in Indigenous communities: guidelines for health workers, clinicians, consumers and carers.* Cairns: Queensland Health.

Janca, A., Z. Lyons, S. Balaratnasingam, D. Parfitt, S. Davison and J. Laugharne (2015). Here and Now Aboriginal Assessment: background, development and preliminary evaluation of a culturally appropriate screening tool. *Australasian Psychiatry* 23(3): 287–92. DOI: 10.1177/1039856215584514.

Kwan, B. and D. Nease (2013). The state of the evidence for integrated behavioral health in primary care. In M.R. Talen and A. Burke Valeras, eds. *Integrated behavioral health in primary care: evaluating the evidence, identifying the essentials*, 65–98. New York: Springer New York. DOI: 10.1007/978-1-4614-6889-9_5.

Langham, E., J. McCalman, V. Matthews, R. Bainbridge, B. Nattabi, I. Kinchin et al. (2017). Social and emotional wellbeing screening for Aboriginal and Torres Strait Islanders within primary health care: a series of missed opportunities? *Frontiers in Public Health* 5(159). DOI: 10.3389/fpubh.2017.00159.

Leung, S., N. Brennan, T. Freeburn, W. Waugh and R. Christie (2022). *Youth survey report 2022.* Sydney: Mission Australia.

Martin, M., B. Potter, A. Crocker, G. Wells and I. Colman (2016). Yield and efficiency of mental health screening: a comparison of screening protocols at intake to prison. *PLOS One* 11(5): e0154106–e06. DOI: 10.1371/journal.pone.0154106.

Mathers, C. and D. Loncar (2006). Projections of global mortality and burden of disease from 2002 to 2030. *PLOS Medicine* 3(11): e442. DOI: 10.1371/journal.pmed.0030442.

Matthews, V., J. Bailie, A. Laycock, T. Nagel and R. Bailie (2016). *Priority evidence – practice gaps in Aboriginal and Torres Strait Islander mental health and wellbeing care: final report.* ESP Project. Brisbane: Menzies School of Health Research.

McCalman, J., R. Bainbridge and T. Benveniste (2019). The use and satisfaction with health care services of Aboriginal and Torres Strait Islander students at boarding schools: baseline results. *International Journal of Integrated Care* 19(S1): A435 1–8. DOI: 10.5334/ijic.s3435.

McCalman, J., R. Bainbridge, C. Brown, K. Tsey and A. Clarke (2018). The Aboriginal Australian Family Wellbeing Program: a historical analysis of the conditions that enabled its spread. *Frontiers in Public Health* 6: 26. DOI: 10.3389/fpubh.2018.00026.

McCalman, J., R. Bainbridge, Y. Cadet-James, R. Bailie, K. Tsey, V. Matthews et al. (2020). Systems integration to promote the mental health of Aboriginal and Torres Strait Islander children: protocol for a community-driven continuous quality improvement approach. *BMC Public Health* 20(1): 1810. DOI: 10.1186/s12889-020-09885-x.

McCalman, J., E. Langham, T. Benveniste, M. Wenitong, K. Rutherford, A. Britton et al. (2020). Integrating health care services for Indigenous Australian students at boarding schools: a mixed-methods sequential explanatory study. *International Journal of Integrated Care* 20(1): 8. DOI: 10.5334/ijic.4669.

McGorry, P., T. Bates and M. Birchwood (2013). Designing youth mental health services for the 21st century: examples from Australia, Ireland and the UK. *British Journal of Psychiatry* 202(s54): s30–s35. DOI: 10.1192/bjp.bp.112.119214.

McGorry, P., R. Purcell, I. Hickie and A. Jorm (2007). Investing in youth mental health is a best buy. *Medical Journal of Australia* 187(7). DOI: 10.5694/j.1326-5377.2007.tb01326.x.

Menzies School of Health Research (2014). Mental health clinical audit tool. One21seventy. Darwin: Menzies School of Health Research. https://www.menzies.edu.au/page/Resources/Mental_Health_clinical_audit/

Menzies School of Health Research and One21seventy (2012). Systems assessment tool – all client groups. Darwin: Menzies School of Health Research. https://www.menzies.edu.au/page/Resources/Systems_Assessment_Tool_SAT/

National Aboriginal Community Controlled Health Organisation and Royal Australian College of General Practitioners (2024). *National guide to a preventative health assessment for Aboriginal and Torres Strait Islander people*, 4th edn. Melbourne: RACGP.

Ngo, V., A. Rubinstein, V. Ganju, P. Kanellis, N. Loza, C. Rabadan-Diehl et al. (2013). Grand challenges: integrating mental health care into the non-communicable disease agenda. *PLOS Medicine* 10(5): e1001443. DOI: 10.1371/journal.pmed.1001443.

Ngo, V.K., J.R. Asarnow, J. Lange, L.H. Jaycox, M.M. Rea and C. Landon (2009). Outcomes for youths from racial-ethnic minority groups in a quality improvement intervention for depression treatment. *Psychiatric Services* 60(10): 1357–64. DOI: 10.1176/ps.2009.60.10.1357.

Nguyen, T., T. Tran, H. Tran, T.D. Tran and J. Fisher (2021). Challenges in integrating mental health into primary care in Vietnam. In S. Okpaku, ed. *Innovations in global mental health*, 1249–69. Switzerland: Springer International Publishing. DOI: 10.1007/978-3-030-57296-9_74.

Paradies, Y., J. Ben, N. Denson, A. Elias, N. Priest, A. Pieterse et al. (2015). Racism as a determinant of health: a systematic review and meta-analysis. *PLOS One* 10(9): e0138511. DOI: 10.1371/journal.pone.0138511.

Patel, V., R. Araya, S. Chatterjee, D. Chisholm, A. Cohen, M. De Silva et al. (2007). Treatment and prevention of mental disorders in low-income and middle-income countries. *Lancet* 370(9591): 991–1005. DOI: 10.1016/s0140-6736(07)61240-9.

Prince, J., N. Jeffrey, L. Baird, S. Kingsburra and B. Tipiloura (2018). *Stories from community: how suicide rates fell in two Indigenous communities.* Canberra: Healing Foundation.

Rehm, J. and K. Shield (2019). Global burden of disease and the impact of mental and addictive disorders. *Current Psychiatry Reports* 21(2): 10. DOI: 10.1007/s11920-019-0997-0.

Schierhout, G., T. Nagel, D. Si, C. Connors, A. Brown and R. Bailie (2013). Do competing demands of physical illness in type 2 diabetes influence depression screening, documentation and management in primary care: a cross-sectional analytic study in Aboriginal and Torres Strait Islander primary health care settings. *International Journal of Mental Health Systems* 7(1): 16. DOI: 10.1186/1752-4458-7-16.

Si, D., M. Dowden, C. Kennedy, R. Cox, L. O'Donoghue, H. Liddle et al. (2011). Indigenous community care: documented depression in patients with diabetes. *Australian Family Physician* 40(5): 331–3.

Wang, P., S. Aguilar-Gaxiola, J. Alonso, M. Angermeyer, G. Borges, E. Bromet et al. (2007). Use of mental health services for anxiety, mood, and substance disorders in 17 countries in the WHO world mental health surveys. *Lancet* 370(9590): 841–50. DOI: 10.1016/S0140-6736(07)61414-7.

WellMob: healing our way (n.d.). *Social, emotional and cultural wellbeing online resources for Aboriginal and Torres Strait Islander People.* https://wellmob.org.au.

WHO and Wonca (2008). *Integrating mental health into primary care: a global perspective.* Geneva: World Health Organization and World Organization of Family Doctors (Wonca).

Woolf, S.H. and R. Harris (2012). The harms of screening: new attention to an old concern. *JAMA : The Journal of the American Medical Association* 307(6): 565–6. DOI: 10.1001/jama.2012.100.

World Health Organization (2019). The WHO special initiative for mental health (2019–2023): universal health coverage for mental health. Geneva, Switzerland: World Health Organization. https://apps.who.int/iris/handle/10665/310981.

World Health Organization (2018). *Mental health: strengthening our response.* Key facts. Geneva, Switzerland: World Health Organization.

Yin, X., N. Sun, N. Jiang, X. Xu, Y. Gan, J. Zhang et al. (2021). Prevalence and associated factors of antenatal depression: systematic reviews and meta-analyses. *Clinical Psychology Review* F83(101932). DOI: 10.1016/j.cpr.2020.101932.

Improving cardiovascular health care

Cardiovascular health care and disease

Cardiovascular diseases are a group of disorders of the heart and blood vessels. They include coronary heart disease, cerebrovascular disease, heart failure and rheumatic heart disease (see Chapter 17). Cardiovascular disease (CVD) is largely caused by the combined effect of risk factors that can be modified. Behavioural risk factors, such as smoking, unhealthy diet, physical inactivity and harmful use of alcohol may show up in individuals as raised blood pressure, raised blood glucose, raised blood lipids, and overweight and obesity.[1] Having type 2 diabetes and associated kidney disease can also increase cardiovascular diseases risk,[2] as can overcrowding and poor living conditions that contribute to chronic inflammation (see Chapters 10 and 17), and periodontal disease. The incidence of heart attack, stroke and CVD death rates increase with increasing socio-economic disadvantage.[3] Poor social and emotional wellbeing is linked with higher risk of a CVD event[4] and difficulty making changes to reduce health risks.[5] In 2018–19, for example, two-thirds of Australian Aboriginal and Torres Strait Islander adults reported low or moderate levels of psychological distress and one-third experienced high levels.[6] Most risk factors for cardiovascular disease can be measured in PHC services to show whether clients have an increased risk of heart attack, stroke, heart failure and other complications.[7] Most are amenable to health service interventions.

CVDs are the leading cause of death globally. More than 80 per cent of the deaths are due to heart attacks and strokes, and one-third occur prematurely in people younger than 70 years of age. At least three-quarters of the world's deaths from CVDs occur in low- and middle-income countries, where people have poor access to PHC and therefore less access to screening and disease management.[8]

PHC practitioners have an important role in the prevention and management of CVD through public health advocacy, and by providing timely access to CVD risk assessment and supporting behaviour modification and treatment to reduce the risk of a cardiovascular event. This is

---

1   World Health Organization 2021.
2   Barr, Barzi et al. 2020.
3   Australian Institute of Health and Welfare 2019.
4   Welsh, Korda et al. 2019.
5   Murray, Craigs et al. 2012.
6   Australian Bureau of Statistics 2019.
7   World Health Organization 2021.
8   World Health Organization 2021.

particularly important for clients with existing chronic conditions such as diabetes, chronic kidney disease and chronic inflammation. A holistic whole-of-lifespan approach is important to help people to reduce their risk through healthy eating, regular exercise, minimal use of alcohol and not smoking tobacco, and to monitor and address other risk factors, such as poor social and emotional wellbeing and depression. Public health policies that make healthy choices easy and affordable are essential for motivating people to adopt and sustain healthy behaviours. Broader policy measures are needed to improve living conditions and reduce poverty and healthcare inequity.

Cardiovascular health and Aboriginal and Torres Strait Islander peoples

Preventable heart-related conditions, such as coronary heart disease, heart failure and rheumatic heart disease contribute substantially to poor health and premature death among Aboriginal and Torres Strait Islander peoples, and are a leading cause of preventable illness and death.[9] Large improvements in cardiovascular health have been made in the last two decades, but challenges remain. Since 1998 the mortality rate due to cardiac conditions has halved for Aboriginal and Torres Strait Islander peoples and the delivery of cardiac-related diagnostic services has increased, but those with suspected or confirmed cardiac disease are still less likely to be reviewed by a specialist than non-Indigenous Australians.[10] It is encouraging that the proportion of Aboriginal and Torres Strait Islander peoples accessing Medicare-funded health assessments has increased from 3 per cent in 2004–05 to 29 per cent in 2019–20.[11] Adult health assessments present opportunities to assess cardiovascular disease risk and provide appropriate care.

Emerging evidence shows that high cardiovascular disease risk starts earlier in Aboriginal and Torres Strait Islander peoples compared with non-Indigenous Australians.[12] An estimated 75 per cent of adults younger than 35 years have one or more risk factors for CVD[13] and almost 5 per cent of people aged 25–34 years are at high risk of a cardiovascular event in the next five years, with most under-treated.[14] A study in the Northern Territory found that 30 per cent of Aboriginal and Torres Strait Islander adults with moderate or high risk were younger than 35 years.[15]

---

9   Australian Institute of Health and Welfare 2021.
10   Australian Institute of Health and Welfare 2021, 2022.
11   Australian Institute of Health and Welfare 2021.
12   Agostino, Wong et al. 2020; Barr, Barzi et al. 2020.
13   Agostino, Wong et al. 2020.
14   Calabria, Korda et al. 2018.
15   Matthews, Burgess et al. 2017.

Findings: quality of cardiovascular health care

Cardiovascular preventive health care

Australian and international guidelines for best practice recommend assessing CVD risk in PHC.[16] Risk assessment is based on the combined effects of multiple risk factors and can identify people who do not have symptoms but are at high risk of cardiovascular disease. The Framingham Risk Equation is widely used for predicting risk of a cardiovascular event over the next five years for people who do not have existing cardiovascular disease or are not already known to be at increased risk. The Framingham Equation is now known to overestimate risk in the general Australia population, and was replaced by the Australian CVD Risk Calculator in 2023. Guidelines recommend the following:

- a CVD risk assessment for all adults aged 45 to 79[17]
- for people with diabetes without known CVD, risk should be assessed from ages 35 to 79 years
- people younger than 30 who meet the clinically determined high risk criteria, people with moderate to severe chronic kidney disease who have high albumin levels, and people with a family history of raised cholesterol levels should be assessed as high risk
- reassessment at intervals according to the level of risk identified, or new or worsening risk factors.[18]

There are additional guidelines for Aboriginal and Torres Strait Islander peoples:

- screening for risk factors from the ages of 18 to 29
- people aged 18–29 years with any of the conditions listed for the general population should be considered at high risk
- annual or opportunistic risk assessment from age 30 years at the latest
- screening and assessment as part of an annual health check, opportunistically or at least every two years, with review according to the level of risk identified.[19]

An assessment of a person's cardiovascular risk takes into account their age and sex, smoking status, blood pressure, serum lipids, diabetes status, CVD medicines, socio-economic situation, and history of atrial fibrillation. For people with diabetes, the indicators to be assessed include blood glucose levels, time since diagnosis of diabetes, urine for albumin and protein levels, kidney function, body mass index, and insulin use. Further factors considered when classifying the risk of cardiovascular disease are the coronary artery calcium score, nutrition and physical activity, alcohol use, mental health, social history including ethnicity and community CVD prevalence, and family history of premature cardiovascular disease.[20]

People already known to be at increased risk for cardiovascular disease (for example, due to type 2 diabetes, moderate to severe chronic kidney disease, markedly raised cholesterol

---

16   Commonwealth of Australia as represented by the Department of Health and Aged Care 2023; National Institute for Health and Care Excellence 2023 (2014).

17   Commonwealth of Australia as represented by the Department of Health and Aged Care 2023.

18   Commonwealth of Australia as represented by the Department of Health and Aged Care 2023.

19   Agostino, Wong et al. 2020; Barr, Barzi et al. 2020; Commonwealth of Australia as represented by the Department of Health and Aged Care 2023.

20   Commonwealth of Australia as represented by the Department of Health and Aged Care 2023.

levels or very high blood pressure) should have their conditions managed according to the relevant clinical guidelines.

Study 1: Healthy adults without chronic conditions

A cross-sectional analysis of clinical records for 2,052 people at 97 health centres (2012–2014) was carried out to investigate delivery of CVD risk assessments in Aboriginal and Torres Strait Islander adults. Clients were older than 20 years and had no recorded chronic disease diagnosis.

The study found wide variation in the delivery of CVD risk assessment between different Australian jurisdictions and between PHC services. While some services provided excellent levels of assessments, others provided low levels.[21] Overall, audited records showed these results:

- approximately 23 per cent of eligible clients (n = 478) had a documented CVD risk assessment
- even in the jurisdiction where most CVD risk assessments were recorded, there was wide variation between health services in the proportion of clients with a documented assessment (median 38 per cent; range 0–86 per cent)
- 11 per cent of clients (n = 53) who received an assessment were found with moderate or high risk; almost one-third of these clients were younger than 35 years of age
- health service factors accounted for 48 per cent of the variation in delivery of risk assessments; services with integrated clinical decision support systems that enable automated assessment of risk from information in clients electronic health records were more likely to document CVD risk assessments
- documentation of follow-up varied with respect to the targeted risk factor; fewer than 30 per cent of people with abnormal blood lipid or glucose levels had follow-up management plans recorded.[22]

Study 2: Teenagers and young adults

Another CQI study focused on Aboriginal and Torres Strait Islander people aged 15–34, examining 1,986 client records from 93 PHC services in remote, rural and urban locations. Despite the young age of the survey population, those who received assessments were commonly found to have important CVD risk factors that could be modified.[23]

- Acute care was the main reason for attendance, rather than a preventive healthcare assessment.
- 85 per cent of eligible clients (n = 1,686) had a record of blood pressure, 63 per cent (n = 1,244) had blood glucose recorded, 37 per cent (n = 743) had an assessment of body mass index, and 31 per cent (n = 625) had lipids recorded. Smoking status was recorded for 52 per cent of clients (n = 1,033) (see Figure 16.1).
- Clients aged 25 to 34 years were much more likely to be assessed for risk factors than those aged 15 to 24 years, except for body mass index measurement.

---

21   Matthews, Burgess et al. 2017.
22   Matthews, Burgess et al. 2017.
23   Crinall, Boyle et al. 2017.

Risk factor assessment   Risk factor present   Follow-up

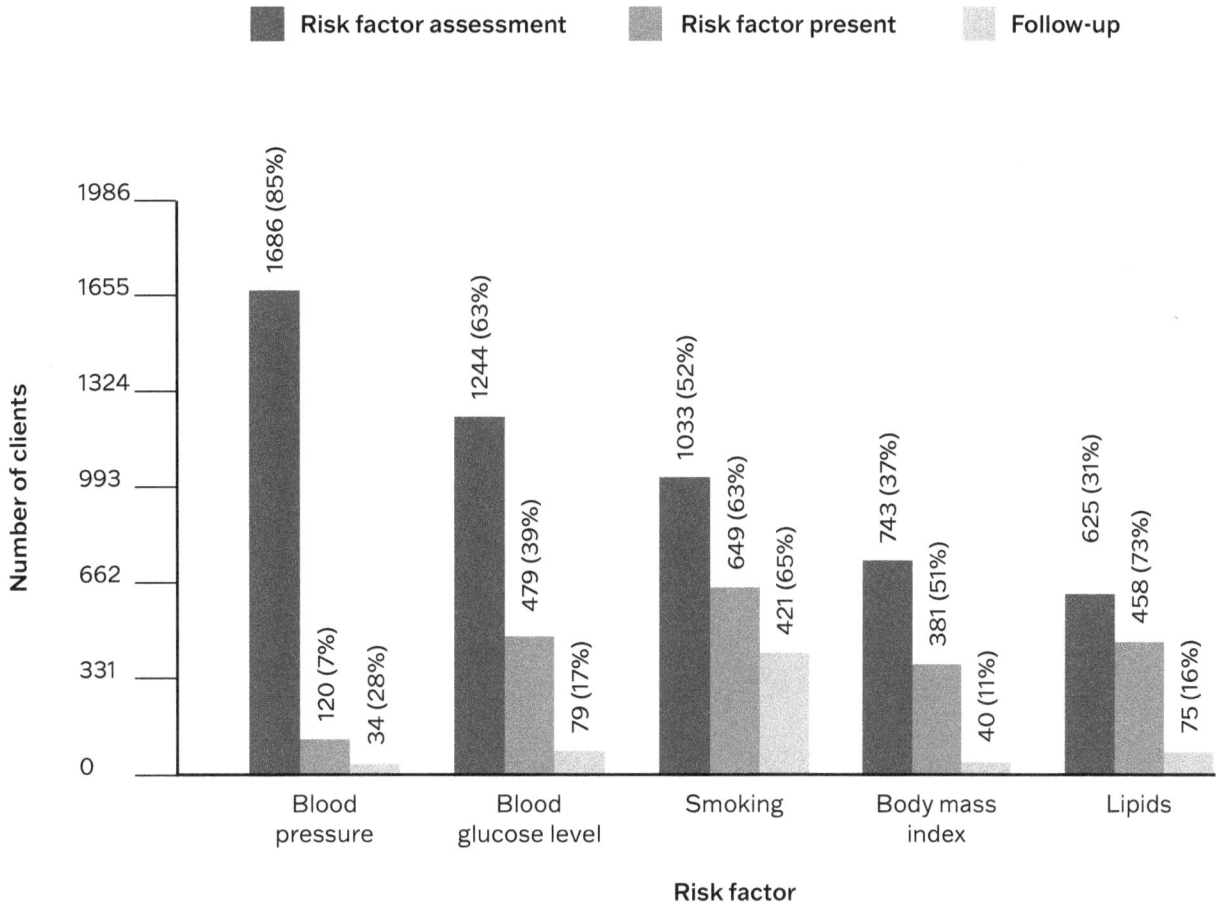

Figure 16.1 Number of clients with documented cardiovascular risk factor assessment and management. Source: Crinall, Boyle et al. 2017.

- Women were more likely to have a record of their blood pressure, blood glucose level and smoking status recorded than men. More women than men were overweight or obese, and men were more likely to have high blood pressure.
- The presence of risk factors was high in those who had a record of assessment, with the exception of blood pressure (7 per cent of clients) (see Figure 16.1).
- Among those clients with abnormal findings, documented follow-up was infrequent except for current smokers (65 per cent) (see Figure 16.1). Brief interventions for smoking and overweight or obesity, and follow-up of abnormal lipid profile were more likely in urban areas than regional or remote areas.[24]

Study 3: Adults with diabetes

Many people with diabetes have an increased CVD risk. A study of clinical records for 1,728 clients with diabetes from 121 health centres (2012–14) in four jurisdictions quantified the extent to which health centre and client characteristics influenced variation in the delivery of CVD risk assessments.[25]

---

24   Crinall, Boyle et al. 2017.
25   Vasant, Matthews et al. 2016.

- 33 per cent of eligible clients had a documented risk assessment, with delivery ranging from 3 to 56 per cent between jurisdictions.
- There were gaps in the recording of CVD risk.
- Health centre characteristics accounted for 70 per cent of the variation in assessments.
- Access to decision support tools and a reporting process for the provision of assessments supported delivery of assessments.
- Women were more likely to have a CVD risk assessment than men – and generally accessed preventive health services more often than men.[26]

Health system factors that appeared to facilitate CVD risk assessments in these health centres were the inclusion of CVD risk assessments into routine adult health checks and standard treatment manuals, and access to a user-friendly electronic cardiovascular risk assessment calculator in clinical information systems.

> Health system factors that appeared to facilitate CVD risk assessments were the inclusion of CVD risk assessments into routine adult health checks and standard treatment manuals, and access to a user-friendly electronic cardiovascular risk assessment calculator in clinical information systems.

Case study: strengthening cardiovascular disease prevention and management as part of holistic care

The CVD risk assessment strategies described above were among the outcomes of an earlier study by Burgess and colleagues, which informed a chronic disease strategy in one Australian jurisdiction (the Northern Territory).[27] The strategy included staff education about the use of CVD risk assessments, outreach support by chronic care educators and CQI facilitators for implementing CVD risk assessments, and a reporting process for delivery of CVD risk assessments and follow-up care.[28]

The strategy was replaced in 2012 by a chronic conditions management model that feeds back actionable data to frontline PHC teams to support CQI.[29] Client data are collected from the electronic health records and uploaded nightly to a centralised data warehouse. Data are then extracted, cleaned and turned into automated reports for the prevention and management of chronic conditions.[30] Box 16.1 outlines the latest version of the model.

---

26   Vasant, Matthews et al. 2016.
27   Burgess, R. Bailie et al. 2011.
28   Vasant, Matthews et al. 2016.
29   Burgess, Sinclair et al. 2015.
30   Productivity Commission 2021.

Box 16.1 The Northern Territory Department of Health Chronic Conditions Management Model

PHC centres receive the following information to feed into CQI activities and clinic meetings.

- Weekly "Recall List" for clinicians that identifies clients who are overdue for care in accordance with their care plans and risk factors.

- Weekly "Full Patient List" for clinicians detailing chronic conditions diagnoses, pathology results, key risk factors, examination findings and care plans. The ability to filter enables at-risk clients to be identified.

- Weekly community "Traffic Light Report" for clinicians and practice managers that compares service performance against chronic conditions program targets and chronic disease key performance indicators, including cardiovascular risk assessment and cardiovascular disease risk-management targets.

- Real-time dashboard (updated monthly) to track trends in regional and Northern Territory–wide service performance against Chronic Conditions Management Model program targets over the past three years. This allows clinicians and practice managers to identify problem areas or disseminate best-practice lessons.[31]

The functional reporting with embedded CQI has resulted in strong engagement from frontline PHC teams and improved delivery of CVD risk assessments. In the first two years of implementation of the chronic conditions management model, population coverage of CVD risk assessments increased from 23 per cent to 58.5 per cent for 7,266 clients. Functional reporting and decision support were also associated with a sustained proportion of high-risk clients achieving clinical targets for CVD risk reduction.[32]

> The functional reporting with embedded CQI has resulted in strong engagement from frontline PHC teams and improved delivery of CVD risk assessments.

During the same period, guidelines for cardiovascular risk assessment were published in the standard treatment manual for PHC practitioners in remote and rural communities,[33] and CQI research and development progressed through the Audit and Best Practice in Chronic Disease (ABCD) program.[34] Clinical outcomes have been studied to identify improvements, trends over time and to inform policymaking and ongoing investment in both primary and secondary prevention.[35]

---

31   Productivity Commission 2021.
32   Burgess, Sinclair et al. 2015.
33   Remote Primary Health Care Manuals 2022.
34   J. Bailie, Schierhout et al. 2014a.
35   Burgess, Sinclair et al. 2015; Coffey, Zhao et al. 2020; Matthews, Burgess et al. 2017.

The Chronic Conditions Management Model and systems development, a comprehensive CQI strategy[36] and increased workforce investment have been integral to the Northern Territory's strategic and sustained approach to chronic conditions prevention and management.

Key messages for improving cardiovascular health care

This CQI research and other relevant studies identify clear priorities and strategies for improving cardiovascular risk assessment, follow-up and management in PHC. Patterns of cardiovascular care delivery in Aboriginal and Torres Strait Islander PHC communities may to some extent reflect care delivery in international settings.

For primary prevention of cardiovascular disease, these are the key actions to take:

- increase awareness of the risk factors for and understanding of cardiovascular disease in the community, including among teenagers and young adults

- link clients and families with health promotion programs that support health (for example, to support healthy eating, regular exercise, not smoking, and social and emotional wellbeing)

- encourage clients and their families to attend PHC centres for preventive health assessments, not just for acute care

- work with individual clients to reduce CVD risk (for example, by not smoking, by losing weight), and to manage identified risk factors (for example, high blood pressure, high cholesterol)

- promote the benefits of CVD risk assessments, particularly amongst groups who are least likely to access PHC (for example, young men)

- work with clients to manage diagnosed cardiac conditions, diabetes and chronic kidney disease.

PHC system changes that can improve cardiovascular care include:

- involving clients and families in CQI processes

- ensuring adequate data are collected about clients to calculate CVD risk

- strengthening systems to enhance follow-up treatment for clients with identified risk factors

- educating PHC teams on the importance of assessing CVD risk, including for young adults

- training PHC practitioners to assess CVD risk and providing appropriate decision-support tools (for example, automated calculators, support from CVD experts, functional reporting of CVD assessment and care)

- routinely calculating CVD risk to inform management plans rather than focusing treatment on individual risk factors

---

36   Copley and Patel 2021.

- training staff to provide interventions that support clients to make lifestyle, behaviour, physical activity and dietary changes to reduce their CVD risk, while respecting the person's age, gender, cultural needs, ethnicity, social and economic circumstances and communication needs

- training and supporting PHC teams in using CQI processes to improve cardiovascular care.

There is also work that can be done at the policy level:

- advocate for policies and programs that support people to adopt and sustain healthy behaviours, such as nutritious food choices, increased physical activity, smoking cessation and reduced alcohol intake

- include cardiovascular risk assessment as a key performance indicator for PHC services

- provide transparent performance reporting to PHC teams and benchmark them against comparable services to lever internal motivation of clinical staff

- support the use of CQI in PHC services.

Improving cardiovascular care in Aboriginal and Torres Strait Islander PHC

Our studies show the need to improve the delivery of cardiovascular risk assessment for Aboriginal and Torres Strait Islander peoples. This is consistent with other research that shows under-treatment, with up to half of Aboriginal and Torres Strait Islander people found to be at high CVD risk not receiving recommended medication.[37] Improved preventive care, CVD risk assessment and best-practice management need to come together to help reduce the CVD events and related deaths that currently occur in our Aboriginal and Torres Strait Islander population, on average, about 10–20 years earlier than in non-Indigenous Australians.[38] Particular concerns are the risk of heart disease for young adults, poorer PHC access by men, and the need to ensure access to CVD risk factor screening and CVD risk assessments in line with best-practice clinical guidelines.

Recent developments are encouraging. Increased uptake of preventive health assessments by Aboriginal and Torres Strait Islander people has increased opportunities for early CVD risk assessment, prevention and management. The updated *Australian guideline for assessing and managing cardiovascular disease risk 2023* recommends commencing risk factor screening and CVD risk assessment at an earlier age for Aboriginal and Torres Strait Islander peoples (as outlined above),[39] and resources for supporting Aboriginal and Torres Strait Islander clients and communities to prevent and manage CVD risk can be found online. A consistent approach to risk assessment and management from an early age needs to be combined with increased

---

37   Calabria, Korda et al. 2018.
38   Australian Institute of Health and Welfare 2015.
39   Commonwealth of Australia as represented by the Department of Health and Aged Care 2023; Agostino, Wong et al. 2020.

health service capacity to deliver CVD prevention and care as part of holistic, culturally safe PHC. Use of CQI can support and sustain improvements in CVD care.

Within PHC services, practice infrastructure and systems need to be strengthened to increase follow-up care and self-management support for clients with identified CVD risk factors and diagnosed CVD.[40] This may require overcoming barriers such as lack of staff time and capacity, inadequate numbers of Aboriginal and Torres Strait Islander staff to guide and deliver culturally appropriate care, and poor availability of culturally appropriate services for Aboriginal and Torres Strait Islander clients who need referral to other providers. Understanding of the competing cultural, family and personal responsibilities, and the logistical challenges that can delay clients accessing specialist and hospital care is crucial when planning referral and communicating with clients about their care needs.[41]

At a higher policy level, incentives designed to increase the delivery of preventive health assessments (for example, specific Medicare rebates) need to be complemented with increased resources for providing follow-up care and management, particularly growing self-management support capacity within Aboriginal and Torres Strait Islander PHC services.[42]

Practitioners working with Aboriginal and Torres Strait Islander clients need to take account of non-behavioural risk factors when calculating risk and planning CVD management. Having diabetes, chronic kidney disease or chronic inflammation may increase CVD risk. Poor social and emotional wellbeing, linked with a history of disempowerment, ongoing racism and hardship, and grieving also place many Aboriginal and Torres Strait Islander clients at higher risk of a cardiac event, or less able to make changes to reduce their CVD risks.[43] Crowded housing and poor living conditions, linked to higher rates of infection, may affect CVD risk in some communities. Poor oral health, experienced by many Aboriginal and Torres Strait Islander people,[44] is another risk factor.[45] CVD risk scores are likely to underestimate real CVD risk for many Aboriginal and Torres Strait Islander people.[46]

> Take account of non-behavioural risk factors when calculating risk and planning CVD management.

Prevention approaches that are community led and that take account of historical, cultural and socio-economic factors and community-identified health priorities are crucial,[47] and require strong engagement between communities and PHC services. Within PHC teams, there is need to increase the Aboriginal and Torres Strait Islander clinical workforce, with emphasis on self-management support.[48] At the higher system level, strategies are needed to address the social and cultural determinants of health – including racism,[49] income and

---

40   Thompson, Haynes et al. 2016.
41   Katzenellenbogen, Haynes et al. 2015.
42   J. Bailie, Schierhout et al. 2014b.
43   Australian Bureau of Statistics 2019.
44   Australian Health Ministers' Advisory Council 2017.
45   Humphrey, Fu et al. 2008.
46   Agostino, Wong et al. 2020.
47   Katzenellenbogen, Haynes et al. 2015.
48   Smith, Kirkham et al. 2019.
49   Paradies, Ben et al. 2015.

employment, education, housing and food security[50] – in order to reduce the inequalities in cardiovascular health experienced by Aboriginal and Torres Strait Islander communities.

References

Agostino, J.W., D. Wong, E. Paige, V. Wade, C. Connell, M.E. Davey et al. (2020). Cardiovascular disease risk assessment for Aboriginal and Torres Strait Islander adults aged under 35 years: a consensus statement. *Medical Journal of Australia* 212(9): 422–7. DOI: 10.5694/mja2.50529.

Australian Bureau of Statistics (2019). *National Aboriginal and Torres Strait Islander health survey, 2018–19*. ABS cat. no. 4715.0. Canberra: ABS.

Australian Health Ministers' Advisory Council (2017). *Aboriginal and Torres Strait Islander Health Performance Framework 2017 report*. Canberra: Australian Government.

Australian Institute of Health and Welfare (2022). *Australia's health 2022: data insights*. Australia's health series. Canberra: AIWH. DOI: 10.25816/vs-vr80.

Australian Institute of Health and Welfare (2021). *Better cardiac care measures for Aboriginal and Torres Strait Islander people: sixth national report 2021*. Cat. no. IHW 263. Canberra: AIWH.

Australian Institute of Health and Welfare (2019). *Indicators of socioeconomic inequalities in cardiovascular disease, diabetes and chronic kidney disease*. Cat. No. CDK 12. Canberra: AIHW.

Australian Institute of Health and Welfare (2015). *Cardiovascular disease, diabetes and chronic kidney disease – Australian facts: Aboriginal and Torres Strait Islander people*. Cardiovascular, diabetes and chronic kidney disease series no. 5. Cat. no. CDK 5. Canberra: AIHW.

Bailie, J., G. Schierhout, F. Cunningham, J. Yule, A. Laycock and R. Bailie (2014a). *Quality of primary health care for Aboriginal and Torres Strait Islander People in Australia. Key research findings and messages for action from the ABCD National Research Partnership Project*. Brisbane: Menzies School of Health Research.

Bailie, J., G. Schierhout, M. Kelaher, A. Laycock, N. Percival, L. O'Donoghue et al. (2014b). Follow-up of Indigenous-specific health assessments – a socioecological analysis. *Medical Journal of Australia* 200(11): 653–7. DOI: 10.5694/mja13.00256.

Barr, E., F. Barzi, A. Rohit, J. Cunningham, S. Tatipata, R. McDermott et al. (2020). Performance of cardiovascular risk prediction equations in Indigenous Australians. *Heart* 106(16): 1252. DOI: 10.1136/heartjnl-2019-315889.

Burgess, C., R. Bailie, C. Connors, R. Chenhall, R. McDermott, K. O'Dea et al. (2011). Early identification and preventive care for elevated cardiovascular disease risk within a remote Australian Aboriginal primary health care service. *BMC Health Services Research* 11: 24. DOI: 10.1186/1472-6963-11-24.

Burgess, C., G. Sinclair, M. Ramjan, P. Coffey, C. Connors and L. Katekar (2015). Strengthening cardiovascular disease prevention in remote Indigenous communities in Australia's Northern Territory. *Heart, Lung and Circulation* 24(5): 450–7. DOI: 10.1016/j.hlc.2014.11.008.

Calabria, B., R. Korda, R. Lovett, P. Fernando, T. Martin, L. Malamoo et al. (2018). Absolute cardiovascular disease risk and lipid-lowering therapy among Aboriginal and Torres Strait Islander Australians. *Medical Journal of Australia* 209(1): 35–41. DOI: 10.5694/mja17.00897.

Coffey, C., Y. Zhao, J. Condon, S. Li and S. Guthridge (2020). Acute myocardial infarction incidence and survival in Aboriginal and non-Aboriginal populations: an observational study in the Northern Territory of Australia, 1992–2014. *BMJ Open* 10(10): e036979. DOI: 10.1136/bmjopen-2020-036979.

Commonwealth of Australia as represented by the Department of Health and Aged Care (2023). *Australian guideline for assessing and managing cardiovascular disease risk 2023*. Canberra: Department of Health and Aged Care.

Copley, K. and L. Patel (2021). *The Northern Territory Continuous Quality Improvement Strategy*. Darwin: Aboriginal Medical Service Alliance Northern Territory.

---

50   Australian Institute of Health and Welfare 2019.

Crinall, B., J. Boyle, M. Gibson-Helm, D. Esler, S. Larkins and R. Bailie (2017). Cardiovascular disease risk in young Indigenous Australians: a snapshot of current preventive health care. *Australian and New Zealand Journal of Public Health* 41(5): 460–6. DOI: 10.1111/1753-6405.12547.

Humphrey, L., R. Fu, D. Buckley, M. Freeman and M. Helfand (2008). Periodontal disease and coronary heart disease incidence: a systematic review and meta-analysis. *Journal of General Internal Medicine* 23(12): 2079–86. DOI: 10.1007/s11606-008-0787-6.

Katzenellenbogen, J., E. Haynes, J. Woods, D. Bessarab., A. Durey, L. Dimer et al. (2015). *Information for action: improving the heart health story for Aboriginal people in Western Australia (BAHHWA report).* Perth: Western Australian Centre for Rural Health, University of Western Australia.

Matthews, V., C. Burgess, C. Connors, E. Moore, D. Peiris, D. Scrimgeour et al. (2017). Integrated clinical decision support systems promote absolute cardiovascular risk assessment: an important primary prevention measure in Aboriginal and Torres Strait Islander primary health care. *Frontiers in Public Health* 5: 233. DOI: 10.3389/fpubh.2017.00233.

Murray, J., C. Craigs, K. Hill, S. Honey and A. House (2012). A systematic review of patient reported factors associated with uptake and completion of cardiovascular lifestyle behaviour change. *BMC Cardiovascular Disorders* 12(1): 120. DOI: 10.1186/1471-2261-12-120.

National Institute for Health and Care Excellence 2023 (2014). *Cardiovascular disease: risk assessment and reduction, including lipid modification CG181*. London: NICE.

Paradies, Y., J. Ben, N. Denson, A. Elias, N. Priest, A. Pieterse et al. (2015). Racism as a determinant of health: a systematic review and meta-analysis. *PLOS One* 10(9): e0138511. DOI: 10.1371/journal.pone.0138511.

Productivity Commission (2021). *Innovations in care for chronic health conditions*. Productivity Reform case study. Canberra: Commonwealth of Australia.

Remote Primary Health Care Manuals, ed. (2022). *CARPA standard treatment manual for remote and rural practice*. Alice Springs, NT: Flinders University. https://www.remotephcmanuals.com.au/home.html.

Smith, G., R. Kirkham, C. Gunabarra, V. Bokmakarray and C. Burgess (2019). "We can work together, talk together": an Aboriginal health care home. *Australian Health Review* 43(5): 486–91. DOI: 10.1071/AH18107.

Thompson, S., E. Haynes, J. Woods, D. Bessarab, L.A. Dimer, M. Wood et al. (2016). Improving cardiovascular outcomes among Aboriginal Australians: lessons from research for primary care. *SAGE Open Medicine* 4: 1–12. DOI: 10.1177/2050312116681224.

Vasant, B., V. Matthews, C. Burgess, C. Connors and R. Bailie (2016). Wide variation in absolute cardiovascular risk assessment in Aboriginal and Torres Strait Islander people with type 2 diabetes. *Frontiers in Public Health* 4: 37. DOI: 10.3389/fpubh.2016.00037.

Welsh, J., R. Korda, G. Joshy and E. Banks (2019). Primary absolute cardiovascular disease risk and prevention in relation to psychological distress in the Australian population: a nationally representative cross-sectional study. *Frontiers in Public Health* 7: 126. DOI: 10.3389/fpubh.2019.00126.

World Health Organization (2021). Cardiovascular diseases. https://www.who.int/health-topics/cardiovascular-diseases#tab=tab_1.

Improving care for acute rheumatic fever and rheumatic heart disease

Acute rheumatic fever and rheumatic heart disease

Acute rheumatic fever (ARF) and rheumatic heart disease (RHD) are preventable conditions associated globally with poverty, crowded housing and poor living conditions.[1] ARF is caused by an autoimmune response to infection with streptococcal bacteria that are often found in skin sores and sore throats. It can cause inflammation of the heart, often resulting in permanent damage to the heart valves, usually because of recurrences. RHD is the long-term condition caused by permanent damage to one or more of the heart valves following ARF. The heart valve or valves may become narrowed, obstructing the flow of blood or failing to close properly or both. This can lead to heart failure and the need for cardiac surgery, or stroke, and often leads to premature death.

RHD is a serious public health problem in low- and middle-income countries and among marginalised communities in high-income countries, including Indigenous populations. In 2018, some 30 million people were thought to be affected by RHD globally. RHD disproportionately affects girls and women; where endemic, it is a significant cause of poor maternal health outcomes.[2]

People affected by ARF and RHD need to have ongoing active engagement with the healthcare system for many years. This means the role of PHC practitioners in the prevention, screening, diagnosis, management and referral for ARF and RHD is crucial. Where RHD control programs are in place, practitioners may also be responsible for ARF and RHD notifications.

ARF/RHD and recommended care for Aboriginal and Torres Strait Islander peoples

RHD data show one of the greatest inequities in disease rates between Indigenous and non-Indigenous Australians, with rates of ARF and RHD in some Aboriginal and Torres Strait Islander communities among the highest documented globally.[3] A recent study found the age standardised ARF incidence (for people younger than 45 years) was 124 times higher and

---

1   Coffey, Ralph and Krause 2018.
2   World Health Organization 2018.
3   Ralph, de Dassel et al. 2018.

RHD prevalence (for those younger than 55 years) was 61 times higher among Aboriginal and Torres Strait Islander people compared with non-Indigenous Australians, with substantially higher rates in northern, remote Australian regions.[4] The number and rate of ARF notifications increased between 2016 and 2022, and almost half (46 per cent) of diagnoses were children aged 5 to 14 years.[5] These data provide compelling evidence of the need to improve living environments, disease awareness and management.

Recommended prevention and treatment

ARF can be prevented through improving living conditions and prompt antibiotic treatment for streptococcal infections. The recommended treatment of ARF and RHD is as follows:

- People diagnosed with ARF or RHD are assigned a RHD priority classification (1–4) based on disease severity. The classification guides recommended disease management.
- People who have had ARF need benzathine benzylpenicillin G injections every 4 weeks for a minimum of 5 years after the last episode or until age 21 (whichever occurs later), to avoid recurrences and prevent RHD progression.
- Continued secondary prevention (prophylaxis) to age 35 is recommended for moderate RHD and to age 40 or lifelong for severe cases, especially in people requiring heart valve surgery.
- Administration of more than 80 per cent of a client's prescribed benzathine benzylpenicillin G injections substantially reduces the risk of ARF recurrence, thereby reducing the risk of early death from RHD.[6]

Comprehensive PHC advice, resources and clinical guidelines are available on the RHD Australia website.[7] The World Heart Federation guidelines for diagnosis of RHD were updated in 2023.[8]

Findings: quality of acute rheumatic fever and rheumatic heart disease prevention and care

The data presented below on the quality of ARF/RHD care come mainly from six research papers and reports from the ABCD research program. The studies collectively analysed 5,209 client records from PHC centres, which were audited between 2008 and 2014. Most PHC centres were in geographically remote locations in northern Australia. Stakeholders participated in data interpretation to identify priority evidence-to-practice gaps and factors influencing improvement. Information on the application of CQI for ARF and RHD care and on clinical audit processes and audit findings are reported elsewhere.[9] We provide a brief overview of key findings below.

---

4 Katzenellenbogen, Bond-Smith et al. 2020b.
5 Australian Institute of Health and Welfare 2022.
6 RHDAustralia (ARF/RHD writing group) 2020.
7 Download guidelines from ARF and RHD Guidelines n.d.
8 Rwebembera, Marangou et al. 2024.
9 J. Bailie, Matthews et al. 2016; Katzenellenbogen, Bond-Smith et al. 2020a; Quinn, Girgis et al. 2019; Ralph, Fittock et al. 2013.

Across the studies, patterns and priorities for improvement could be identified.

- Secondary prevention: the majority of clients did not receive levels of secondary prevention known to offer best protection from ARF recurrence. From 2008 to 2014, the proportion of clients receiving more than 80 per cent of their scheduled benzathine benzylpenicillin G injections did not improve. PHC centres with high scores for "systematic processes of follow-up" were significantly better at administering the injections at recommended levels.[10]
- Management plans and education: some 70 to 80 per cent of clients had a disease management plan in place. However, clients' RHD priority classification, the provision of education about secondary prevention and follow-up action plans for clients with low rates of benzathine benzylpenicillin G injections were not consistently recorded. Only 12 per cent of clients with poor adherence to benzathine benzylpenicillin G injections had action plans. Provision of health education appeared low, even among people younger than 25 years, for whom secondary prevention has the most potential to improve outcomes. These findings indicate a need for better systems to translate secondary prevention guidelines into quality care.[11]
- Overall delivery of ARF/RHD prevention and care: there were improvements in overall service delivery. PHC centre mean delivery of care went from 42 per cent in 2008 to 66 per cent in 2012, but the upward trend was not sustained. There was large variation in service delivery between health centres, and this variation did not reduce over time, despite sustained CQI activities[12] (see Figure 17.1)
- Client age: children younger than 15 years received a higher level of ARF/RHD care compared with adults in all age groups. Most clients younger than 25 years (88.5 per cent) had RHD (as opposed to ARF), and 20 per cent had RHD without a documented history of ARF, indicating earlier missed diagnosis or asymptomatic cases of ARF. Many older people were found to have been prescribed penicillin, in contradiction to guidelines.[13]

Figure 17.1 shows the trend over the audit years for service delivery for up to nine best-practice indicators for rheumatic heart disease care (present in the rheumatic heart disease audit tool): a record of the rheumatic heart disease classification in the health summary; a record of current and of complete acute rheumatic fever and rheumatic heart disease management plans; a record of planned frequency of injections (if the client had been prescribed injections); whether 80 per cent or more of injections had been received (if the client had been prescribed regular injections and there was a record of planned frequency); a record of active recall if less than 80 per cent of injections had been received; timely doctor and specialist review, and echocardiogram (according to recommended schedule based on the rheumatic heart disease classification); and record of client education (provided within the last 12 months).

---

10 Quinn, Girgis et al. 2019.
11 J. Bailie, Matthews et al. 2016; Katzenellenbogen, Bond-Smith et al. 2020a; Quinn, Girgis et al. 2019.
12 J. Bailie, Matthews et al. 2016; Ralph, Fittock et al. 2013.
13 Katzenellenbogen, Bond-Smith et al. 2020a.

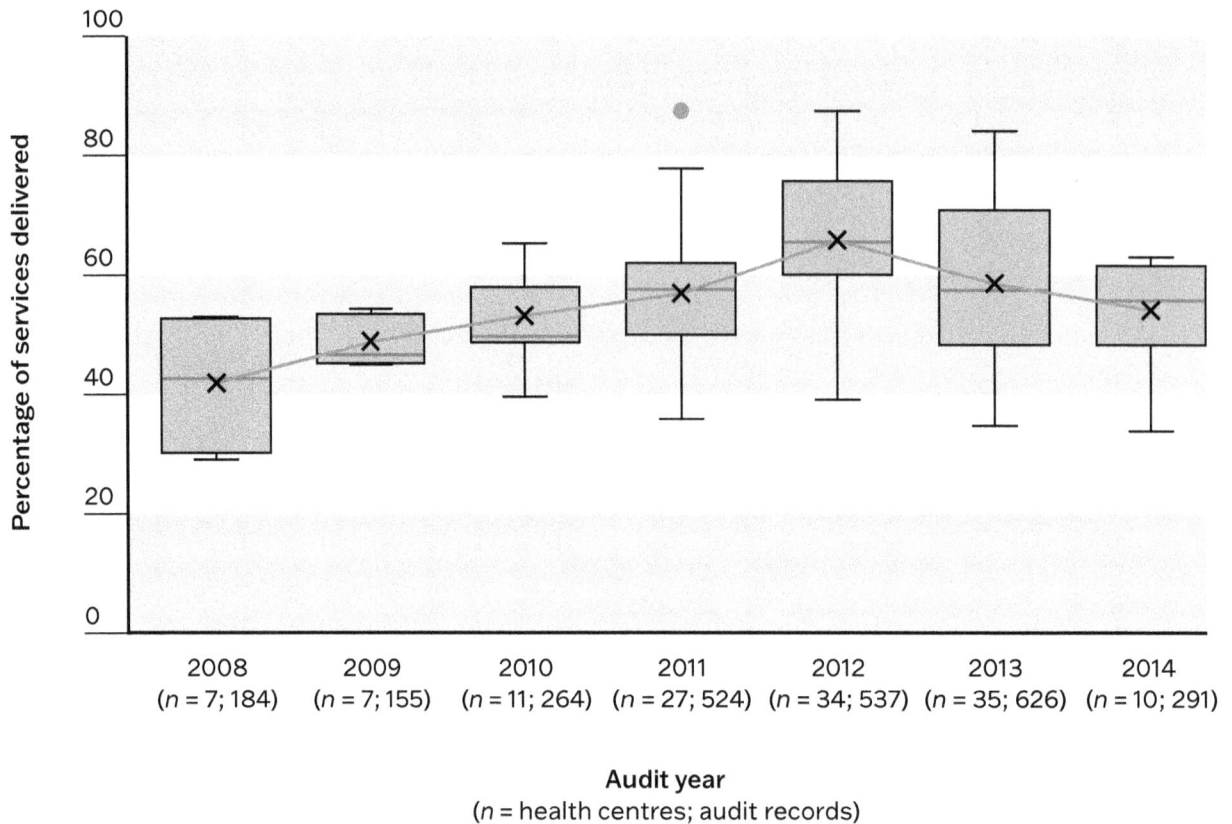

Figure 17.1 Trends in overall RHD care. Source: J. Bailie, Matthews et al. 2016.

> **Key messages for improving acute rheumatic fever and rheumatic heart disease care**
>
> This CQI research identifies clear priorities and strategies for improving PHC for ARF/RHD, and includes stakeholder interpretation of CQI data. Patterns of ARF/RHD care delivery in Aboriginal and Torres Strait Islander PHC communities are likely to reflect, at least to some extent, care delivery in international settings where ARF/RHD persist.
>
> These are the messages for action:
>
> - Educate PHC teams on the importance of the injection schedule to manage ARF/RHD, on best-practice guidelines and on use of client information systems. Clarify roles for RHD care, including RHD-related responsibilities for selected nursing staff.
>
> - Aim to provide at least 80 per cent of planned benzathine benzylpenicillin G injections. This requires good follow-up systems and flexible options for delivery, such as outreach services. Pain management for reducing discomfort from injections should be considered.
>
> - Accurately record ARF diagnosis, care and management plans in client records.
>
> - Notify all cases as required by regional and national guidelines.

- Develop transition care to support children with ARF and RHD through adolescence, and develop strategies to engage young adults who are affected.

- Provide culturally appropriate client, family and community education to improve health literacy.

- Increase the focus on primary prevention (not included in audits), such as facilities for washing, wastewater and rubbish removal, reducing household crowding, improving nutrition and dust control, and strengthening school-based education and prevention measures.

- Use CQI to sustain and strengthen health promotion strategies and clinical care.

Improving ARF/RHD care in Aboriginal and Torres Strait Islander PHC

Our studies show that systems are inadequate to translate secondary prevention guidelines into quality care. In addition, the low number of clients with a recorded RHD priority classification (30 per cent of 1,081 audits in one study) suggests that this classification is rarely used to guide management.[14]

ARF and RHD occur mostly amongst people living in remote locations, where poor housing infrastructure and crowded living contribute to the transmission of infections.[15] PHC centres are typically understaffed and have a high turnover of staff. A workforce study in the Northern Territory found that only 20 per cent of nurses and Aboriginal healthcare providers remained working at surveyed remote clinics 12 months after commencing. Half left within four months.[16] Embedding change in care delivery systems, providing staff training and maintaining knowledge in ARF/RHD management and use of information systems is very challenging but even more critical under these circumstances.[17] The trial of a multi-strategy RHD intervention in 10 remote communities found that long-term PHC system–strengthening strategies, with more linkages between PHC teams and communities, are essential to improve adherence to secondary prevention.[18]

> Long-term PHC system–strengthening strategies, with more linkages between PHC teams and communities, are essential to improve adherence to secondary prevention.

Early prevention should include comprehensive skin and throat programs in high-risk communities.[19] Transitioning children with ARF safely to adulthood without rheumatic heart damage requires tailored care. Engaging and valuing local navigators to address language and

---

14   Katzenellenbogen, Bond-Smith et al. 2020a.
15   McDonald, R. Bailie et al. 2009.
16   Russell, Zhao et al. 2017.
17   Read, Mitchell et al. 2018.
18   Ralph, de Dassel et al. 2018.
19   Wyber, Noonan et al. 2020.

cultural barriers has been recommended as a sustainable alternative to transition coordinators in mainstream programs.[20]

Cultural competence of healthcare teams, including appropriate communication styles that empower clients and their families with knowledge about their health conditions and treatment,[21] is critically important when tackling diseases of disparity such as RHD. Clinicians' competency in communicating influences health outcomes for Aboriginal and Torres Strait Islander people,[22] and multiple Australian studies of CQI in ARF and RHD care have highlighted the importance of communicating with clients in local languages and using culturally appropriate educational resources for improving RHD prevention and management.[23] Culturally competent and well-prepared PHC teams, strong community engagement and Aboriginal and Torres Strait Islander leadership are key to improvement.[24]

References

ARF and RHD Guidelines (n.d.). Clinical guidelines. https://www.rhdaustralia.org.au/.

Australian Institute of Health and Welfare (2022). *Acute rheumatic fever and rheumatic heart disease in Australia 2016–2020*. Cat. no. CVD 95. Canberra: AIHW, Australian Government.

Bailie, J., V. Matthews, A. Laycock and R. Bailie. (2016). *Aboriginal and Torres Strait Islander acute rheumatic fever and rheumatic heart disease care: final report*. ESP Project. Brisbane: Menzies School of Health Research.

Coffey, P., A. Ralph and V. Krause (2018). The role of social determinants of health in the risk and prevention of group A streptococcal infection, acute rheumatic fever and rheumatic heart disease: a systematic review. *PLOS Neglected Tropical Diseases* 12(6): e0006577–e77. DOI: 10.1371/journal.pntd.0006577.

Haynes, E., M. Marawili, B. Marika, A. Mitchell, J. Phillips, D. Bessarab et al. (2019). Community-based participatory action research on rheumatic heart disease in an Australian Aboriginal homeland: evaluation of the "On track watch" project. *Evaluation and Program Planning* 74: 38–53. DOI: 10.1016/j.evalprogplan.2019.02.010.

Katzenellenbogen, J., D. Bond-Smith, A. Ralph, M. Wilmot, J. Marsh, R. Bailie et al. (2020a). Priorities for improved management of acute rheumatic fever and rheumatic heart disease: analysis of cross-sectional continuous quality improvement data in Aboriginal primary health care centres in Australia. *Australian Health Review* 44(2): 212–21. DOI: 10.1071/AH19132.

Katzenellenbogen, J., D. Bond-Smith, R. Seth, K. Dempsey, J. Cannon, I. Stacey et al. (2020b). Contemporary incidence and prevalence of rheumatic fever and rheumatic heart disease in Australia using linked data: the case for policy change. *Journal of the American Heart Association* 9(19): e016851–e51. DOI: 10.1161/JAHA.120.016851.

McDonald, E., R. Bailie, J. Grace and D. Brewster (2009). A case study of physical and social barriers to hygiene and child growth in remote Australian Aboriginal communities. *BMC Public Health* 9(1): 346. DOI: 10.1186/1471-2458-9-346.

Mitchell, A., S. Belton, V. Johnston, W. Gondarra and A. Ralph (2019). "That heart sickness": young Aboriginal people's understanding of rheumatic fever. *Medical Anthropology* 38(1): 1–14. DOI: 10.1080/ 01459740.2018.1482549.

---

20   Mitchell, Belton et al. 2018.
21   Mitchell, Belton et al. 2019.
22   Mitchell, Belton et al. 2019.
23   J. Bailie, Matthews et al. 2016; Haynes, Marawili et al. 2019; Katzenellenbogen, Bond-Smith et al. 2020a; Mitchell, Belton et al. 2019; Ralph, de Dassel et al. 2018; Read, Mitchell et al. 2018.
24   Wyber, Noonan et al. 2020, Haynes, Marawili et al. 2019, download resources from The Kids Research Institute Australia 2024.

Mitchell, A., S. Belton, V. Johnston and A. Ralph (2018). Transition to adult care for Aboriginal children with rheumatic fever: a review informed by a focussed ethnography in northern Australia. *Australian Journal of Primary Health* 24(1): 9–13. DOI: 10.1071/PY17069.

Quinn, E., S. Girgis, J. Van Buskirk, V. Matthews and J. Ward (2019). Clinic factors associated with better delivery of secondary prophylaxis in acute rheumatic fever management. *Australian Journal of General Practice* 48(12): 859–65. DOI: 10.31128/ajgp-07-19-4987.

Ralph, A., J. de Dassel, A. Kirby, C. Read, A. Mitchell, G. Maguire et al. (2018). Improving delivery of secondary prophylaxis for rheumatic heart disease in a high-burden setting: outcome of a stepped-wedge, community, randomized trial. *Journal of the American Heart Association* 7(14): e009308. DOI: 10.1161/jaha.118.009308.

Ralph, A., M. Fittock, R. Schultz, D. Thompson, M. Dowden, T. Clemens et al. (2013). Improvement in rheumatic fever and rheumatic heart disease management and prevention using a health centre-based continuous quality improvement approach. *BMC Health Services Research* 13: 525. DOI: 10.1186/1472-6963-13-525.

Read, C., A. Mitchell, J. de Dassel, C. Scrine, D. Hendrickx, R. Bailie et al. (2018). Qualitative evaluation of a complex intervention to improve rheumatic heart disease secondary prophylaxis. *Journal of the American Heart Association* 7(14): e009376. DOI: 10.1161/JAHA.118.009376.

RHDAustralia (ARF/RHD writing group) (2020). *The 2020 Australian guideline for prevention, diagnosis and management of acute rheumatic fever and rheumatic heart disease*, 3rd edn. Darwin: Menzies School of Health Research.

Russell, D., Y. Zhao, S. Guthridge, M. Ramjan, M. Jones, J.S. Humphreys et al. (2017). Patterns of resident health workforce turnover and retention in remote communities of the Northern Territory of Australia, 2013–2015. *Human Resources for Health* 15(1): 52. DOI: 10.1186/s12960-017-0229-9.

Rwebembera, J., J. Marangou, J. Mwita, A. Mocumbi, C. Mota, E. Okello et al. (2024). 2023 World Heart Federation guidelines for the echocardiographic diagnosis of rheumatic heart disease. *Nature Reviews Cardiology* 21(4): 250–63. DOI: 10.1038/s41569-023-00940-9.

The Kids Research Institute Australia (2024). RHD endgame strategy. https://endrhd.telethonkids.org.au/RHD-Endgame-Strategy/.

World Health Organization (2018). *Seventy-first World Health Assembly, rheumatic fever and rheumatic heart disease: report by the Director-General*. Geneva, Switzerland: World Health Organization.

Wyber R., K. Noonan, C. Halkon, S. Enkel, A. Ralph, A. Bowen et al. (2020). *RHD endgame strategy: the blueprint to eliminate rheumatic heart disease in Australia by 2031*. END RHD Centre of Research Excellence. Perth: Telethon Kids Institute. https://endrhd.telethonkids.org.au/RHD-Endgame-Strategy/.

Improving the quality of care for sexually transmissible infections

Sexual health and sexually transmissible infections

Best practice for sexual and reproductive health in primary health care (PHC) is part of a client-centred, holistic approach to health and human rights. It includes contraception services and maternal care, and covers unsafe abortion, sexually transmissible infections and cancers related to reproduction, sexual violence, and the sexual and reproductive health needs of adolescents.[1] This chapter is about improving services for the prevention and control of sexually transmissible infections (STIs).

More than 1 million STIs are acquired every day worldwide, and the majority are asymptomatic. Each year, there are an estimated 374 million new infections with one of four curable STIs: chlamydia, gonorrhoea, syphilis and trichomoniasis.[2] More than 500 million people are estimated to have genital infection with herpes simplex virus, while an estimated 300 million women have a human papillomavirus (HPV) infection: the primary cause of cervical cancer and preventable with vaccination.[3] STIs are associated with significant morbidity in both women and men (for example, tubal infertility, pelvic inflammatory disease, ectopic pregnancy)[4] and also increase the risk of HIV transmission and acquisition.[5] STIs can have other serious consequences beyond the direct effect of the infection, such as mother-to-child transmission resulting in stillbirth, neonatal death, low birth weight and prematurity, sepsis and inherited abnormalities.[6]

Preventive care for STIs includes counselling and behavioural interventions: education, pre- and post-test counselling, condom promotion, and interventions that target high-risk groups (for example, sex workers, men who have sex with men, people who inject drugs) and young people.[7]

Chlamydia, gonorrhoea, syphilis and trichomoniasis are generally curable with a single course of antibiotics, while antivirals can slow the effects of herpes, HIV and hepatitis B.

---

1   Temmerman, Khosla and Say 2014.
2   Rowley, Vander Hoorn et al. 2019; World Health Organization 2018.
3   de Sanjosé, Diaz et al. 2007; World Health Organization 2023.
4   World Health Organization 2023.
5   Ward and Rönn 2010.
6   World Health Organization 2024.
7   World Health Organization 2024.

In low- and middle-income countries, diagnostic tests are often unavailable or are too expensive (except for rapid testing for syphilis and HIV). As a result, diagnosis and management are often based on recognisable signs and symptoms. This commonly leads to over-treatment and missed treatment (as a majority of STIs have no symptoms). Screening strategies are important. Treatment for the sexual partners of people with STIs is essential.[8] PHC should aim to raise public awareness and reduce stigma around STIs and to prevent, diagnose and treat STIs effectively. Training PHC workers to provide these interventions is key.

Improving STI care for Aboriginal and Torres Strait Islander peoples

Chlamydia, gonorrhoea and syphilis are readily treatable STIs that continue to occur at high rates in Australia. They are notifiable STIs in Australia, along with donovanosis. High rates of STIs within Aboriginal and Torres Strait Islander communities are influenced by the social and structural determinants of health, which include access to high-quality PHC that, by definition, is culturally appropriate.[9] The notification rates for chlamydia are nearly three times higher among Aboriginal and Torres Strait Islander peoples compared to non-Indigenous Australians; comparative infection rates for gonorrhoea and syphilis are higher again.[10] Young people aged 15–29 years are the most affected group, with the highest incidence among 15- to 19-year-olds.[11] Identified risk factors for STIs are living in a community with high STI rates; age (being sexually active when younger than 35 years old, especially younger than 25 years); having an STI within the past year, having a new sexual partner; or having more than one partner in the past six months. Drug or alcohol use can be a risk factor for multiple sexual partners or unsafe sex.[12]

Aboriginal and Torres Strait Islander peoples living in remote and very remote areas experience much higher rates of STIs compared to those in urban and regional areas.[13] A decade-long infectious syphilis epidemic has affected almost 4,000 mainly rural young Indigenous people in Queensland, Northern Territory, Western Australia and South Australia.[14] Despite remote communities experiencing endemic rates of STIs for well over two decades,[15] relatively recent estimates put annual STI testing coverage in remote communities at only 20 per cent, with lower rates in men than in women.[16]

The National Aboriginal Community Controlled Health Organisation and the Royal Australian College of General Practitioners guidelines for preventive health recommend annual testing for chlamydia (15- to 29-year-old age group) and gonorrhoea (15- to 39-year-old age group) among Aboriginal and Torres Strait Islander clients attending primary healthcare centres.[17] Clinical guidelines for communities in the Northern Territory and central Australia recommend

8   World Health Organization 2024.
9   Ward, Crooks and Russell 2016.
10   The Kirby Institute 2020.
11   Silver, Guy et al. 2015; The Kirby Institute 2022.
12   Remote Primary Health Care Manuals 2022.
13   Nattabi, Matthews et al. 2017; The Kirby Institute 2018.
14   Communicable Diseases Network of Australia 2021.
15   Ward, Hengel et al. 2020.
16   Hengel, Wand et al. 2017.
17   National Aboriginal Community Controlled Health Organisation and Royal Australian College 2024.

at least annual STI testing, prompt treatment, partner notification and testing, repeat testing after a positive result and treatment, education and positive health messages, particularly for those younger than 35 years.[18]

The *CARPA standard treatment manual* recommends two standard STI tests a year for men and women, and for sexually active young people (with consent). Testing can be done at these times:

- as part of another consultation (opportunistic), if the client is between 15 and 35 years old
- as part of an adult health check
- as part of community-wide screening
- if symptoms and risk factors suggest STI
- if requested by the client – even if it has not been long since the last check.

Doing STI work in a culturally sensitive way is crucial. Experienced and respected Aboriginal and Torres Strait Islander health practitioners, health councils, and respected community members are important sources of help for non-Indigenous staff.[19]

Findings: quality of STI care

Preventive health audits of 16,086 client records were conducted at 137 Aboriginal and Torres Strait Islander PHC centres between 2005–06 and 2014 (see Chapter 11). The audits involved government- and community-controlled, urban, regional and remote health centres. Testing and counselling data for sexually transmissible infections were analysed, looking for the levels of variation in testing for chlamydia, syphilis and gonorrhoea, and in discussions about sexual health. Overall, the audited preventive health records showed that there were several areas of STI care where improvement is needed:

- 68 per cent of clients had attended the PHC centres in the last six months, 49 per cent for acute care and only 8 per cent specifically for sexual health
- clients aged 20–24 and 25–29 years were more than three times more likely to be tested than clients in other age groups
- women received higher levels of testing for sexually transmitted infections compared with men (a 45 per cent greater chance of being tested)
- women having a Pap smear test were more than four times more likely to have STI testing and counselling than women attending for other types of care.[20]

Recent surveillance reports about STIs indicate that these findings about the quality of preventive care for sexual health are still relevant for focusing improvement efforts.[21]

The CQI research found that adherence to clinical guidelines for sexual health testing and counselling varied widely between PHC centres, ranging from 0 per cent to 100 per cent in some years or cycles. Overall, service delivery for sexual health testing and counselling services improved over time, from a median of 27 per cent in 2005/06 to 54 per cent in 2014 (see Figure 18.1). There were several factors accounting for the variation:

---

18   Northern Territory Department of Health 2019; Remote Primary Health Care Manuals 2022.
19   Remote Primary Health Care Manuals 2022.
20   Nattabi, Matthews et al. 2017.
21   The Kirby Institute 2020, 2022.

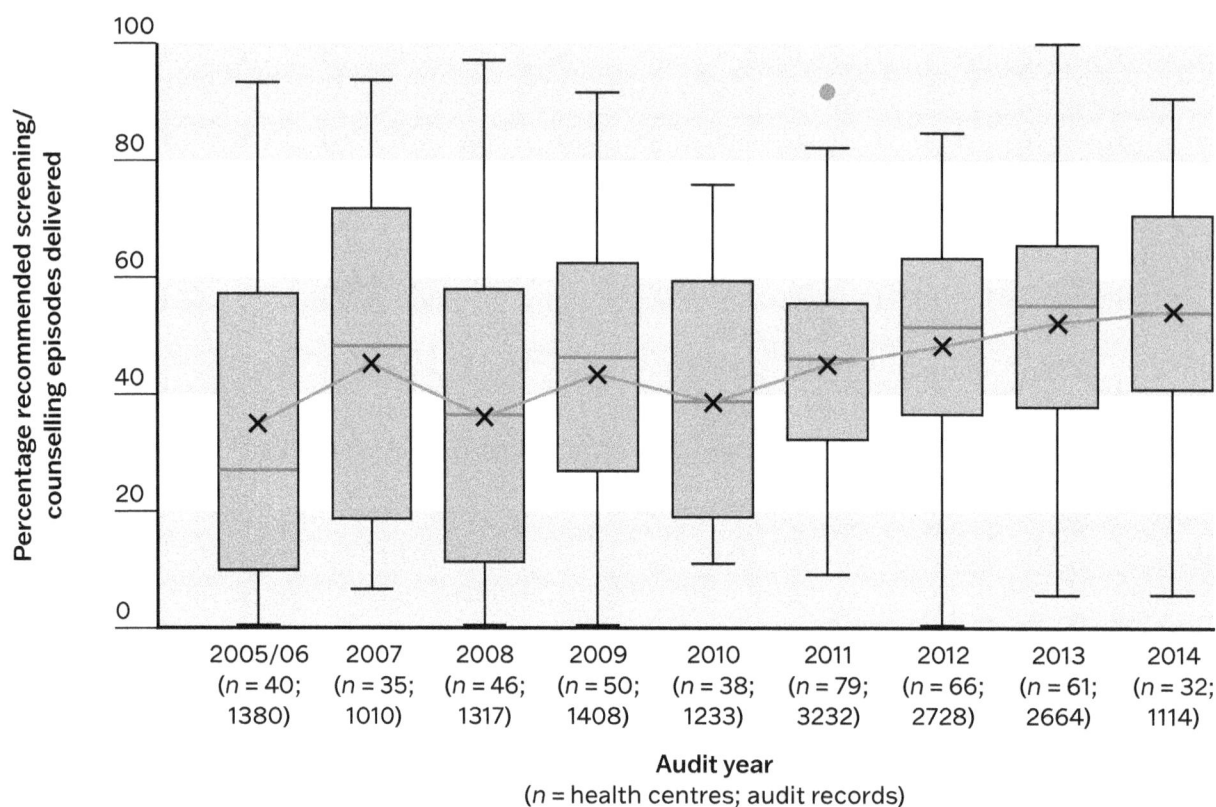

Figure 18.1a Sexual health–related service delivery over time (including nucleic acid amplification tests for gonorrhoea and chlamydia, syphilis screen and reproductive health discussion): mean percentage of STI testing and counselling delivered, by audit year. Source: Nattabi, Matthews et al. 2017.

- whether or not adult health checks were provided by the PHC centre: individuals undergoing an adult health check were three times more likely to be tested for STIs
- whether or not the centre had participated in one to two CQI cycles compared with just conducting a baseline audit (see Figure 18.1b)
- whether or not there was policy support and infrastructure for CQI. There were higher levels of service delivery in the two jurisdictions that had regional CQI facilitator networks and statewide CQI planning and governance committees.[22]

In the context of a syphilis outbreak among Aboriginal and Torres Strait Islander peoples in Northern Australia, CQI data from 77 PHC services (2012–14) were analysed to examine associations between PHC health centre (or clinic) factors and syphilis-testing performance.[23] The study provided insights to help PHC managers respond to the syphilis outbreak, as follows:

- neither accreditation status nor governance model were associated with syphilis-testing performance
- with respect to Systems Assessment Tool[24] component scores, "Delivery system design" (which refers to the design of the clinic's infrastructure, staffing profile, allocation of

---

22   Nattabi, Matthews et al. 2017.
23   Nattabi, Girgis et al. 2018.
24   Menzies School of Health Research and One21seventy 2012.

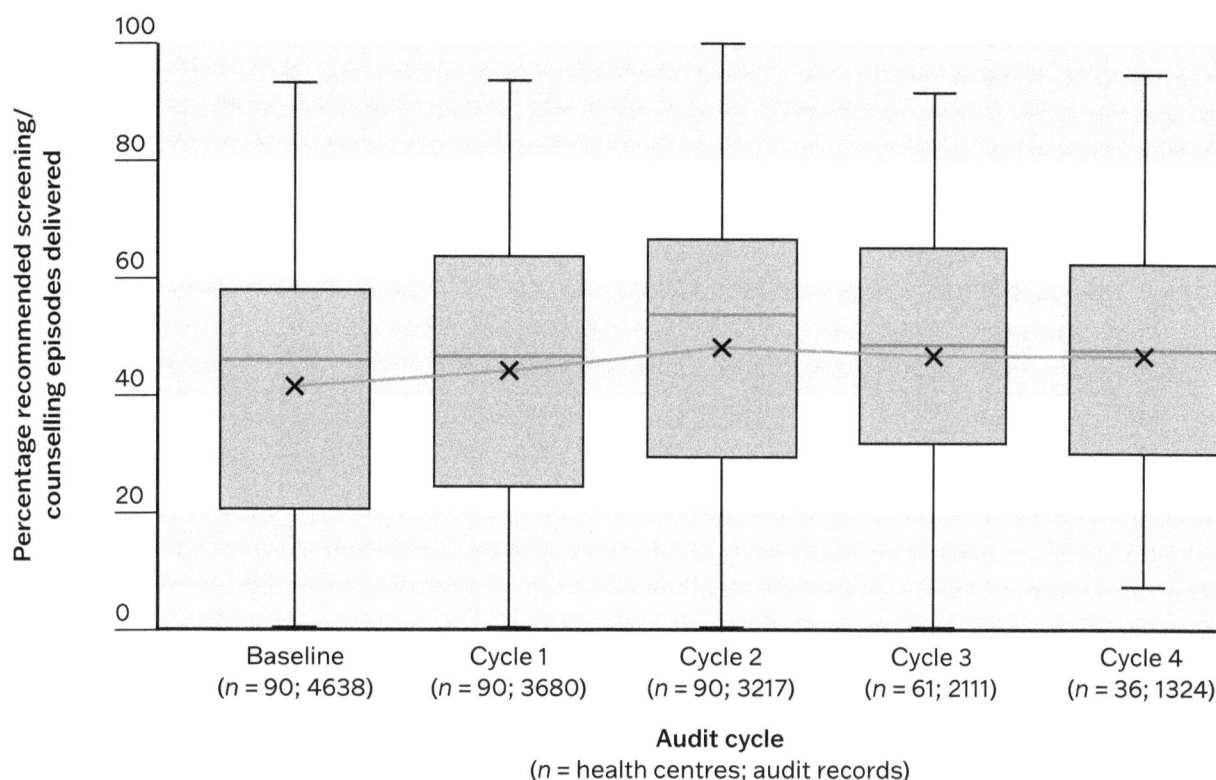

Figure 18.1b Sexual health–related service delivery over time (including nucleic acid amplification tests for gonorrhoea and chlamydia, syphilis screen and reproductive health discussion): mean percentage of STI testing and counselling delivered, by audit cycle. Source: Nattabi, Matthews et al. 2017.

roles and responsibilities, client flow and care processes) was significantly associated with syphilis-testing performance in all clinics

- within "Delivery system design", three items were significantly associated: "Continuity of care", "Team structure and function" and "Care planning"
- "Information systems and design support" was also linked with syphilis-testing performance.[25]

The STRIVE trial

The "STIs in Remote communities, ImproVed and Enhanced primary care" (STRIVE) trial was a stepped wedge cluster-randomised trial with CQI as an intervention. STRIVE was the first large-scale investigation of clinical CQI strategies for the control of STIs in remote Aboriginal community settings. The trial was conducted over three years from 2010 in 67 remote communities in three Australian jurisdictions (Northern Territory, Queensland and Western Australia).[26]

STRIVE established evidence-based tools and processes to drive CQI and showed that a clinic-level sexual health CQI program supported by regional sexual health coordinators could

---

25   Nattabi, Girgis et al. 2018.
26   Ward, McGregor et al. 2013.

improve care systems and STI testing rates. The trial found that simple but reproducible actions increased testing and retesting for STIs.

"Now that sexual health is integrated into the adult health check, through the men's and women's checks, that has been the single most [important change]. Putting in recalls for sexual health in the [client care information system] has actually improved it. Making sure that I'm auditing so that we know if somebody's not being followed up. Then we ask the hard questions why and follow that through." – sexual health coordinator A[27]

"There's things like putting recalls on for test for reinfection, using the STI template which is embedded in [the electronic client information system] and things like that, as a prompt to help better sexual health delivery." – sexual health coordinator B[28]

Context-specific CQI tools and audit reports helped teams to use data for improvement.

"I've done the stats, my system assessments tools … that's a very powerful tool because the clinic [team] will sit back and go, 'oh, wow' … They'll look at the spider graphs and they really get into that visual stuff to find out their strengths and weaknesses and how they can improve." – sexual health coordinator C.[29]

Over the trial period, testing coverage improved by almost 40 per cent overall, and aspects of the CQI program became normalised in clinical practice. There was no change in prevalence of STIs over the three-year time frame. This was mainly because baseline testing was so low.[30]

Sexual health (STI/BBV) clinical audit tool

The above findings about quality of care for STI testing resulted from the use a preventive health audit tool. A sexual health audit tool[31] was developed, piloted and refined by service providers in four Australian jurisdictions. Released by Menzies School of Health Research in 2014, the tool is intended to be used in conjunction with the Systems Assessment Tool and the preventive health and youth health audit tools (see Chapters 5, 11 and 14).

The purpose of the sexual health audit is to determine the management of a sexually transmissible infection (STI) or bloodborne virus (BBV) episode from the time the client first presents to the health centre for assessment of symptoms and diagnosis through to laboratory investigations, treatment and follow-up care.

27   Gunaratnam, Schierhout et al. 2019, 3.
28   Gunaratnam, Schierhout et al. 2019, 4.
29   Gunaratnam, Schierhout et al. 2019, 3.
30   Hengel, Bell et al. 2018; Ward, Guy et al. 2019.
31   Menzies School of Health Research and One21 seventy 2014. Download from https://www. menzies.edu.au/page/Resources/.

Key messages for improving the delivery of STI care in PHC

The patterns of sexual healthcare delivery for STIs in Aboriginal and Torres Strait Islander PHC communities are likely to have similarities with care delivery in other settings internationally, and in populations that experience a high burden of STIs. This CQI research identifies priorities for improvement and offers messages for improving the delivery of sexual health care in PHC.

At the health centre and community level, these actions can be undertaken for improvement:

- integrate STI testing into routine care and community screening (for example, cervical screening, contraception and adult healthcare checks)

- set up clinical information systems to flag clients for follow-up treatment, and to recall clients for retesting

- increase STI testing efforts for groups with high incidence rates (for example, young people 15–19 years old) and groups with lower testing rates (for example, men); this may require tackling barriers to accessing sexual health care for these groups

- record the delivery of sexual health care accurately in client records to ensure effective screening and treatment for clients and their partners, and to provide data for CQI

- put STI notification systems in place and train staff to keep STI notifications up to date

- adapt CQI tools and reports as needed to support improvement in STI testing and care; CQI tools should be adaptable for responding to the local context, to a risk environment such as a syphilis outbreak, or to an update to clinical guidelines

- encourage ownership of, and management support for, CQI processes for sexual health care.

At the regional or area level, these activities can support improvement efforts:

- coordinate sexual health care and CQI support across communities and PHC centres

- encourage compliance with STI notifications and other high-level information systems for improving STI care

- promote CQI as a tool to identify and act on areas for improvement in sexual health services

- encourage local ownership of, and management support for, CQI processes for sexual health care (this is relevant at regional and local levels)

- invest in CQI infrastructure and support.

Improving STI care in Aboriginal and Torres Strait Islander PHC

Improving knowledge and awareness of STIs among communities and health professionals is essential for improving sexual health care and reducing the rate and consequences of STIs. While common STIs are easily detected and easily treated, a high proportion of STIs are asymptomatic. Therefore, diagnosis rates depend on testing that mainly occurs in PHC services.[32] This requires PHC staff to be aware of the STI risk factors and the current guidelines on testing and treatment, and skilled in communicating with clients and providing culturally safe care. This in turn highlights the need for these elements:

- a stable workforce that includes Aboriginal and Torres Strait Islander practitioners
- training in cultural safety for non-Indigenous staff
- a team mix that enables culturally appropriate care (for example, male practitioners providing care for men)
- measures that ensure privacy and confidentiality, particularly in smaller communities (for example, family members may work in the health centre).[33]

Our findings showed that a high proportion of the variation in quality of care was explained by health centre factors rather than client factors, suggesting that structural and organisational developments are needed to provide high-quality sexual health care. In addition to the measure suggested above, organisational-level strategies such as multidisciplinary clinical teams, refined professional roles and structural changes (for example, changes in clinic hours, outreach services) could increase the capacity of PHC staff to provide high-quality care and ensure that STI prevention and management services are always available. Barriers such as workload pressures and competing work priorities should also be considered.[34]

> A high proportion of the variation in quality of care was explained by health centre factors rather than client factors.

There have been a number of interventions to improve the quality of sexual health care for Aboriginal and Torres Strait Islander clients attending PHC services. In addition to the ABCD program (the source of our audit findings) and the STRIVE project they include, for example, the Sexual Health Quality Improvement program (SHIMMER) in New South Wales.[35] Across these interventions, the use of CQI was shown to increase STI testing rates. Findings supported the integration of STI testing into general medical consultations and adult health checks, and health promotion programs that encourage people to present more frequently to PHC services and request STI testing.[36]

Community health promotion for STIs should include knowledge of risk factors and the important role of condoms, the need for timely testing and treatment, and the potential long-term consequences of STIs. Client and community approaches must be culturally safe,

---

32   Ward, Hengel et al. 2020.
33   Nattabi, Matthews et al. 2017.
34   Nattabi, Matthews et al. 2017.
35   Graham, Guy et al. 2015.
36   Graham, Guy et al. 2015.

and gender and age appropriate. This may involve, for example, peer-based approaches and outreach services in places where young people meet. Resources should present an Aboriginal and Torres Strait Islander perspective and any approach used should aim to counter shame and STI-related stigma. Resources for PHC staff doing STI work with different groups are available through the Australian Indigenous Health*InfoNet*.[37]

> Approaches must be culturally safe, and gender and age appropriate.

CQI research findings about the positive association between cervical screening test and STI testing in female clients highlights the value of integrating STI testing and counselling with other aspects of care. Cervical screening among Aboriginal and Torres Strait Islander women is important given that the incidence of and mortality from cervical cancer is higher compared to non-Aboriginal women,[38] but also because cervical screening provides an opportunity for STI testing.[39] From 2017, CQI activities have needed to monitor the possible effect of changes in Australia's cervical cancer screening program on STI testing rates among women, as the introduction of a primary human papillomavirus (HPV) test every five years has replaced the requirement for Pap tests every two years.[40]

A national surveillance and research network for STIs and bloodborne viruses in Aboriginal and Torres Strait Islander PHC services (ATLAS) has been established to augment the Australian National Notifiable Diseases Surveillance System. The ATLAS network analyses de-identified client records to help improve understanding of patterns of infection, testing and care, risk and protective behaviours, and returns data to participating health services every six months for use in CQI processes.[41]

References

Australian Indigenous Health*InfoNet* (n.d.). Edith Cowan University. https://healthinfonet.ecu.edu.au/.

Bowden, F., M. Currie, H. Toyne, C. McGuiness, L. Lim, J. Butler et al. (2008). Screening for Chlamydia trachomatis at the time of routine Pap smear in general practice: a cluster randomised controlled trial. *Medical Journal of Australia* 188(2): 76–80. DOI: 10.5694/j.1326-5377.2008.tb01526.x.

Bradley, C., B. Hengel, K. Crawford, S. Elliott, B. Donovan, D. Mak et al. (2020). Establishment of a sentinel surveillance network for sexually transmissible infections and blood borne viruses in Aboriginal primary care services across Australia: the ATLAS project. *BMC Health Services Research* 20(1): 769. DOI: 10.1186/s12913-020-05388-y.

Communicable Diseases Network of Australia (2021). *Multijurisdictional syphilis outbreak surveillance report: February 2021*. Canberra: Department of Health.

Condon, J., X. Zhang, P. Baade, K. Griffiths, J. Cunningham, D. Roder et al. (2014). Cancer survival for Aboriginal and Torres Strait Islander Australians: a national study of survival rates and excess mortality. *Population Health Metrics* 12(1): 1. DOI: 10.1186/1478-7954-12-1.

de Sanjosé, S., M. Diaz, X. Castellsagué, G. Clifford, L. Bruni, N. Muñoz et al. (2007). Worldwide prevalence and genotype distribution of cervical human papillomavirus DNA in women with normal cytology: a meta-analysis. *Lancet Infectious Diseases* 7(7): 453–9. DOI: 10.1016/S1473-3099(07)70158-5.

---

37   Australian Indigenous HealthInfoNet. n.d. https://healthinfonet.ecu.edu.au/.
38   Condon, Zhang et al. 2014.
39   Bowden, Currie et al. 2008.
40   Nattabi, Matthews et al. 2017.
41   Bradley, Hengel et al. 2020.

Graham, S., R. Guy, H. Wand, J. Kaldor, B. Donovan, J. Knox et al. (2015). A sexual health quality improvement program (SHIMMER) triples chlamydia and gonorrhoea testing rates among young people attending Aboriginal primary health care services in Australia. *BMC Infectious Diseases* 15(1): 370. DOI: 10.1186/s12879-015-1107-5.

Gunaratnam, P., G. Schierhout, J. Brands, L. Maher, R. Bailie, J. Ward et al. (2019). Qualitative perspectives on the sustainability of sexual health continuous quality improvement in clinics serving remote Aboriginal communities in Australia. *BMJ Open* 9(e026679). DOI: 10.1136/bmjopen-2018-026679.

Hengel, B., S. Bell, L. Garton, J. Ward, A. Rumbold, D. Taylor-Thomson et al. (2018). Perspectives of primary health care staff on the implementation of a sexual health quality improvement program: a qualitative study in remote Aboriginal communities in Australia. *BMC Health Services Research* 18(1): 230. DOI: 10.1186/s12913-018-3024-y.

Hengel, B., H. Wand, J. Ward, A. Rumbold, L. Garton, D. Taylor-Thomson et al. (2017). Patient, staffing and health centre factors associated with annual testing for sexually transmissible infections in remote primary health centres. *Sexual Health* 14(3): 274–81. DOI: 10.1071/SH16123.

Menzies School of Health Research and One21seventy (2014). Sexual health (STI/BBV) clinical audit tool. Brisbane: Menzies School of Health Research. https://www.menzies.edu.au/page/Resources/.

Menzies School of Health Research and One21seventy (2012). Systems assessment tool – all client groups. Darwin: Menzies School of Health Research.

National Aboriginal Community Controlled Health Organisation and Royal Australian College of General Practitioners (2024). *National guide to a preventative health assessment for Aboriginal and Torres Strait Islander people*, 4th edn. Melbourne: RACGP.

Nattabi, B., S. Girgis, V. Matthews, R. Bailie and J. Ward (2018). Clinic predictors of better syphilis testing in Aboriginal primary health care: a promising opportunity for primary health care service managers. *Australian Journal of Primary Health* 24(4): 350–8. DOI: 10.1071/PY17148.

Nattabi, B., V. Matthews, J. Bailie, A. Rumbold, D. Scrimgeour, J. Ward et al. (2017). Wide variation in sexually transmitted infection testing and counselling at Aboriginal primary health care centres in Australia: analysis of longitudinal continuous quality improvement data. *BMC Infectious Diseases* 17(1). DOI: 10.1186/s12879-017-2241-z.

Northern Territory Department of Health (2019). *NT Guidelines for the management of sexually transmitted infections in the primary health care setting*, 5th edn. Darwin: Northern Territory Government.

Remote Primary Health Care Manuals (2022). *CARPA standard treatment manual for remote and rural practice*. Alice Springs, NT: Flinders University. https://remotephcmanuals.com.au/document/35499.html.

Rowley, J., S. Vander Hoorn, E. Korenromp, N. Low, M. Unemo, L. Abu-Raddad et al. (2019). Chlamydia, gonorrhoea, trichomoniasis and syphilis: global prevalence and incidence estimates, 2016. *Bulletin of the World Health Organization* 97(8): 548–62P. DOI: 10.2471/BLT.18.228486.

Silver, B., R. Guy, H. Wand, J. Ward, A. Rumbold, C. Fairley et al. (2015). Incidence of curable sexually transmissible infections among adolescents and young adults in remote Australian Aboriginal communities: analysis of longitudinal clinical service data. *Sexually Transmitted Infections* 91(2): 135–41. DOI: 10.1136/sextrans-2014-051617.

Temmerman, M., R. Khosla and L. Say (2014). Sexual and reproductive health and rights: a global development, health, and human rights priority. *Lancet* 384(9941): e30–e31. DOI: 10.1016/S0140-6736(14)61190-9.

The Kirby Institute (2022). *Blood borne viral and sexually transmissible infections in Aboriginal and/or Torres Strait Islander peoples 2021*. Sydney: University of New South Wales.

The Kirby Institute (2020). *National update on HIV, viral hepatitis and sexually transmissible infections in Australia: 2009–2018*. Sydney: University of New South Wales.

The Kirby Institute (2018). *Bloodborne viral and sexually transmissible infections in Aboriginal and Torres Strait Islander people: annual surveillance report 2018*. Sydney: University of New South Wales.

Ward, H. and M. Rönn (2010). Contribution of sexually transmitted infections to the sexual transmission of HIV. *Current Opinion in HIV & AIDS* 5(4): 305–10. DOI: 10.1097/COH.0b013e32833a8844.

Ward, J., L. Crooks and D. Russell (2016). *High level summit on rising HIV, sexually transmissible infections (STI) and viral hepatitis in Aboriginal and Torres Strait Islander communities – final report 2016.* Adelaide: South Australian Health and Medical Research Institute.

Ward, J., R. Guy, A. Rumbold, S. McGregor, H. Wand, H. McManus et al. (2019). Strategies to improve control of sexually transmissible infections in remote Australian Aboriginal communities: a stepped-wedge, cluster-randomised trial. *Lancet Global Health* 7(11): e1553–e63. DOI: 10.1016/S2214-109X(19)30411-5.

Ward, J., B. Hengel, D. Ah Chee, O. Havnen and J. Boffa (2020). Setting the record straight: sexually transmissible infections and sexual abuse in Aboriginal and Torres Strait Islander communities. *Medical Journal of Australia* 212(5): 205–7.e1. DOI: 10.5694/mja2.50492.

Ward, J., S. McGregor, R. Guy, A. Rumbold, L. Garton, B. Silver et al. (2013). STI in remote communities: improved and enhanced primary health care (STRIVE) study protocol: a cluster randomised controlled trial comparing "usual practice" STI care to enhanced care in remote primary health care services in Australia. *BMC Infectious Diseases* 13(1): 425. DOI: 10.1186/1471-2334-13-425.

World Health Organization (2024, 21 May). Sexually transmitted infections (STIs): Key facts. https://www.who.int/news-room/fact-sheets/detail/sexually-transmitted-infections-(stis).

World Health Organization (2018). *Report on global sexually transmitted infection surveillance, 2018.* Geneva, Switzerland: WHO.

Improving eye health care

Eye health care

In primary health care (PHC), best practice for eye care is part of a client-centred, holistic approach to child health, preventive care and the management of chronic conditions such as diabetes. When linked with eye care referral processes and appropriate and accessible treatment, regular eye examinations and vision assessments can help to identify and refer eye problems earlier, preventing vision loss.

Poorer people suffer far more blindness and visual impairment than wealthier populations. This is partly due to untreated diseases, such as corneal infections, and to the persistence of infectious diseases linked to poor living conditions, such as trachoma.[1] Trachoma is generally found in dry and dusty environments, where transmission of the infecting organism – Chlamydia trachomatis – is enabled by household crowding, limited access to and use of water, and poor waste disposal systems. It is a major cause of preventable blindness globally and is endemic in 44 countries, with children having more frequent and longer lasting episodes of infection than adults.[2] Multiple trachoma infections can lead to an eyelid abnormality called trichiasis. While the underlying causes of trachoma and associated blindness are socio-economic and environmental, a related cause of visual impairment from trachoma and other causes is lack of access to ophthalmic services that can help to prevent or treat a variety of conditions that can lead to blindness. In low-income countries, only a small fraction of those who need eye care services get them.[3]

PHC practitioners have an important role in vision screening, referral to eye care services and case management. They support and coordinate clients' timely access to comprehensive eye examinations and specialist eye care, particularly for clients with chronic conditions such as diabetes. The critical nature of this role is more apparent in rural and remote locations where specialist eye health services are typically provided by visiting practitioners, and where a shortage of optometric and ophthalmic services often results in lower rates of eye examinations.[4]

---

1   Sommer, Taylor et al. 2014.
2   World Health Organization 2022.
3   Sommer, Taylor et al. 2014.
4   Kelaher, Ferdinand and Taylor 2012; Taylor and Stanford 2010.

Aboriginal and Torres Strait Islander peoples

Aboriginal and Torres Strait Islander people, as a population, face higher rates of vision loss than other Australians.[5] Many cases of vision loss (94 per cent) are avoidable, preventable or treatable.[6] Over the past decade and more, the gap in eye health and vision for Aboriginal and Torres Strait Islander people has halved through the collective efforts of individuals, organisations and governments. However, too many Aboriginal and Torres Strait Islander people still experience avoidable vision loss and blindness, and those who have lost vision often find it difficult to access the support and services they need.[7]

The factors that contribute to eye health are complex. They may include past eye health, access to eye health services, the complexity of the health system and continuity of care, and medical factors (for example, low birth weight, diabetes, high blood pressure). Having diabetes can lead to diabetic retinopathy and accelerate the development of cataracts. Living conditions (for example, housing and sanitation facilities), environmental conditions (for example, dust, access to water, assess to good food), health behaviours (for example, diet, alcohol and tobacco use), education and income are also linked with eye health.[8]

Aboriginal and Torres Strait Islander adults older than 40 years with diabetes form 72 per cent of those requiring an eye examination in any year.[9] In addition, Australia is the only high-income country in the world where trachoma is endemic. Trachoma currently occurs in remote and very remote communities in the Northern Territory, South Australia and Western Australia. In 2014, jurisdictions identified 160 communities as being at risk or potentially at risk of trachoma; 115 communities were identified as being at risk in 2019;[10] and 92 in 2021.[11] While the risk and prevalence of trachoma have declined, elimination will be difficult unless living conditions are improved.

The national guide on eye and vision assessments for Aboriginal and Torres Strait Islander peoples[12] makes these recommendations:

- People with diabetes should have a recorded annual visual acuity assessment with a dilated eye examination or retinal photograph. This includes the use of retinal photography by trained PHC staff combined with review by an ophthalmologist.[13]
- Adults aged over 40 years with no diagnosed major chronic disease should have a recorded visual acuity assessment, and, for those who lived in trachoma endemic areas as children, a trichiasis assessment every two years.

---

5   Taylor and Stanford 2010.

6   Taylor, Keeffe et al. 2009.

7   Vision 2020 Australia 2019.

8   Australian Institute of Health and Welfare 2020; Taylor, Anjou et al. 2012.

9   Tapp, Boudville et al. 2015.

10   The Kirby Institute 2015, 2020.

11   The Kirby Institute and WHO Collaborating Centre in Neglected Tropical Diseases 2022.

12   National Aboriginal Community Controlled Health Organisation and Royal Australian College 2024.

13   National Health and Medical Research Council 2008.

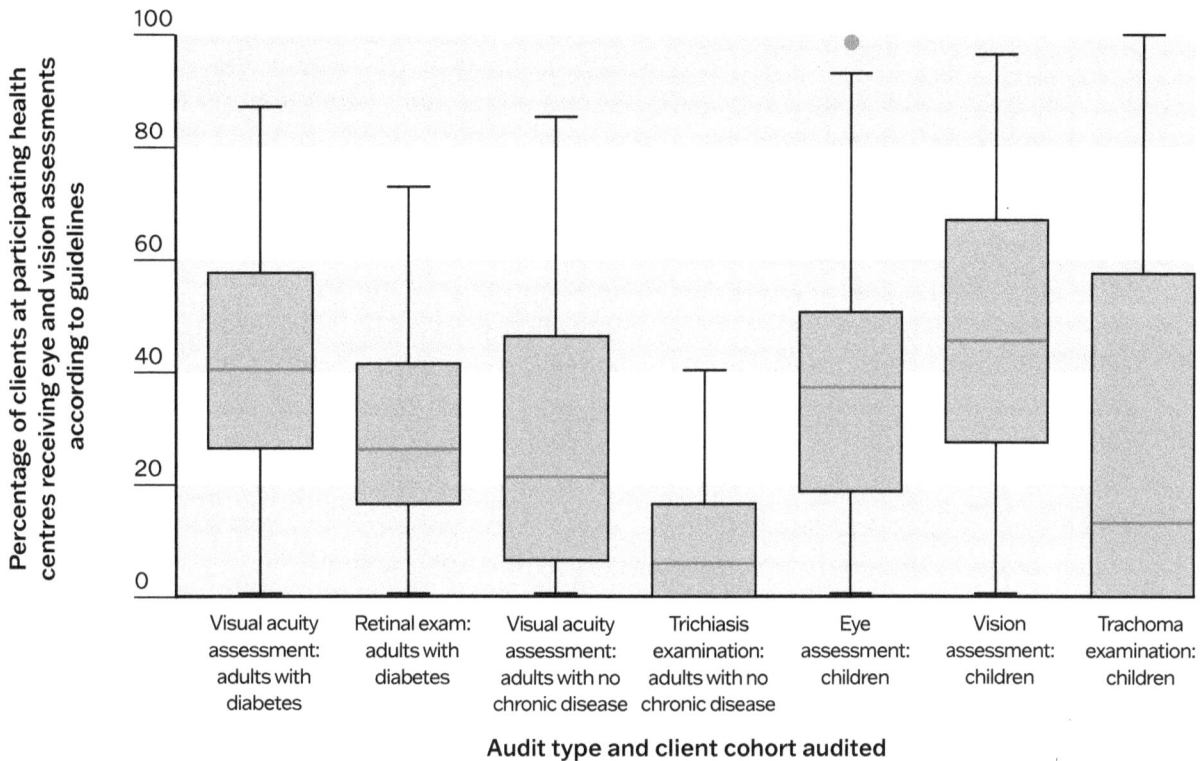

Figure 19.1 Variation in delivery of eye and vision assessments to Aboriginal and Torres Strait Islander clients across participating health centres. Source: Burnett, Morse et al. 2016.

- Infants and children should have these checks:
  - a general eye examination before 3 months of age and again between 3 and 6 months of age
  - screening for visual acuity as part of a routine health assessment at or before starting school, for children aged 3–5 years
  - a record of any parental concern around vision, and an eye examination and visual acuity assessment every one to two years, as part of a routine health check
  - a recorded annual trachoma examination if living in at-risk regions for trachoma; this is part of the annual health check and annual screening done by public health teams for children living in endemic areas.[14]

Findings: quality of eye health care

Three standardised audit tools were used to collect data about the delivery of eye and vision services: those for type 2 diabetes, preventive health and child health. Information on the application of CQI for these aspects of PHC are reported and cited in Chapters 10–12. Our research on the quality of eye care analysed data from 124 PHC centres and 15,175 client records audited between 2005 and 2012.[15]

---

14   National Aboriginal Community Controlled Health Organisation and Royal Australian College 2024.
15   Burnett, Morse et al. 2016.

The research found that the delivery of recommended eye and vision assessments varied widely between PHC centres and between different aspects of eye care (see Figure 19.1). While some centres provided excellent levels of assessments, others provided low levels. Overall, audited records across three client groups (total *n* = 7,320 clients) showed routine eye and vision assessments for adults and children were not being recorded at the recommended levels:

- *Adults with diabetes:* 46 per cent had a visual acuity assessment and 33 per cent had received a retinal examination within the previous 12 months.
- *Adults with no diagnosed major chronic disease:* 31 per cent of 759 clients had had a visual acuity assessment recorded within the last two years. Only 13 per cent of 2,829 records examined showed that clients had received an examination for trichiasis; it was unknown how many had lived in areas where trachoma was endemic when they were children.
- *Children:* 49 per cent of 4,909 children had a vision assessment recorded within the past 12 months; 45 per cent had had an eye examination and 25 per cent of 893 of children in affected areas had had a recorded examination for trachoma.[16]

Key messages for improving the delivery of eye care in PHC

A shared challenge for many PHC teams and for populations worldwide is that specialist eye health services are not delivered by local staff. Trachoma screening is generally provided by visiting public health teams, while retinal examinations are often done by visiting or off-site eye practitioners, particularly in under-served rural and remote areas.[17]

The patterns of eye care delivery in Aboriginal and Torres Strait Islander PHC communities are likely to be consistent with eye care delivery in other settings internationally, and in populations that experience a high burden of chronic illness. This CQI research identifies priorities for improvement and offers messages for improving the delivery of eye care in PHC:

- eye health and vision loss screening should be done in PHC services when resources are available (for example, retinal cameras and trained PHC staff)

- systems need to be in place to support coordination between external or visiting eye care services and programs and PHC centres:

  - when possible, integrate specialist eye health services (such as retinal examinations) provided by visiting or off-site eye practitioners around routine PHC delivery

  - ensure that examinations conducted by external providers and specialised programs, such as trachoma screening, are recorded in client files

- client records need to include accurate recording of the delivery of eye care; this is important for supporting coordinated and holistic care, and for providing data for CQI with the aim of improving client care

---

16   Burnett, Morse et al. 2016.
17   Sommer, Taylor et al. 2014.

- PHC practitioners require knowledge about the risk of vision loss for patients with diabetes and in trachoma affected areas, and skills to conduct and record visual acuity assessments and eye examinations
- clients' chronic disease management plans should include regular visual acuity assessment and eye examinations
- clients with diabetes, their carers and families need to be aware of the increased risk of vision loss, and clients should be encouraged to access eye care services and to report vision issues.

Improving eye health care in Aboriginal and Torres Strait Islander PHC

Overall, routine eye and vision assessments for Aboriginal and Torres Strait Islander adults and children attending PHC centres are not generally being recorded at the recommended levels, with considerable variation between health centres. There is continuing need to significantly increase the percentage of Aboriginal and Torres Strait Islander people with diabetes who receive the recommended eye examinations, and to increase eye health and vision loss screening generally. Good vision is important in its own right, but people with diabetes need good vision to look after medications, check their blood glucose levels and feet, and to attend healthcare appointments unassisted.[18] Around 60 per cent of vision loss amongst Aboriginal and Torres Strait Islander people can be addressed through access to affordable glasses, and those with vision loss due to cataract or diabetic eye disease require culturally sensitive treatment pathways.[19]

The higher likelihood of clients with diabetes to have a visual acuity assessment recorded (46 per cent) than adults with no diagnosed major chronic disease (31 per cent)[20] may be due to several factors. It may reflect stricter adherence to routine screening and regular monitoring for clients with diabetes through their chronic disease management plans, or practitioners' knowledge of the risk of vision loss for clients with diabetes. Higher rates of testing for people with diabetes may be because annual visual acuity assessments are recommended for people with diabetes, whereas for other adults the recommended frequency for eye examinations may be every two years or less often. It could be that clients with diabetes report issues with their vision or have a higher level of engagement in their health care. Action needs to be taken by PHC teams based on interpretation of local CQI data, while recognising the need to increase delivery of eye health services across all at-risk groups.

Action needs to be taken by PHC teams based on interpretation of local CQI data, while recognising the need to increase delivery of eye health services across all at-risk groups.

18   Taylor 2017.
19   Vision 2020 Australia 2019.
20   Burnett, Morse et al. 2016.

Until recently, retinal examinations largely relied on services being provided by visiting or off-site eye practitioners. A Medical Benefits Scheme item enabling visual acuity testing and retinal photography to be done by PHC practitioners as part of a health assessment (MBS 715) was introduced in 2016.[21] Use of retinal photo-screening integrated with primary care, image grading, and reporting systems has improved screening outcomes among other Australians who have diabetes.[22] This strategy is expected to increase rates of examinations in Aboriginal and Torres Strait Islander PHC centres.

The low level of recording of trachoma examinations in this research – 40 per cent of children from the Northern Territory and fewer than 10 per cent of children in other at-risk areas – is not consistent with the screening rates of 63 to 92 per cent recorded by the National Trachoma Surveillance and Reporting Unit in 2014,[23] or more recent screening rates (for example, 95 per cent overall in at-risk communities in 2021).[24] Not all remote communities are at risk, which complicates comparisons. Nonetheless, these earlier CQI results indicate a failure to record the trachoma examinations conducted by the jurisdictional trachoma screening programs in children's clinical records held by PHC services, rather than a failure to screen. This suggests a need for better coordination and communication between external service providers and PHC teams. The living conditions that underly trachoma transmission in remote communities must also be addressed through a reliable and easily accessible clean water supply to households alongside raised community awareness, better supply of housing, and training of PHC staff to screen for trachoma and trichiasis.

Since this CQI research was undertaken, considerable progress has been made. Mandatory inclusion of vision tests is now included in adult health assessments. A five-year plan for Aboriginal and Torres Strait Islander eye health and vision (2019–2024) is being implemented. The plan has four action areas: enhanced service delivery through service expansion and flexible and community-led models; strengthened regional partnerships and local supports; embedded eye health in Indigenous community-controlled health services and other PHC organisations; a multifaceted strategy to eliminate trachoma.[25]

As in other areas of PHC, a priority is equitable outcomes and access to high-quality eye health and vision care services for Aboriginal and Torres Strait Islander peoples. Aboriginal and Torres Strait Islander peoples should be empowered to shape and lead how they receive services. Ongoing CQI research will examine whether policy support and increased resources for eye health and vision screening have had a significant effect on rates of recorded eye assessments and eye health.

21 Taylor 2017.
22 Askew, Schluter et al. 2009; Crossland, Askew et al. 2016.
23 The Kirby Institute 2015.
24 The Kirby Institute and WHO Collaborating Centre in Neglected Tropical Diseases 2022.
25 Vision 2020 Australia 2019.

References

Askew, D., P. Schluter, G. Spurling, C. Maher, P. Cranstoun, C. Kennedy et al. (2009). Diabetic retinopathy screening in general practice: a pilot study. *Australian Family Physician* 38(8): 650–6.

Australian Institute of Health and Welfare (2020). *Indigenous eye health measures 2020.* Cat. no. IHW 231. Canberra: AIHW.

Burnett, A., A. Morse, T. Naduvilath, A. Boudville, H.R. Taylor and R. Bailie (2016). Delivery of eye and vision services in Aboriginal and Torres Strait Islander primary health care centers. *Frontiers in Public Health* 4: 276. DOI: 10.3389/fpubh.2016.00276.

Crossland, L., D. Askew, R. Ware, P. Cranstoun, P. Mitchell, A. Bryett et al. (2016). Diabetic retinopathy screening and monitoring of early stage disease in Australian general practice: tackling preventable blindness within a chronic care model. *Journal of Diabetes Research* 8405395. DOI: 10.1155/2016/8405395.

Kelaher, M., A. Ferdinand and H. Taylor (2012). Access to eye health services among indigenous Australians: an area level analysis. *BMC Ophthalmology* 12(1): 51. DOI: 10.1186/1471-2415-12-51.

National Aboriginal Community Controlled Health Organisation and Royal Australian College of General Practitioners (2024). *National guide to a preventative health assessment for Aboriginal and Torres Strait Islander People*, 4th edn. Melbourne: RACGP.

National Health and Medical Research Council (2008). *Guidelines for the management of diabetic retinopathy*. Canberra: Australian Diabetes Society for the Department of Health and Ageing.

Sommer, A., H. Taylor, T. Ravilla, S. West, T. Lietman, J. Keenan et al. (2014). Challenges of ophthalmic care in the developing world. *JAMA Ophthalmology* 132(5): 640–4. DOI: 10.1001/jamaophthalmol.2014.84.

Tapp, R., A. Boudville, M. Abouzeid, M. Anjou and H. Taylor (2015). Impact of diabetes on eye care service needs: the National Indigenous Eye Health Survey. *Clinical and Experimental Ophthalmology* 43(6): 540–3. DOI: 10.1111/ceo.12499.

Taylor, H. (2017). A game changer for eye care for diabetes. *Medical Journal of Australia* 206(1): 8–9. DOI: 10.5694/mja16.00647.

Taylor, H., M. Anjou, A. Boudville and R. McNeil (2012). *The roadmap to close the gap for vision: full report*. Melbourne: Indigenous Eye Health Unit, Melbourne School of Population Health.

Taylor, H., J. Keeffe, A. Arnold, R. Dunn, S. Fox, N. Goujon et al. (2009). *National Indigenous Eye Health Survey, minum barreng (tracking eyes)*. Melbourne: School of Population Health, University of Melbourne.

Taylor, H. and E. Stanford (2010). *Provision of Indigenous eye health services*. Melbourne: School of Population Health Indigenous Eye Health Unit, University of Melbourne.

The Kirby Institute (2020). *Australian Trachoma Surveillance Report 2019*. Sydney: University of New South Wales.

The Kirby Institute (2015). *Australian Trachoma Surveillance Report 2014*. Sydney: University of New South Wales.

The Kirby Institute and WHO Collaborating Centre in Neglected Tropical Diseases (2022). *Australian Trachoma Surveillance Report 2021*. Sydney: University of New South Wales.

Vision 2020 Australia (2019). *Strong eyes, strong communities: a five year plan for Aboriginal and Torres Strait Islander eye health and vision 2019–2024*. Melbourne: Vision 2020. https://www.vision2020australia.org.au/resources/strong-eyes-strong-communities/.

World Health Organization (2022). *Trachoma*. Fact sheets. https://www.who.int/news-room/fact-sheets/detail/trachoma.

Part III Summary

Applying lessons learnt from CQI implementation

Part III has shared findings and messages from implementing CQI in key areas of clinical PHC over more than a decade, using an innovative approach developed and refined through rigorous research and a commitment to long-term research-policy-service partnerships in PHC. The approach was implemented at scale and involved 175 PHC services and centres in five Australian jurisdictions.

There is limited literature reporting the effectiveness of CQI for improving PHC. Available studies tend to focus on single CQI interventions. What sets the work presented here apart from other CQI programs was the opportunity to study what happened when comparable CQI tools and processes were implemented across varied PHC settings over time. The ABCD CQI research program provided evidence that the sustained use of CQI can improve the delivery of evidence-based PHC. It showed that participatory CQI approaches can be adapted for identifying and acting on improvement priorities across settings. The program also demonstrated the benefits of sustained policy, training and system support for CQI (summarised in Chapter 9, Table 9.1). Further, a participatory approach with diverse PHC stakeholders was used to review and synthesise the findings and identify lessons from this extensive CQI program in comprehensive PHC.[1]

Consistent themes

Some consistent themes emerged from the experiences of implementing CQI across key areas of clinical PHC, particularly the importance of these actions:

- adhering to evidence-based best-practice clinical guidelines
- increasing follow-up of abnormal clinical results in all areas of care
- inquiring about behavioural risks to each client's health, and providing brief interventions as required
- ascertaining social and emotional risk factors and, when risks are identified, providing brief intervention and support (for example, around living environment, family relationships)
- improving documentation of care provided
- establishing better referral systems (within services and externally) and service options

---

1   Conte, Laycock et al. 2024; Laycock, Conte et al. 2020.

- overcoming barriers to the delivery of high-quality care that occur in these areas:
  - clinical information systems (for example, improving the ability to generate data for client follow-up and recall)
  - the PHC workforce (for example, strategies to reduce high staff turnover)
  - staff skills and training (for example, recruiting teams with the right mix of roles and skills, providing professional development, supervision and support)
  - community engagement (for example, in service delivery design, CQI).

Implementing improvement

Important lessons have been learnt about implementing CQI in PHC. Improvement efforts need to focus on strengthening systems at different levels of the health system.

At the PHC centre service or practice level, these are the essential actions:

- accurately recording care delivery in client records – a pre-requisite for high-quality data about clinical performance
- ensuring PHC teams, managers and community members participate in CQI – they are more likely to see its benefits and to take ownership of the processes; CQI needs to be everybody's business
- making improvement strategies context-specific – that is, responsive to social, cultural economic and environmental context
- allocating time and resourcing staff at all levels and in all roles in PHC services and practices to participate in CQI training and activities
- keeping on going with CQI in PHC. Teams that implemented consecutive CQI cycles observed measurable improvements in the data: the quality of care improved.

The integrated nature of PHC can extend the benefits of improvement interventions, because system changes targeting one group of clients frequently flow on to benefit other groups. Changes targeting one aspect of care can contribute to holistic, client-centred care overall. Some individual and team experiences of implementing CQI are shared in Part II.

At the district and regional level, these are the essential actions:

- using CQI tools and processes to enable PHC services and practices to identify and act on local priorities for improvement, in addition to meeting reporting requirements
- using CQI to strengthen systems for tackling the social, cultural, structural and environmental determinants of health
- working with communities to incorporate client perspectives on care into the measures of quality used in CQI
- allocating funding for CQI roles or functions and for staff working at different levels to participate in CQI training and activities
- investing in data literacy and data analysis skills at all levels of the health system to build understanding and capacity in generating and using data to inform improvement
- investing in resources to improve data quality and to monitor trends in best-practice care, the effect of CQI and whole-of-systems responses to quality issues.

The CQI approach described in Chapters 9–19 reflects internationally accepted principles for the effective implementation of CQI and responds to PHC improvement challenges that prevail across countries and populations, such as the provision of high-quality maternal and child health care and the prevention and management of chronic diseases. The findings and messages from this innovative CQI work in Aboriginal and Torres Strait islander PHC may have ongoing relevance for improving the quality of PHC in other settings.

References

Conte, K., Laycock, A., Bailie, J., Walke, E., Onnis, L., Feeney et al. (2024). Producing knowledge together: a participatory approach to synthesising research across a large-scale collaboration in Aboriginal and Torres Strait Islander health. *Health Research Policy and Systems* 22(1): 3. DOI: 10.1186/s12961-023-01087-2.

Laycock, A., K. Conte, K. Harkin, J. Bailie, V. Matthews, F. Cunningham et al. (2020). *Improving the quality of primary health care for Aboriginal and Torres Strait Islander Australians: messages for action, impact and research*. Centre for Research Excellence in Integrated Quality Improvement 2015–2019. Lismore, NSW: University Centre for Rural Health, University of Sydney.

Strengthening systems for PHC equity

High-quality PHC is, by definition, equitable and fair (as described in Chapter 1). Fairness underpins the concept of social justice, whereby everybody in society has equal rights, including the right to good health. The United Nations has characterised equity-related determinants of health, which enable or hinder people in achieving their health potential, as social, economic and environmental.[1] Cultural determinants of health are interrelated with equity-related determinants for many Indigenous peoples and other groups for whom cultural identity is centred on rights and linked to good health and wellbeing.[2]

In Part I (Chapter 3), we highlighted the link between quality of care and equity, describing health equity and CQI as a "natural fit". An equity focus is essential in CQI, as poor-quality care accounts for more deaths globally than lack of access to care, with the most disadvantaged populations having the worst outcomes.[3] Part II described some of the CQI tools and processes for improving PHC. In Part III, we wrote about CQI achievements and challenges, drawing on experiences in Aboriginal and Torres Strait Islander PHC in Australia and on international literature to identify key findings and messages for improving PHC quality. Some are messages for PHC practices, teams and communities. Others are targeted at promoting action at higher levels of the health system (for example, policymakers, regional health authorities) and in other systems that influence the social, cultural, structural and environmental determinants of health. At the heart of these messages is the recognition that globally, and within countries, there is much work to be done to improve PHC quality and to achieve equitable health care and fairer health outcomes.

Improving health equity involves simultaneously dealing with the institutional or structural bias in systems that perpetuate injustice and poor health outcomes (for example, based on ethnicity, race, wealth, gender, disability), and issues such as poverty and unfair wages, lack of access to land and resources intrinsic to survival, and poor access to high-quality education, housing and health care.[4] Organisations and individuals involved in PHC can contribute actions that advance these necessary reforms. Health services are ideally positioned to implement strategies to address both the indirect and direct determinants of health (for example, policies and training to address institutionalised racism and other forms of discrimination), and link with other agencies and sectors to integrate service delivery and promote wellbeing.[5]

---

1   Bell, Grobicki and Hamelmann 2014.
2   Bourke, Wright et al. 2018; Lowitja Institute 2020; Verbunt, Luke et al. 2021.
3   Hirschhorn, Magge and Kiflie 2021; Kruk 2018.
4   Carson, Dunbar et al. 2007; Paradies, Ben et al. 2015.
5   Wyatt, Laderman et al. 2016. Download the Institute's health equity self-assessment tool: http://ihi.org/resources.

Services can also partner with consumer groups, community organisations and researchers to identify and bridge gaps in knowledge and services involving equity-related issues, including ways to deal with systemic racism, and avoidable and unfair differences in the quality of care provided to different groups. PHC teams using CQI can strengthen care systems and sustain the gains made through service initiatives. Everyone involved in CQI, including PHC clients and communities, researchers and service providers as well as program managers and funding bodies, should be an advocate for more equitable policies and practices. In Part IV, we explore how these actions can come together in a comprehensive PHC approach for greater healthcare equity, concluding with considerations for future directions in CQI.

References

Bell, R., L. Grobicki and C. Hamelmann (2014). *Ensure healthy lives and well-being for all: addressing social, economic and environmental determinants of health and the health divide in the context of sustainable human development.* Denmark: United Nations Development Programme.

Bourke, S., A. Wright, J. Guthrie, L. Russell, T. Dunbar and R. Lovett (2018). Evidence review of Indigenous culture for health and wellbeing. *International Journal of Health, Wellness and Society* 8(4): 11–27. DOI: 10.18848/2156-8960/CGP/v08i04/11-27.

Carson, B., T. Dunbar, R. Chenhall and R. Bailie, eds (2007). *Social determinants of Indigenous health.* Sydney: Allen & Unwin.

Hirschhorn, L., H. Magge and A. Kiflie (2021). Aiming beyond equality to reach equity: the promise and challenge of quality improvement. *BMJ* 374: n939. DOI: 10.1136/bmj.n939.

Lowitja Institute (2020). *Culture is key: towards cultural determinants-driven health policy – final report.* Melbourne: Lowitja Institute. DOI: 10.48455/k9vd-zp46.

Kruk, M., A. Gage, C. Arsenault, K. Jordan, Leslie, H., S. Roder-Dewan et al. (2018). High-quality health systems in the Sustainable Development Goals era: time for a revolution. *Lancet Global Health* 6(11): E1196–E252.

Paradies, Y., J. Ben, N. Denson, A. Elias, N. Priest, A. Pieterse et al. (2015). Racism as a determinant of health: a systematic review and meta-analysis. *PLOS One* 10(9): e0138511. DOI: 10.1371/journal.pone.0138511.

Verbunt, E., J. Luke, Y. Paradies, M. Bamblett, C. Salamone, A. Jones et al. (2021). Cultural determinants of health for Aboriginal and Torres Strait Islander people – a narrative overview of reviews. *International Journal for Equity in Health* 20(1): 1–181. DOI: 10.1186/s12939-021-01514-2.

Wyatt, R., M. Laderman, L. Botwinick, K. Mate and J. Whittington (2016). Achieving health equity: a guide for health care organizations. *IHI White Paper.* Cambridge, MA: Institute for Health Care Improvement.

Multi-level systems approaches

Throughout this book we have advocated the use of systems thinking in CQI: analysing how parts of a healthcare system work together to support PHC, and how parts of a system can be changed to produce better outcomes.[1] Systems thinking helps in understanding how care systems interact to influence quality of care for clients. Systems thinking also encourages teams to consider the wider contexts in which PHC services operate: the resources available and the historical, social, economic and environmental circumstances that influence people's health and wellbeing across the life course.[2] Examples are the positive health effects of a secure food supply and employment opportunities, or the negative effects of discrimination on health and wellbeing. While these types of determinants of health may not be within the sphere of control of a PHC service or practice, they will be of concern, and the intersectoral action required to improve outcomes can be influenced and facilitated by PHC services.[3]

> The intersectoral action required to improve outcomes can be influenced or facilitated by PHC services.

Healthcare equity has been advanced when system-strengthening efforts take account of various determinants of health (for example, social, economic, cultural, structural, political, environmental), and when these efforts are applied on a wide scale and at different levels of the system. In systems thinking, everyone's actions count, and – while it requires societal and political commitment and collective effort to create change – the quality improvement efforts of PHC professionals and communities make important contributions. These contributions are strengthened when CQI efforts are sustained through policy and funding commitment at a higher system level. This chapter uses real-world examples to illustrate how multi-level and intersectoral systems approaches to CQI can be used to improve the quality of comprehensive PHC, as part of a broader systems approach to improving health and wellbeing.

---

1   McCalman, Jongen and Bainbridge 2017; Peters, Tran and Adam 2013.
2   Bainbridge, McCalman et al. 2019.
3   National Aboriginal Community Controlled Health Organisation 2021.

A systems framework for CQI in PHC services

In Chapter 3, we introduced a systems framework that illustrates the potential for PHC services to support and extend CQI efforts in two dimensions: vertically across the health system and horizontally across sectors (Figure 3.1). The framework demonstrates these features:

- vertical integration, referring to the use of CQI across all levels of health systems from community engagement and client care (base of diagram) to jurisdiction/provincial and national levels (top of diagram)
- horizontal integration, referring to the incorporation of CQI into evidence-based clinical care (left of diagram) and linkages and advocacy for influencing the social and cultural determinants of health (right of diagram)
- within PHC services, the conditions that support an integrated systems approach to improvement are trained and supported staff, engaged and active service users, strong management systems and a culture of CQI, resourcing and cost-effectiveness.[4]

While the contexts in which PHC operates vary widely, the health of populations is always influenced by a range of determinants, which are in turn influenced by many factors including collective action. And while quality improvement strategies and tools differ, CQI is inherently participatory and requires partnering with other agencies and groups (or teams) to monitor and mobilise action on social, cultural, economic, political and environmental determinants.

The framework in action

In the following examples, people working in different sectors or at different levels of the health system came together in a systems approach to quality improvement. The supportive conditions identified in the framework can be identified to varying degrees within these examples.

Example: community engagement improves ear health

After a review of child ear health data, the child health team at Yadu Health Aboriginal Corporation identified the need to increase screening (otoscopy and tympanometry) rates to enable early identification and management of middle ear disease. The team worked with staff at local schools and childcare centres to set up outreach clinics and trained several colleagues in screening techniques. During consultations, a video otoscope was used to spark conversations about healthy ears with children and their parents or carers. Letters advising families of screening results and next steps were followed up with phone calls and home visits as needed, and the child health team worked with other PHC practitioners to provide children with ongoing ear care. A new referral process was put in place to increase families' access to visiting specialist services at the regional hospital. Senior managers also negotiated for an ear specialist to deliver care at the PHC service twice a year, reducing the need for families to undertake the 1,600-kilometre return journey to the capital city for treatment.

---

4   Heyeres, McCalman et al. 2016; McCalman, R. Bailie et al. 2018.

Early outcomes included increased staff skills and confidence in ear health care, significant increases in ear health screening, multiple pathways for families to access ear health services, greater community interest in ear health and care, and stronger health service/community connections.[5]

Example: partnerships improve cancer care

A quality improvement initiative is supporting Aboriginal community controlled PHC services in Dharawal Country in New South Wales to deliver evidence-based holistic cancer prevention, support and care. Illawarra Aboriginal Medical Service partnered with health support organisations at the national and state level and with university researchers to evaluate the cancer care training needs of staff and to document case studies of best-practice cancer care reflecting Aboriginal practices and values. The information from this initiative was used to develop a manual and training materials to help teams to continually improve and monitor the quality of cancer prevention programs and cancer care, as well as palliative care, advanced care planning and grief support for families and carers.[6]

Example: access to data enhances improvement

In some large organisations, key performance indicator reports or data dashboards are prepared centrally and sent to health services to support their CQI programs. PHC teams can see the areas of care where they are doing well and not so well, data trends over time, and how their health centre's indicators are benchmarked against regional averages. CQI facilitators generally aim to involve as many staff as possible in reviewing reports and interpreting data, including those who live in the local community. An inclusive approach brings contextual knowledge and a range of perspectives to data interpretation, goal setting and improvement planning.[7]

Example: clients' priorities improve healthy ageing supports

Communities and PHC services in the Torres Strait are working with researchers to develop a framework to facilitate healthy ageing. Elderly residents join yarning circles to talk about what it means to them to age well and what their priorities are as they age. CQI methods are then used to audit existing community and health services to identify gaps in holistic care for older people and act on the priorities. Outcomes from the community engagement process include a quality framework of best-practice screening and assessment with a toolbox of resources to support healthy ageing. The resources are designed to be implemented in local communities and PHC services.[8]

---

5   National Aboriginal Community Controlled Health Organisation 2018.
6   Trees, Levett et al. 2022.
7   National Aboriginal Community Controlled Health Organisation 2018.
8   James Cook University 2019.

Example: partnerships to combat environmental determinants of health

In parts of northern Australia, the convergence of excessive heat, poor housing, energy insecurity and chronic disease has reached critical levels. Uninsulated, poorly ventilated houses are becoming dangerously hot as climate change increases temperatures, and poor energy efficiency means that more electricity is needed to keep homes thermally safe. This increases financial stress on already disadvantaged communities; most households are disconnected from the electricity supply more than ten times a year. Extreme heat causes significant health problems and makes existing conditions worse, and, when the power goes off, people cannot safely store medications or use vital health equipment, such as machines to help them breathe or home dialysis equipment.

A multi-sectoral response is needed. Indigenous community leaders are involving health professionals, architects, engineers, researchers and others in advocating for climate-resilient, energy-efficient public housing that is co-designed with communities or retrofitted to reflect their cultural practices and accumulated knowledge of how to live in hot climates. Healthcare leaders are raising clinicians' awareness of the need to be cognisant of the direct effects of heat on their clients' health and health risks, care management and capacity for self-care, and are joining calls for legislative protections for safe housing and energy security in remote communities.[9]

The CQI tools described in Box 20.1 were developed to support a systems approach to improving social and environmental determinants of health in rural and remote Australian communities. They were created and piloted through multi-phase and iterative processes that involved a series of consultations with community members and relevant stakeholders. The tools can be used in conjunction with clinical audit tools to promote a holistic, systems-thinking approach to CQI.

A similar approach was used to develop the Good Food Systems Tool described in Chapter 5, which supports community-driven decision-making to tackle inequities in food supply and food access for remote Indigenous communities.[10]

---

9   Quilty, Frank Jupurrurla et al. 2022; Quilty and Jupurrurla 2022.
10   Brimblecombe, van den Boogaard et al. 2015.

Box 20.1 A cross-sector initiative to develop CQI tools

Some of the common factors underlying poor child health are crowded housing, and inadequate access to health hardware, health resources and services. A CQI initiative aimed to identify the factors underlying high rates of poor child health in remote Aboriginal communities and develop indicators and CQI tools. The project brought together people from different knowledge systems, backgrounds and disciplines, allowing for diverse perspectives to be reflected in the physical and social factors identified and in the two tools developed.

- The Healthy Community Assessment Tool[11] assessed whether communities had the infrastructure and programs that enabled community members to make healthy lifestyle choices. Indicators such as water supply, food supply, waste disposal, sport and recreational facilities, early childhood education and childcare services were included.

- The Household Assessment Tool[12] was initiated by a health service manager for use in an early intervention program aiming to prevent progression from growth faltering to failure to thrive among infants. Social and environmental indicators placing children at greater risk of poor health and development outcomes were included (for example, housing functionality, hygiene and child safety, crowding, food security, social environment, school attendance). Household-level indicators aimed to match the objectives and performance indicators in service agreements between government and community agencies.

Linking PHC staff and community members with people beyond the health sector had several benefits.

- Different perspectives were incorporated in addition to evidence-based indicators already in the public domain: scientific (for example, biological plausibility), lay perceptions and Aboriginal perspectives.

- The indicators were seen as meaningful and appropriate by community residents (and other key stakeholders).

- The tools were co-designed with community members and can be used by health practitioners, health promotion officers, community leaders, environmental health and housing officers, and other government officers.[13]

---

11   McDonald, R. Bailie and Michel 2013.
12   McDonald, R. Bailie and Morris 2014.
13   McDonald, R. Bailie and Morris 2014.

A multi-level, system-wide approach to improvement

CQI is particularly effective in improving the standard of care when applied system-wide.[14] When Ferlie and Shortell examined quality strategies in the United States and the United Kingdom more than two decades ago, they found that efforts relying on narrow, single-level program changes were largely unsuccessful. The health systems researchers argued that system changes are needed concurrently at four levels to achieve and sustain quality improvement:

- individual level (for example, education, leadership development at all levels, guideline use)
- group or team level (for example, clinical audits, team development, guideline use)
- organisation level (for example, CQI, organisational learning, organisational culture)
- larger system or policy environment in which an organisation operates (for example, national improvement policies, accrediting agencies, legal systems, funding policies).[15]

It is now widely accepted that "for CQI to add value, have impact and realise its potential, it [needs] to be managed at multiple levels".[16] In Australia, for example, efforts to tackle entrenched health inequality for Aboriginal and Torres Strait Islander peoples have featured multi-level investment in CQI. While there are different CQI program approaches across jurisdictions, and different levels of maturity in the use of CQI across services, national level policy and funding agreements require that PHC services use CQI processes to monitor improvement efforts and enhance the quality of service delivery.[17] This high-level policy and funding approach helps to sustain CQI processes at the PHC service and practice level. A comparative case study published in 2017 found that consistent and sustained policy and multi-level infrastructure support for CQI in the Northern Territory (as outlined in the following example) enabled wide-scale and ongoing improvement in quality of care, compared with jurisdictions where CQI efforts were generally smaller in scale and more fragmented.[18] The authors concluded that it was not sufficient for improvement initiatives to rely on local service managers and clinicians, as their efforts are strongly mediated by higher system-level influences.

> **Example: sustained commitment to CQI at multiple levels**
>
> **Larger system level**
>
> A five-year National Framework for Continuous Quality Improvement in Primary Health Care for Aboriginal and Torres Strait Islander People 2018–23[19] was developed in Australia as a joint initiative of the National Aboriginal Community Controlled Health Organisation and affiliates, with support from the Commonwealth Department of Health. The framework is complemented by a Model of Aboriginal and Torres Strait Islander Community-Controlled Comprehensive Primary Health Care,[20] which specifies the use of CQI in each of the four domains of core services:

---

14   J. Bailie, Matthews et al. 2017; Shortell, Bennett and Byck 1998; Tricco, Ivers et al. 2012.
15   Ferlie and Shortell 2001.
16   Sollecito and Johnson 2019, 314.
17   National Aboriginal Community Controlled Health Organisation 2018.
18   R. Bailie, Matthews et al. 2017.
19   National Aboriginal Community Controlled Health Organisation 2018.
20   National Aboriginal Community Controlled Health Organisation 2021.

governance; community health promotion and empowerment; clinical services; policy direction and partnerships.

Organisation level

In the Northern Territory, a CQI strategy[21] is governed by a steering committee representing key stakeholders. Community-controlled and government-managed health services participate in the strategy, which aims to ensure CQI is part of core business for every PHC service. There has been sustained investment in building CQI knowledge and skills and providing health services with tools and strategies for engaging in CQI. Processes to support the use of data for CQI were established through a data working group and collaboratives.

Group or team level

Two coordinators provide program management and leadership, CQI expertise and support to facilitators employed by health services, who provide practical support in planning and implementing CQI. All PHC teams have access to CQI training, a range of data sources and opportunities to participate in CQI processes.

Individual level

Feedback about quality of care to PHC staff, members of governing boards, clients and communities is tailored to identified needs. Managers and members of multidisciplinary PHC teams have access to CQI and cultural safety training, CQI collaboratives and other professional development. There is high workforce turnover, particularly in remote communities, however a core of CQI leaders and community champions endures.[22]

For CQI to add value, have effect and realise its potential, it needs to be managed at multiple levels.

Using CQI data for wide-scale improvement

Despite developments in CQI theory and practice, there is little evidence about how to engage stakeholders in wide-scale CQI processes to inform system strengthening. Yet bringing together CQI data from multiple PHC centres has scope to engage stakeholders in identifying common priorities for improving care, and interventions that target change at different health-system levels. To this end, our CQI research network conducted an interactive data dissemination process targeting people in diverse PHC roles at different levels of the health system. The CQI data had been collected over 10 years and represented more than 60,000 de-identified clinical audits of client records and 492 systems assessments from 175 PHC centres across five Australian jurisdictions.[23]

---

21   Copley and Patel 2021.
22   Copley and Patel 2021.
23   Laycock, J. Bailie et al. 2017.

Interactive dissemination

Aggregated data

Child health

Chronic illness care

Preventive care

Maternal health

Mental health

Acute rheumatic fever and rheumatic heart disease care

Stakeholder feedback…

… report refinement

Final report

Other products

Phase 1

Phase 2

Phase 3

Identify priority evidence–practice gaps

Identify barriers, enablers and strategies for improvement

Provide feedback on draft final report

Developmental evaluation

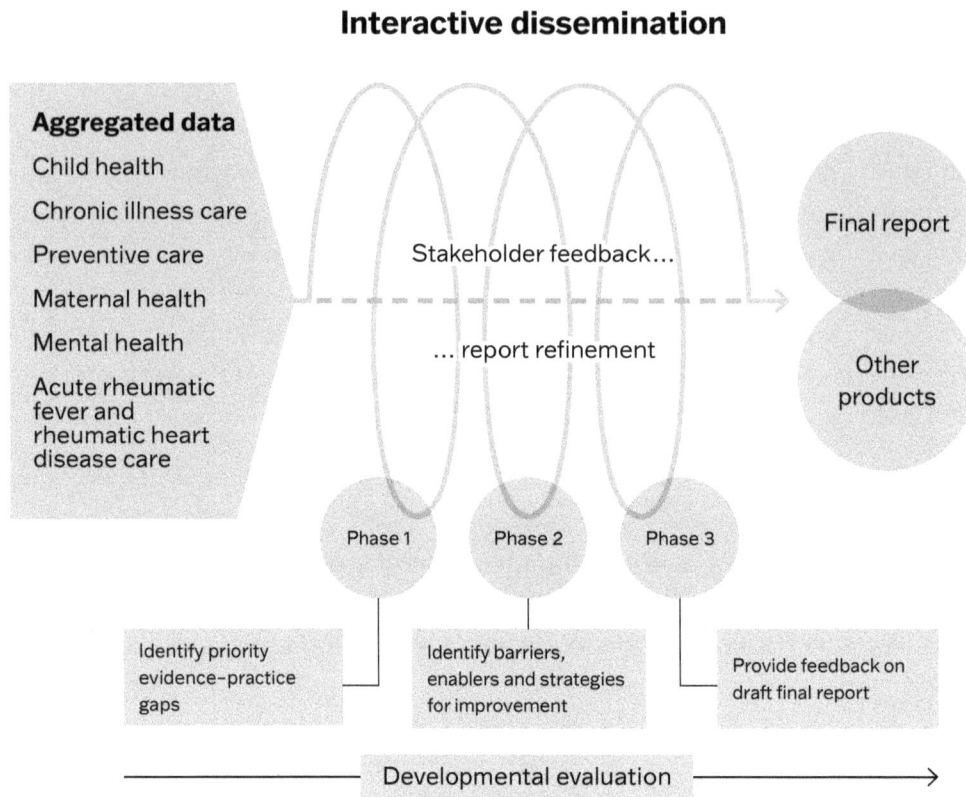

Figure 20.1 Engaging stakeholders in identifying priority evidence–practice gaps, barriers and strategies for improvement (ESP) project. Source: Laycock, Harvey et al. 2018.

- Aggregated CQI data reports were distributed by email through the existing ABCD National Research Partnership network (described in Chapter 9) and a snowballing recruitment technique was used to invite wider participation.
- Stakeholders were invited to use aggregated CQI data reports to identify the evidence-to-practice gaps, barriers and enablers most critical to improving health outcomes in key areas of clinical care, and to suggesst improvement strategies.
- Feedback was obtained through online surveys. A phased reporting and feedback process was used, culminating in a final report and other outputs (for example, journal articles, summaries) (see Figure 20.1).
- The process was used to generate findings for child health, maternal health, preventive care, chronic illness, mental health, and acute rheumatic fever and rheumatic heart disease care. (Key findings are reported in Part III.[24])

People who responded to the project surveys included Aboriginal and Torres Strait Islander health practitioners, nurses, doctors and other health practitioners, CQI facilitators, policymakers, PHC managers, governing board members and researchers.[25]

---

24   C. Bailie, Matthews et al. 2016; J. Bailie, Matthews et al. 2017; J. Bailie, Laycock et al. 2016; Gibson-Helm, J. Bailie et al. 2018.

25   For a breakdown of respondents' roles and numbers see Laycock, Harvey et al. 2018.

The commonly identified evidence-to-practice gaps across all the data could be grouped into five categories:

- follow-up of abnormal findings
- assessment and counselling for lifestyle risk factors
- emotional wellbeing screening and support
- treatment adherence (for example, taking medications) and self-management
- physical checks and investigations.

Synthesising the findings to identify messages for greater impact

When the priority evidence-to-practice gaps in each area of PHC (for example, child health, chronic illness care) were mapped according to these five categories, three improvement needs were common to all areas:

- follow-up of abnormal findings
- risk factor inquiry and provision of brief interventions
- social and emotional wellbeing support.

This finding suggested that improving these care processes would improve the quality of care for clients with a range of health conditions and care needs. Survey data about system barriers to improving the three gaps were analysed; these data reflected participants' contextual and professional knowledge and their experience working in Aboriginal and Torres Strait Islander PHC. Pareto analysis was used to identify the "vital few" system barriers to improvement in each of the categories. (For an explanation of Pareto analysis, see Chapter 5). The findings are summarised in Figure 20.2.

As illustrated in Figure 20.2, the "vital few" barriers to improvement were identified as clinical information systems, workforce, staff skills and training, financial resources and community engagement. The findings suggested that focusing improvement efforts on these aspects of PHC would increase the effect for improving people's health.

The analysis also reinforced the importance of multi-level action across the health system to improve PHC performance, and the need to bring communities, policymakers and practitioners together to plan system improvement. As project participants reflected:

"At the micro level [the process] can start conversations ... on a macro level, it provides this large scale, very hard to argue with evidence for why action is needed, and support from the wider health system, government and funders." – researcher

"I see the role of data as bringing strategic people closer to the frontline practitioners, and then saying, 'We need to do something about this, help us and we will help you.'" – senior manager[26]

---

26   Laycock, Harvey et al. 2018.

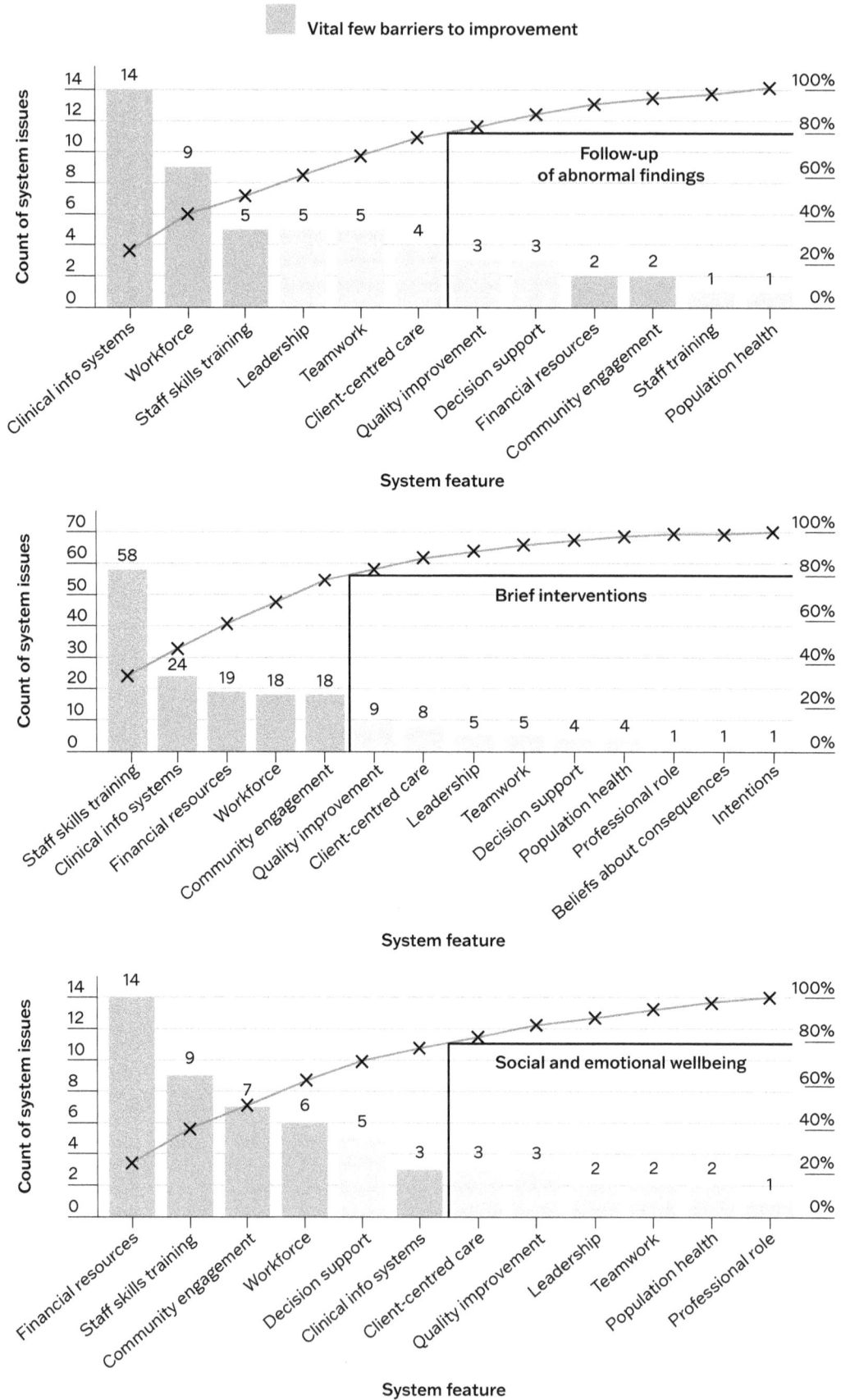

Figure 20.2 Using Pareto analysis to identify the "vital few" system barriers to wide-scale improvement: follow-up of abnormal findings, brief interventions, social and emotional wellbeing. Source: Matthews, J. Bailie et al. 2017.

Summary

This chapter has provided examples of a systems approach to CQI in PHC. The varied examples illustrate the benefit of people in complementary roles and at different system levels being involved in quality improvement. High-level policy support and action for CQI help to build sustainability of CQI processes at the health service and community level. Concurrent action at different system levels and across sectors has more potential to create synergy for change than efforts that are narrow in focus, due in large part to the interconnectedness of the systems that affect health. Strengthening systems in one area of health can reduce pressure on other systems; bridging a common evidence-to-practice gap can improve the quality of clinical care for clients with a range of health conditions.

A systems approach to CQI is situated within a broader systems approach to health services and health services research. It is important to acknowledge that not all system improvements are amenable to a classic CQI approach. Health systems research is a diverse and innovative field of research, and a range of mechanisms are required to improve health systems and other systems that affect health, such as legislation, justice, education, food production and social welfare. CQI is one key element in the coordinated and sustained action required to achieve improvement in population health outcomes and health equity.

References

Bailie, C., V. Matthews, J. Bailie, P. Burgess, K. Copley, C. Kennedy et al. (2016). Determinants and gaps in preventive care delivery for Indigenous Australians: a cross-sectional analysis. *Frontiers in Public Health* 4(34). DOI: 10.3389/fpubh.2016.00034.

Bailie, J., A. Laycock, V. Matthews and R. Bailie (2016). System-level action required for wide-scale improvement in quality of primary health care: synthesis of feedback from an interactive process to promote dissemination and use of aggregated quality of care data. *Frontiers in Public Health* 4(86). DOI: 10.3389/fpubh.2016.00086.

Bailie, J., V. Matthews, A. Laycock, R. Schultz, C. Burgess, D. Peiris et al. (2017). Improving preventive health care in Aboriginal and Torres Strait Islander primary care settings. *Globalization and Health* 13: 48. DOI: 10.1186/s12992-017-0267-z.

Bailie, R., V. Matthews, S. Larkins, S. Thompson, P. Burgess, T. Weeramanthri et al. (2017). Impact of policy support on uptake of evidence-based continuous quality improvement activities and the quality of care for Indigenous Australians: a comparative case study. *BMJ Open* 7(10). DOI: 10.1136/bmjopen-2017-016626.

Bainbridge, R., J. McCalman, M. Redman-MacLaren and M. Whiteside (2019). Grounded theory as systems science: working with Indigenous nations for social justice. In Antony Bryant and Kathy Charmaz, eds. *The Sage handbook of current developments in grounded theory*, 611–29. Thousand Oaks, CA: SAGE Publications.

Brimblecombe, J., C. van den Boogaard, B. Wood, S. Liberato, J. Brown, A. Barnes et al. (2015). Development of the good food planning tool: a food system approach to food security in Indigenous Australian remote communities. *Health Place* 34: 54–62. DOI: 10.1016/j.healthplace.2015.03.006.

Copley, K. and L. Patel (2021). *The Northern Territory continuous quality improvement strategy*. Darwin: Aboriginal Medical Service Alliance Northern Territory.

Ferlie, E.B. and S.M. Shortell (2001). Improving the quality of health care in the United Kingdom and the United States: a framework for change. *Milbank Quarterly* 79(2): 281–315.

Gibson-Helm, M., J. Bailie, V. Matthews, A. Laycock, J. Boyle and R. Bailie (2018). Identifying evidence–practice gaps and strategies for improvement in Aboriginal and Torres Strait Islander maternal health care. *PLOS One* 13(2): e0192262. DOI: 10.1371/journal.pone.0192262.

Heyeres, M., J. McCalman, K. Tsey and I. Kinchin (2016). The complexity of health service integration: a review of reviews. *Frontiers in Public Health* 4: 223. DOI: 10.3389/fpubh.2016.00223.

James Cook University (2019). Plan for healthy ageing in the Torres Strait. *James Cook University*. https://www.jcu.edu.au/news/releases/2019/july/plan-for-healthy-ageing-in-the-torres-strait.

Laycock, A., J. Bailie, V. Matthews, F. Cunningham, G. Harvey, N. Percival et al. (2017). A developmental evaluation to enhance stakeholder engagement in a wide-scale interactive project disseminating quality improvement data: study protocol for a mixed-methods study. *BMJ Open* 7: e016341. DOI: 10.1136/bmjopen-2017-016341.

Laycock, A., G. Harvey, N. Percival, F. Cunningham, J. Bailie, V. Matthews et al. (2018). Application of the i-PARIHS framework for enhancing understanding of interactive dissemination to achieve wide-scale improvement in Indigenous primary health care. *Health Research Policy and Systems* 16(117). DOI: 10.1186/s12961-018-0392-z.

Matthews, V., J. Bailie, A. Laycock, R. Bailie (2017). The vital few: key barriers to widescale improvement in Aboriginal & Torres Strait Islander primary health care. Presentation. 10th Health Services and Research Policy Conference, 1–3 November 2017, Gold Coast, Queensland.

McCalman, J., R. Bailie, R. Bainbridge, K. McPhail-Bell, N. Percival, D. Askew et al. (2018). Continuous quality improvement and comprehensive primary health care: a systems framework to improve service quality and health outcomes. *Frontiers in Public Health* 6: 76. DOI: 10.3389/fpubh.2018.00076.

McCalman, J., C. Jongen and R. Bainbridge (2017). Organisational systems' approaches to improving cultural competence in health care: a systematic scoping review of the literature. *International Journal for Equity in Health* 16(78). DOI: 10.1186/s12939-017-0571-5.

McDonald, E., R. Bailie and T. Michel (2013). Development and trialling of a tool to support a systems approach to improve social determinants of health in rural and remote Australian communities: the healthy community assessment tool. *International Journal for Equity in Health* 12(15). DOI: 10.1186/1475-9276-12-15.

McDonald, E., R. Bailie and P. Morris (2014). Participatory systems approach to health improvement in Australian Aboriginal children. *Health Promotion International* 32: 62–72. DOI: 10.1093/heapro/dau003.

National Aboriginal Community Controlled Health Organisation (2021). *Core Services and Outcomes Framework: the Model of Aboriginal and Torres Strait Islander Community-Controlled Comprehensive Primary Health Care*. Canberra, ACT: NACCHO. https://csof.naccho.org.au.

National Aboriginal Community Controlled Health Organisation (2018). *National Framework for continuous quality improvement in primary health care for Aboriginal and Torres Strait Islander people 2018–2023*. Canberra: NACCHO.

Peters, D., N. Tran and T. Adam (2013). *Implementation research in health: a practical guide*. Geneva, Switzerland: World Health Organization.

Quilty, S., N. Frank Jupurrurla, R. Bailie and R. Gruen (2022). Climate, housing, energy and Indigenous health: a call to action. *Medical Journal of Australia* 217(1): 9–12. DOI10.5694/mja2.51610.

Quilty, S. and N. Jupurrurla (2022). How climate change is turning remote Indigenous houses into dangerous hot boxes. *The Conversation*, 17 June. https://theconversation.com/how-climate-change-is-turning-remote-indigenous-houses-into-dangerous-hot-boxes-184328.

Shortell, S., C. Bennett and G. Byck (1998). Assessing the impact of continuous quality improvement on clinical practice: what it will take to accelerate progress. *Milbank Quarterly* 7(4): 593–624.

Sollecito, W. and J. Johnson (2019). *McLaughlin and Kaluzny's continuous quality improvement in health care*. Burlington, MA: Jones & Bartlett Learning.

Trees, J., T. Levett, K. Wynn and R. Ivers (2022). Ngununggula: the story of a cancer care team for Aboriginal people. *International Journal of Whole Person Care* 9(1): 50–1.

Tricco, A., N. Ivers, J. Grimshaw, D. Moher, L. Turner, J. Galipeau et al. (2012). Effectiveness of quality improvement strategies on the management of diabetes: a systematic review and meta-analysis. *Lancet* 379(9833): 2252–61. DOI: 10.1016/S01406736(12)60480-2.

Centralising respect, equity and justice in health research

This chapter draws with permission on the work of the Aboriginal and Torres Strait Islander Reference Committee of the Centre for Research Excellence: Strengthening Systems for Indigenous Health Care Equity (CRE-STRIDE).

Previous chapters have demonstrated how research evidence is key to advancing the theory and practice of continuous quality improvement. The principles of respect, equity and justice that underpin primary health care and CQI are central to quality improvement research. In this chapter, we describe important concepts and approaches in equity- and justice-focused research, drawing on international literature and our experience in Aboriginal and Torres Strait Islander health research to illustrate how these concepts and approaches can be put into CQI research practice.

The chapter starts with an introduction to equity- and systems-focused health research, identifying the need for approaches that shift power in research, enabling the "researched" to become researchers into their priority concerns and determine appropriate action for health improvement. We refer to methodologies developed by Indigenous research leaders in response to Indigenous peoples' experience with Euro-Western research – methodologies that align with Indigenous rights and reflect Indigenous ways of knowing, being and doing. Some of the generalisable principles embedded in these methodologies are illustrated through the research guidance provided by the Aboriginal and Torres Strait Islander Reference Committee of our Australian research collaboration, the Centre for Research Excellence: Strengthening Systems for Indigenous Health Care Equity (CRE-STRIDE). The second part of the chapter describes other participatory research approaches that respect and draw on the knowledge and lived experiences of research participants. These approaches have proved appropriate in our CQI research, empowering primary healthcare staff by building competence and confidence to sustain CQI.

Equity- and systems-focused health research

Many studies identify health inequities and their causes. Progressing a health equity agenda through research acknowledges the power imbalances that prevail in research (for example, between academic institutions and participating communities) and the inequalities that exist across the health system and other systems influencing the determinants of health. While research approaches and methods vary, health research that progresses an equity agenda commonly seeks to achieve these goals:

- advance the priorities and aspirations of groups who experience health and other inequities
- harness the knowledge and strengths that communities and research participants bring, and empower those groups through research processes
- provide a platform for advocacy and transformative change – that is, positive changes in attitudes, systems and behaviours.[1]

Much quality improvement work is, by definition, concerned with healthcare equity. CQI aims to inform and sustain system changes that benefit those most in need and reduce health inequity between population groups. Research into health systems and CQI informs this endeavour. An important component of health systems research is finding ways to overcome systemic (sometimes called structural) inequities. Systemic inequities are embedded in the systems, laws, policies and practices that support unjust treatment based on intentional or unconscious prejudice. This is the experience of many poor people, and many Indigenous peoples and people of colour in countries that were colonised. Systemic inequities lead to poorer health and wellbeing for those who experience continuing discrimination and for society more generally.[2] Thus, equity- and systems-focused health research has a critical role in improving health equity and social justice.

> Equity- and systems-focused health research has a critical role in improving health equity and social justice.

Earlier chapters have referred to CRE-STRIDE. CRE-STRIDE is one example of a research collaboration working to strengthen systems for more equitable health outcomes through quality improvement research in Aboriginal and Torres Strait Islander health. Collaboration members have built evidence for policy, system and research reform while championing the importance of equity- and community-driven health policy. Various methodologies have been used by research teams involved in the collaboration, including emancipatory and transformational methodologies designed to support action for social justice.[3] CRE-STRIDE's approach to research is described in the next chapter.

Research concepts and approaches for Indigenous healthcare equity

Overcoming Indigenous healthcare inequity and injustice is a critical global health issue. Indigenous peoples comprise 5 per cent of the of the world's population yet make up 15 per cent of the world's extreme poor, with many communities having limited or no access to health and social services.[4] Improving the availability and quality of PHC for Indigenous peoples are critical equity issues.

---

1   R. Bailie, Matthews et al. 2017; Bainbridge, McCalman et al. 2019; Hernández, Ruano et al. 2017; McCalman, Bainbridge et al. 2018; Mertens 2021.

2   Braveman, Arkin et al. 2022.

3   Bainbridge, McCalman et al. 2019.

4   Amnesty International 2021.

Indigenous peoples are also among the most researched communities in the world,[5] without corresponding improvements in health.[6] Over the past two decades, efforts to reform Indigenous health research in several countries have acknowledged the prevailing power imbalances in academic research and taken steps to increase Indigenous community engagement and control of research. In the following pages we identify some key concepts and approaches being used to deliver healthcare equity and other benefits to Indigenous peoples through research.

The need to decolonise research

The history of research for Indigenous peoples is tied to the history of colonisation. As Indigenous peoples were colonised by European nations, Indigenous societies and cultures were studied from the perspective of those with more power and privilege, and with different systems of knowledge.[7] Indigenous lands, peoples and resources were observed through a lens of European values, beliefs and prejudices, ignoring extensive Indigenous knowledges developed over millennia and dehumanising Indigenous people as objects of scientific research.[8]

The effect and role of Euro-Western research in colonising Indigenous peoples and research has been well documented by Indigenous academics.[9] While experiences of colonisation differ between colonised countries, there is common recognition that Euro-Western research paradigms contributed to racism and ongoing oppression.[10] For example, colonisers used research to perpetrate inaccurate stereotyping of Indigenous peoples[11] and to help justify policies that dispossessed people of their lands and freedom, repressed language use, cultural practices and spiritual beliefs, and removed children from their families.[12] Much present-day research is conducted in the context of continuing colonial power imbalances. The decolonisation of research shifts these power imbalances to centre the concerns, knowledges and worldviews of Indigenous peoples.

> The decolonisation of research shifts these power imbalances to centre the concerns, knowledges and worldviews of Indigenous peoples.

As Indigenous peoples demand greater control over research that involves their communities, there is increasing recognition that Indigenous cultures, knowledges and experience can inform solutions to remedy health inequities.[13] Some academic systems are working towards greater Indigenous inclusion in research leadership, while policy guidelines for research in Indigenous contexts increasingly reflect the need for communities and researchers to work in partnership

---

5   Tuhiwai Smith 1999.
6   Bainbridge, Tsey et al. 2015; Harfield, Pearson et al. 2020.
7   Laycock, Walker et al. 2011.
8   Tuhiwai Smith 1999.
9   For a concise list, see Ryder, Mackean et al. 2020.
10   Rix, Wilson et al. 2019.
11   Thambinathan and Kinsella 2021.
12   Anderson, Baum and Bentley 2004; Laycock, Walker et al. 2011.
13   Coalition of Aboriginal and Torres Strait Islander Peak Organisations and Australian Governments 2020.

to identify research needs and to design, conduct and translate research in ways that benefit Indigenous peoples.[14] Continuing purposeful effort is required to decolonise research.

Adopting core values in research

The decolonisation of research requires researchers to examine the values that shape their practice. Values underpin every aspect of research including researcher–participant relationships, the research questions, how research is conducted, what constitutes knowledge and who owns it, how power and knowledge are shared, and other ethical decisions and behaviours.

In some countries, Indigenous peoples have identified core values to be upheld when conducting research that involves their communities. For example, in Australia, guidelines for ethical research in Aboriginal and Torres Strait Islander health are structured around six core values: spirit and integrity, cultural continuity, equity, reciprocity, respect and responsibility, as described in Table 21.1. The guidelines are adopted as government policy and companion guidelines have been developed for keeping research on track to uphold these values.[15] Australian human research ethics committees use these guidelines when assessing projects involving Indigenous peoples.

Table 21.1 The six core values for ethical research in Aboriginal and Torres Strait Islander health.

Spirit and integrity	The central value that binds the other five values together. Spirit is about the ongoing connection and continuity between Aboriginal and Torres Strait Islander peoples' past, current and future generations. Integrity is about the respectful and honourable behaviours that hold Aboriginal and Torres Strait Islander values and cultures together.
Cultural continuity	Research can harm Aboriginal and Torres Strait Islander peoples' and communities' knowledge, cultures, languages and identity. This value is about research being conducted in a way that protects the rights of Aboriginal and Torres Strait Islander peoples to uphold, enjoy and protect their knowledge, cultures, languages and identity, as individuals and as communities.
Equity	Aboriginal and Torres Strait Islander people and communities have experienced inequities as a result of discrimination and marginalisation. Aboriginal and Torres Strait Islander peoples recognise the equal value of all individuals. One of the ways that this is shown is in commitment to fairness and justice. Equity affirms and recognises Aboriginal and Torres Strait Islander peoples' right to be different.

---

14   Harfield, Pearson et al. 2020; National Health and Medical Research Council 2018a, b.
15   National Health and Medical Research Council 2018b.

Reciprocity	Aboriginal and Torres Strait Islander peoples' way of shared responsibility and obligation is based on diverse kinship networks. This keeps ways of living and family relationships strong. These responsibilities also extend to caring for country and all within it, and involve sharing benefits from the air, land and sea, redistribution of resources, and sharing food and housing.
Respect	Respect is expressed as having regard for the welfare, rights, knowledge, skills, beliefs, perceptions, customs and cultural heritage (both individual and collective) of people involved in research. Within Aboriginal and Torres Strait Islander cultures, respect is reinforced through, and in turn strengthens, dignity. A respectful relationship promotes trust and cooperation.
Responsibility	All Aboriginal and Torres Strait Islander communities recognise the same most important (core) responsibilities. These responsibilities involve caring for Country and all within it, kinship bonds, caring for others, and the maintenance of cultural and spiritual awareness. The main responsibility is to do no harm to any person or any place. Sometimes these responsibilities may be shared so that others may also be held accountable.

Source: National Health and Medical Research Council 2018a, b.

Articulating values can strengthen understanding of what is important to groups involved in research and support ethical practice. It has additional importance when different knowledge systems come together in a research project, when researchers have had minimal experience working in cross-cultural contexts, and when participants have had negative experiences of research.

Decolonising and Indigenous research methodologies

Decolonising research methodologies emerged from Indigenous scholarship in response to the lack of engagement with Indigenous philosophies within Euro-Western research. There has been a growing body of influential literature since the Māori academic Linda Tuhiwai Smith (Ngāti Awa and Ngati Porou) published a groundbreaking book on the topic in 1999.[16] Smith advocated for Indigenous intellectual sovereignty of research involving Indigenous people and interests,[17] articulating the benefits of making Indigenous cultural protocols, values and behaviours integral to research methodology. Concurrently in Australia, First Nations scholar, Lester-Irabinna Rigney (Narungga, Kaurna and Ngarrindjeri Nations) defined Indigenist research as culturally safe and respectful research based on three principles: resistance as vital for emancipation; political integrity, with Indigenous Australians setting their own political agenda while simultaneously engaging in research and the Indigenous struggle; and

---

16   Tuhiwai Smith 1999.
17   Rix, Wilson et al. 2019.

privileging of Indigenous voices in research.[18] Scholars in various colonised nations have progressed work to centre the politics of Indigenous identity, experiences and cultural action in their research approaches.[19]

Some Euro-Western methods that consider Indigenous critiques of research practices and integrate the values, expectations and cultures of Indigenous communities may support research decolonisation. Grounded theory, for example, is a methodology committed to social justice that may serve as a decolonising method.[20]

Indigenous research methodologies reference the theories and principles that Indigenous peoples have been developing and practising for millennia. In this respect, all Indigenous methodologies have a decolonising intent, empowering Indigenous peoples to represent experiences and realities consistent with cultural understandings.[21] As described by the Aboriginal and Torres Strait Islander leaders in our quality improvement research collaborative, CRE-STRIDE:

> [Indigenous research methodologies] are embodied in our culture that sees, knows and feels Country and connection of kin. They reflect a complex and integrated system of knowledge and beliefs. These practices and systems have sustained our culture and continue to provide resilience for our communities against challenges brought about by the impact of colonisation.[22]

Descriptions of Indigenous methodologies differ based on cultural and geographical contexts and experiences of the Indigenous theorist, but there is a common essence. Indigenous research methodologies are based on Indigenous ways of knowing, being and doing, and are enacted through principles of relationality, respect and reciprocity (see Box 21.1).

Box 21.1 Theoretical principles informing Indigenous methodologies

Noonuccal scholar Karen Martin-Booran Mirraboopa identified these principles:

Recognition of our worldviews, our knowledges and our realities as distinctive and vital to our existence and survival;

Honouring our social mores as essential processes through which we live, learn and situate ourselves as Aboriginal people in our own lands and when in the lands of other Aboriginal people;

Emphasis of social, historical and political contexts which shape our experiences, lives, positions and futures;

Privileging the voices, experiences and lives of Aboriginal people and Aboriginal lands.[23]

---

18   Rigney 1999, 2001.
19   Archibald, Lee Morgan and de Santolo 2019; Hughes and Barlo 2021; Martin-Booran Mirraboopa 2003; Watego, Whop et al. 2021.
20   Bainbridge, McCalman et al. 2019; Jongen, Langham et al. 2019.
21   Moreton-Robinson and Walter 2009.
22   Indigenous Reference Committee 2020, 2.
23   Martin-Booran Mirraboopa 2003, 205.

Indigenous research methodologies reference the theories and principles that Indigenous peoples have been developing and practising for millennia.

Indigenous knowledge is at the core of Indigenous peoples' rights to survival, dignity and wellbeing.[24] Indigenous knowledge systems involve living well with, and being in relationship with, the natural world while building upon the experiences of earlier generations, informing the practice of current generations, and evolving in the context of contemporary society.[25] Thus, the wellbeing of communities is understood to be inextricably linked to Indigenous rights and to the social, cultural, historical and environmental determinants of health.

> Our knowledge systems are holistic and relational. Our health encompasses our relationship to Country, culture, spirituality, community and family. With this relationality comes responsibility ... to look after Country and each other.[26]

The holistic understanding of health embodied in many Indigenous knowledge systems can inform *holistic* healthcare systems and comprehensive models of care.[27] Because the construction of knowledge is holistic, adaptive, multilayered and continuous over millennia, the traditional knowledge and expertise of Indigenous communities can also inform responses to biodiversity risks, land and natural resources management, food security, disaster risk reduction and other issues critical to planetary and human health and survival.[28] Much Indigenous health research occurs at the interface of knowledge systems.

The holistic understanding of health embodied in many Indigenous knowledge systems can inform *holistic* healthcare systems and comprehensive models of care.

Martin Nakata, a leading academic from the Torres Strait Islands, described the intersection of Euro-Western and Indigenous research methodologies as a "cultural interface", where researchers generate new stories, methodologies and approaches.[29] First Nations people of Canada have described this process as "two-eyed seeing".[30] The Yolŋu people of Arnhem Land in Australia's north describe the concept of Ganma, relating the coming together of two knowledge systems to the convergence of river water and seawater in a coastal lagoon.

> In coming together, the streams of water mix across the interface of the two currents and foam is created. This foam represents a new kind of knowledge. The forces of the stream combine and lead to deeper understanding and truth. Essentially, Ganma is a place where knowledge is (re)created.[31]

---

24   United Nations 2007.
25   Government of Canada 2022.
26   CRE-STRIDE 2022.
27   Panaretto, Wenitong et al. 2014.
28   Jones, Reid and Macmillan 2022.
29   Nakata 2010.
30   Roher, Yu et al. 2021.
31   Kelly 2008; Laycock, Walker et al. 2011, 50; Yunggirringa and Garnggulkpuy 2007.

Within each of these examples, Indigenous Elders and leaders describe knowledge as relational, with knowledge-sharing processes embodying mutual respect, shared benefits, reciprocity and discovery. The bringing together of Indigenous knowledge and Euro-Western science is enabling more comprehensive understandings of health, illness and healing, while challenging researchers to straddle the knowledge divide and act as agents at the cultural interface.[32] Indigenous and non-Indigenous researchers are required to locate themselves within the community context and to immerse research inquiries within culture and place, while fulfilling the roles and obligations of relationships in research.[33] This is a complex space requiring careful negotiation, relationship building and continuous learning – particularly given the historical dominance of biomedical knowledge and marginalisation of Indigenous knowledge in research and health care.[34]

Participatory and system-focused research approaches

The previous pages have identified some important issues and approaches for improving Indigenous healthcare equity through research, with references for further reading. Lessons learnt as Indigenous peoples seek redress from the ongoing impact of colonisation are relevant for working with groups who are oppressed and those who have historically been marginalised or discriminated against.[35] The following pages describe participatory research approaches that are used more broadly in equity-focused health and CQI research.

Participatory action research and community-based participatory research

Participatory action research has been used to develop the CQI tools (Chapter 5) and much of the evidence presented in this book (as outlined in Chapter 9). Participatory action research and community-based participatory research seek to capture and incorporate the perspective(s) of the people who are most affected by the research, positioning participants as experts in their own lives and knowledges. Research is conducted "with" or "by" people, in contrast to research "on" or "for" people, thereby facilitating shared leadership and ownership of research.[36] Together, researchers and participants engage in collective, self-reflective inquiry so they can understand and improve upon their practices and situation.[37]

The theory and practice of both these forms of research have roots in the Indigenous de-colonial community-capacity-building practices and social movements documented in the 1960s and 1970s, rather than the academic world.[38] In Australia, Aboriginal participatory action research is a transformative Indigenous research methodology that has contributed to the conceptualisation of Indigenous social and emotional wellbeing and a strength-based Indigenous psychology. This distinguishes Aboriginal participatory action research from its Euro-Western adaptation.[39]

---

32   Durie 2004; Ryder, Mackean et al. 2020.
33   Barlo, Boyd et al. 2021; CRE-STRIDE 2022.
34   Cass, Lowell et al. 2002; Rix, Wilson et al. 2019.
35   Maguire 2013.
36   Braun, Browne et al. 2014; Doyle, Cleary et al. 2017.
37   Baum, MacDougall and Smith 2006.
38   Hall and Tandon 2017.
39   Dudgeon, Bray et al. 2020.

Central to the methodology of participatory action research is engagement in cycles of reflection, planning, acting, further observation and reflection, then new plans and action. In this respect, its processes align with CQI cycles, such as plan-do-study-act. Within the broader framework of participatory action research, community-based participatory research focuses on issues identified by the community, empowering community members in research and prioritising opportunities to build on the community's strengths and resources.[40] Both approaches foster co-learning and capacity building between partners, with translation into action as part of the research process.

Participatory action research and community-based participatory research have potential to mobilise community action on health inequities and the social and environmental determinants of health.[41] As the implementation of findings is integral to the research, these approaches have greater likelihood of bringing about sustainable changes compared with traditional research approaches.[42] Bainbridge and colleagues propose that participatory action research approaches can strengthen relationships between Indigenous and non-Indigenous researchers and research users to maximise the benefits of knowledge and expertise brought by all stakeholders.[43]

Co-design and co-production

Co-design, co-production and co-creation are related concepts. They refer to participatory processes whereby target users are involved from the start of an initiative. The "users" build and test the program or product together with the designers, service providers or researchers.

As with participatory action research, co-design and co-production (or co-creation) are intrinsically linked with the concept of empowerment. In primary healthcare research, the underlying principles are that clients and communities have expert knowledge of their lives, environment and needs, and that meaningful collaboration will result in greater benefits. These benefits may include services that are better tailored to the local setting and clients' needs, and the experiential learning of all who are involved.

Relationships are the foundation of co-design and co-production. Together, stakeholders with productive relationships can frame the right research questions, design research for real-world environments and commit to implementing the research and the findings.[44] In settings where researchers are working with minority or disempowered groups, co-production supports the use of appropriate research methodologies and strengths-based approaches (described below). In Indigenous health research, it supports critical reflexivity and has potential to deepen non-Indigenous co-researchers' knowledge and understanding of local, place-based cultural practices. Effective research starts with striving to understand complex health issues from community perspectives and asking the right questions. It involves reporting findings in formats determined by the community, working together to locate solutions, and engaging service managers and policymakers to facilitate the use of findings for policy and system change. Positive relationships are critical.

---

40   Frerichs, Lich et al. 2016; Leung, Chan et al. 2004.
41   Baum 2016; Frerichs, Lich et al. 2016.
42   Braun, Browne et al. 2014; Smith, Devine and Preston 2020.
43   Bainbridge, Tsey et al. 2015.
44   Jackson and Greenhalgh 2015.

> Relationships are the foundation of co-design and co-production.

Research co-design with Indigenous participants and minority groups must be culturally safe. Every group and context are unique. Depending on the historical context, issues such as power inequalities, racism, privilege based on dominant societal culture and unconscious bias need to be addressed as part of the co-design process.[45]

Strengths-based approaches

The strengths-based approach is a philosophy and a way of seeing individuals and communities as resourceful and resilient in the face of adversity. It is a response to problem- or deficit-based approaches that focus on weaknesses, risks or needs as identified by others. A strengths-based approach is centred on solutions and capabilities; it focuses holistically on the interests, desired outcomes, and strengths that people bring to a situation. In applied research, it emphasises the self-determination and personal strengths of individuals as well as wider social and community networks. Community-based participatory research and appreciative inquiry are strengths-based research approaches.

> A strengths-based approach is centred on solutions and capabilities; it focuses holistically on the interests, desired outcomes, and strengths that people bring to a situation.

Strengths-based approaches to knowing, being and doing have enabled the survival of Indigenous communities,[46] with strengths-based practice identified by Aboriginal and Torres Strait Islander primary healthcare practitioners as the way of working with Indigenous people.[47] Strengths-based approaches are compatible with holistic concepts of health and protective factors for wellbeing, with some authors describing culture-based and strengths-based approaches as interrelated.[48]

Strengths-based research approaches are consistent with ethically sound research that achieves mutually beneficial outcomes for researchers and communities.[49] They are more likely to support positive stories and to motivate change than deficit-focused approaches that do not accurately reflect progress.[50] As Thurber writes:

> A strengths-based approach [to research] focuses on the community [or population] of interest and looks at how things are going within that population. It considers who is doing well, who is doing less well, what is working, and what is not working. This

---

45   Wright, Brown et al. 2021.
46   Dudgeon, Bray et al. 2020.
47   Askew, Brady et al. 2020.
48   Fogarty, Lovell et al. 2018.
49   Bainbridge, Whiteside et al. 2013.
50   Fogarty, Lovell et al. 2018; Thurber, Thandrayen et al. 2020.

provides a more accurate story of what is going on, and it gives the community real data to work with.[51]

The aim of strengths-based approaches is not to deny problems or inequities. Strengths need to be understood in relation to constraints (for example, how community-driven responses are constrained by power imbalances), so that the research can support individual and community autonomy and identify pathways for translating findings into action.[52]

Holistic, systems-thinking approaches

Sustainable change requires changes to systems rather than short-term effects. Systems-thinking approaches (as described in Chapter 6) underpin purposeful system change decisions. The CQI tools in Chapter 5, for example, are designed to help primary healthcare teams to use systems thinking when identifying the causes of poor-quality care and planning sustainable improvement strategies.

If CQI and health systems research are to improve equity and health outcomes, research must aim to strengthen systems for PHC, based on understanding how systems intersect and behave to influence health and wellbeing. Systems-thinking and holistic approaches to health (as defined in Chapter 1) are embodied in Indigenous understanding of life, health and human connection and in the many real-world examples of CQI in this book. The previous chapter describes improvement initiatives at different system levels and involving multiple sectors (for example, community health and housing). The next chapter describes a long-term research network focused on multi-level system reform. Holism and the use of systems thinking are common elements across this work (as are the importance of social and cultural determinants of health, and community-driven and people-centred approaches).

Summary

This chapter has described some important concepts, approaches and methodologies for advancing equity- and system-focused CQI research in PHC. It has included Indigenous methodologies that seek to redress power imbalances and ongoing colonisation through research, and participatory and system-focused research approaches that can be used in a variety of settings.

Participatory and collaborative research approaches have led the reform of methodologies used in equity-focused research. These approaches are critical for meaningful engagement, but do not necessarily bring about positive change. Transformational and emancipatory methodologies, such as those described in this chapter, are required to progress an equity agenda[53] and to consciously tackle the unequal power dynamics inherent in academic power structures and much research practice. In our research interactions, we must be sensitive to different worldviews and potential miscommunication, practise cultural safety and genuinely listen to and privilege the voices of those who are traditionally disempowered through research.

---

51   Thurber 2021.
52   Bond 2009; Bulloch, Fogarty and Bellchambers 2019; Fogarty, Lovell et al. 2018.
53   Bainbridge, McCalman et al. 2019.

The next chapter shares lessons learnt by our nationwide research network, which brings together Aboriginal and Torres Strait Islander and non-Indigenous researchers with the common aim of improving healthcare equity through collaborative CQI research.

References

Amnesty International (2021). Indigenous peoples' rights. https://www.amnesty.org/en/what-we-do/indigenous-peoples/.

Anderson, I., F. Baum and M. Bentley, eds (2004). *Beyond bandaids: exploring the underlying social determinants of Aboriginal health*. Papers from the Social Determinants of Aboriginal Health Workshop, Adelaide. Darwin: Cooperative Research Centre for Aboriginal Health.

Archibald, J., J. Lee Morgan and J. de Santolo, eds (2019). *Decolonizing research: indigenous storywork as methodology*. London: Zed Books.

Askew, D.A., K. Brady, B. Mukandi, D. Singh, T. Sinha, M. Brough et al. (2020). Closing the gap between rhetoric and practice in strengths-based approaches to Indigenous public health: a qualitative study. *Australian and New Zealand Journal of Public Health* 44(2): 102–5. DOI: 10.1111/1753-6405.12953.

Bailie, R., V. Matthews, S. Larkins, S. Thompson, P. Burgess, T. Weeramanthri et al. (2017). Impact of policy support on uptake of evidence-based continuous quality improvement activities and the quality of care for Indigenous Australians: a comparative case study. *BMJ Open* 7(10). DOI: 10.1136/bmjopen-2017-016626.

Bainbridge, R., J. McCalman, M. Redman-MacLaren and M. Whiteside (2019). Grounded theory as systems science: working with Indigenous nations for social justice. In A. Bryant and K. Charmaz, eds. *The SAGE handbook of current developments in grounded theory*, 611–29. London: SAGE.

Bainbridge, R., K. Tsey, J. McCalman, I. Kinchin, V. Saunders and F. Watkin (2015). No one's discussing the elephant in the room: contemplating questions of research impact and benefit in Aboriginal and Torres Strait Islander health research. *BMC Public Health* 16: 696. DOI: 10.1186/s12889-015-2052-3.

Bainbridge, R., M. Whiteside and J. McCalman. (2013). Being, knowing and doing: a phronetic approach to constructing grounded theory with Australian Aboriginal partners. *Qualitative Health Research* 23(2): 275–88. DOI: 10.1177/1049732312467853.

Barlo, S., W. Boyd, M. Hughes, S. Wilson and A. Pelizzon (2021). Yarning as protected space: relational accountability in research. *AlterNative: An International Journal of Indigenous Peoples* 17(1): 40–8. DOI: 10.1177/1177180120986151.

Baum, F. (2016). Power and glory: applying participatory action research in public health. *Gaceta Sanitaria* 30(6): 405–7. DOI: 10.1016/j.gaceta.2016.05.014.

Baum, F., C. MacDougall and D. Smith (2006). Participatory action research. *Journal of Epidemiology and Community Health* 60(10): 854–7. DOI: 10.1136/jech.2004.028662.

Bond, C. (2009). Starting at strengths . . . an Indigenous early years intervention. *Medical Journal of Australia* 191(3): 175–7.

Braun, K., C. Browne, L. Ka'opua, B. Kim and N. Mokuau (2014). Research on indigenous elders: from positivistic to decolonizing methodologies. *Gerontologist* 54(1): 117–26. DOI: 10.1093/geront/gnt067.

Braveman, P., E. Arkin, D. Proctor, T. Kauh and N. Holm (2022). Systemic and structural racism: definitions, examples, health damages, and approaches to dismantling. *Health Affairs* 41(2): 171–7. DOI: 10.1377/hlthaff.2021.01394.

Bulloch, H., W. Fogarty and K. Bellchambers (2019). *Aboriginal health and wellbeing services: putting community-driven, strengths-based approaches into practice*. Melbourne: Lowitja Institute.

Cass, A., A. Lowell, M. Christie, P.L. Snelling, M. Flack, B. Marrnganyin et al. (2002). Sharing the true stories: improving communication between Aboriginal patients and healthcare workers. *JAMA: The Journal of the American Medical Association* 176(10): 466–70. DOI: 10.5694/j.1326-5377.2002.tb04517.x.

Coalition of Aboriginal and Torres Strait Islander Peak Organisations and Australian Governments (2020). *National Agreement on Closing the Gap*. Department of the Prime Minister and Cabinet. Canberra: Commonwealth of Australia.

CRE-STRIDE (2022). Aboriginal and Torres Strait Islander research methodologies and frameworks. https://cre-stride.org/indigenous-research-methodologies-frameworks/.

Doyle, K., M. Cleary, D. Blanchard and C. Hungerford (2017). The Yerin Dilly Bag Model of Indigenist health research. *Qualitative Health Research* 27(9): 1288–301. DOI: 10.1177/1049732317700125.

Dudgeon, P., A. Bray, D. Darlaston-Jones and R. Walker (2020). *Aboriginal participatory action research: an Indigenous research methodology strengthening decolonisation and social and emotional wellbeing.* Discussion paper. Melbourne: Lowitja Institute.

Durie, M. (2004). Understanding health and illness: research at the interface between science and indigenous knowledge. *International Journal of Epidemiology* 33(5): 1138–43. DOI: 10.1093/ije/dyh250.

Fogarty, W., M. Lovell, J. Langenberg and M. Heron (2018). *Deficit discourse and strengths-based approaches: changing the narrative of Aboriginal and Torres Strait Islander health and wellbeing.* Melbourne: Lowitja Institute.

Frerichs, L., K. Lich, G. Dave and G. Corbie-Smith (2016). Integrating systems science and community-based participatory research to achieve health equity. *American Journal of Public Health* 106(2): 215–22. DOI: 10.2105/AJPH.2015.302944.

Government of Canada (2022). What is Indigenous knowledge? https://www.canada.ca/en/impact-assessment-agency/programs/aboriginal-consultation-federal-environmental-assessment/indigenous-knowledge-policy-framework-initiative.html.

Hall, B. and R. Tandon (2017). Participatory research: Where have we been, where are we going? – a dialogue. *Research for All.* DOI: 10.18546/RFA.01.2.12.

Harfield, S., O. Pearson, K. Morey, E. Kite, K. Canuto, K. Glover et al. (2020). Assessing the quality of health research from an Indigenous perspective: the Aboriginal and Torres Strait Islander quality appraisal tool. *BMC Medical Research Methodology* 20(1): 79. DOI: 10.1186/s12874-020-00959-3.

Hernández, A., A. Ruano, B. Marchal, M. San Sebastián and W. Flores (2017). Engaging with complexity to improve the health of indigenous people: a call for the use of systems thinking to tackle health inequity. *International Journal for Equity in Health* 16(1): 26. DOI: 10.1186/s12939-017-0521-2.

Hughes, M. and S. Barlo (2021). Yarning with Country: an Indigenist research methodology. *Qualitative Inquiry* 27(3–4): 353–63. DOI: 10.1177/1077800420918889.

Indigenous Reference Committee, Centre for Research Excellence: Strengthening Systems for Indigenous Health Care Equity (2020). *Indigenous Research Framework.* Lismore, NSW: University Centre for Rural Health, University of Sydney.

Jackson, C. and T. Greenhalgh (2015). Co-creation: a new approach to optimising research impact? *Medical Journal of Australia* 203(7): 283–4. DOI: 10.5694/mja15.00219.

Jones, R., P. Reid and A. Macmillan (2022). Navigating fundamental tensions towards a decolonial relational vision of planetary health. *Lancet Planet Health* 6(10): e834–e41. DOI: 10.1016/S2542-5196(22)00197-8.

Jongen, C., E. Langham, R. Bainbridge and J. McCalman (2019). Instruments for measuring the resilience of Indigenous adolescents: an exploratory review. *Frontiers in Public Health* 7(194). DOI: 10.3389/fpubh.2019.00194.

Kelly, J. (2008). Moving forward together in Aboriginal women's health: a participatory action research exploring knowledge sharing, working together and addressing issues collaboratively in urban primary health care settings. Doctoral thesis, Flinders University, Adelaide.

Laycock, A., D. Walker, N. Harrison and J. Brands (2011). *Researching Indigenous health: a practical guide for researchers.* Melbourne: Lowitja Institute.

Leung, D., S. Chan, C. Lau, V. Wong and T. Lam (2004). Community based participatory research: a promising approach for increasing epidemiology's relevance in the 21st century. *International Journal of Epidemiology* 33(3): 4999–506. DOI: 10.1093/ije/dyh010.

Maguire, A. (2013). Contemporary anti-colonial self-determination claims and the decolonisation of international law. *Griffith Law Review* 22(1): 238–68. DOI: 10.1080/10383441.2013.10854774.

Martin-Booran Mirraboopa, K. (2003). Ways of knowing, being and doing: a theoretical framework and methods for indigenous and indigenist re-search. *Journal of Australian Studies: Voicing Dissent* 27(76): 203–14. DOI: 10.1080/14443050309387838.

McCalman, J., R. Bainbridge, C. Brown, K. Tsey and A. Clarke (2018). The Aboriginal Australian Family Wellbeing Program: a historical analysis of the conditions that enabled its spread. *Frontiers in Public Health* 6: 26. DOI: 10.3389/fpubh.2018.00026.

Mertens, D.M. (2021). Transformative research methods to increase social impact for vulnerable groups and cultural minorities. *International Journal of Qualitative Methods* 20: 16094069211051563. DOI: 10.1177/16094069211051563.

Moreton-Robinson, A. and M. Walter (2009). Indigenous methodologies in social research. In A. Bryman, ed. *Social research methods*, 95–109. Melbourne: Oxford University Press.

Nakata, M. (2010). The cultural interface of Islander and scientific knowledge. *Australian Journal of Indigenous Education* 39: 53–7.

National Health and Medical Research Council (2018a). *Ethical conduct in research with Aboriginal and Torres Strait Islander Peoples and communities: guidelines for researchers and stakeholders* Canberra: Commonwealth of Australia.

National Health and Medical Research Council (2018b). *Keeping research on track II: a companion document to* Ethical conduct in research with Aboriginal and Torres Strait Islander Peoples and communities: guidelines for researchers and stakeholders. Canberra: Commonwealth of Australia. https://www.nhmrc.gov.au/about-us/resources/keeping-research-track-ii.

Panaretto, K., M. Wenitong, S. Button and I. Ring (2014). Aboriginal community controlled health services: leading the way in primary care. *Medical Journal of Australia* 200(11): 649–52. DOI: 10.5694/mja13.00005.

Rigney, L.I. (2001). A first perspective of Indigenous Australian participation in science: framing Indigenous research towards Indigenous Australian intellectual sovereignty. *Kaurna Higher Education Journal* 7: 1–13.

Rigney, L.I. (1999). Internationalization of an Indigenous anticolonial cultural critique of research methodologies: a guide to Indigenist research methodology and its principles. *Journal for Native American Studies* 14(2): 109–21.

Rix, E., S. Wilson, N. Sheehan and N. Tujague (2019). Indigenist and decolonizing research methodology. In Pranee Liamputtong, ed. *Handbook of Research Methods in Health Social Sciences*, 253–67. Singapore: Springer.

Roher, S., Z. Yu, D. Martin and A. Benoit (2021). How is etuaptmumk/two-eyed seeing characterized in Indigenous health research? A scoping review. *PLOS One* 16(7): e0254612. DOI: 10.1371/journal.pone.0254612.

Ryder, C., T. Mackean, J. Coombs, H. Williams, K. Hunter, A.J.A. Holland et al. (2020). Indigenous research methodology – weaving a research interface. *International Journal of Social Research Methodology* 23(3): 255–67. DOI: 10.1080/13645579.2019.1669923.

Smith, R., S. Devine and R. Preston (2020). Recommended methodologies to determine Australian Indigenous community members' perceptions of their health needs: a literature review. *Australian Journal of Primary Health* 26(2): 95. DOI: 10.1071/PY19078.

Thambinathan, V. and E. Kinsella (2021). Decolonizing methodologies in qualitative research: creating spaces for transformative praxis. *International Journal of Qualitative Methods* 20: 16094069211014766. DOI: 10.1177/16094069211014766.

Thurber, K. (2021). Why we need strengths-based approaches to achieve social justice. *Integration and Implementation Insights*, 12 January. https://i2insights.org/2021/01/12/strengths-based-approaches/#katie-thurber.

Thurber, K., J. Thandrayen, E. Banks, K. Doery, M. Sedgwick and R. Lovett (2020). Strengths-based approaches for quantitative data analysis: a case study using the Australian Longitudinal Study of Indigenous Children. *SSM – Population Health* 12: 100637. DOI: 10.1016/j.ssmph.2020.100637.

Tuhiwai Smith, L. (1999). *Decolonizing methodologies: research and Indigenous peoples*. London: Zed Books.

United Nations (2007). United Nations Declaration on the Rights of Indigenous Peoples. https://www.ohchr.org/en/indigenous-peoples/un-declaration-rights-indigenous-peoples.

Watego, C., L. Whop, D. Singh, B. Mukandi, A. Macoun, G. Newhouse et al. (2021). Black to the future: making the case for Indigenist health humanities. *International Journal of Environmental Research and Public Health* 18(16). DOI: 10.3390/ijerph18168704.

Wright, M., A. Brown, P. Dudgeon, R. McPhee, J. Coffin, G. Pearson et al. (2021). Our journey, our story: a study protocol for the evaluation of a co-design framework to improve services for Aboriginal youth mental health and well-being. *BMJ Open* 11(5): e042981–e81. DOI: 10.1136/bmjopen-2020-042981.

Yunggirringa, D. and J. Garnggulkpuy (2007). Yolngu participatory action research. Paper presented at the Moving Forwards Together; Action Learning and Action Research, ALARA Australian Conference, Tauondi College, Adelaide.

Learning from two decades of CQI research in Indigenous PHC

Aboriginal and Torres Strait Islander Australians have demonstrated extraordinary cultural strength, adaptability and resilience across time. Vital for the continuing improvement of health outcomes is research that produces the knowledge, processes, tools and resources to enable communities, health practitioners, other service providers and policymakers to improve health care, prevent disease and support wellbeing. Shifts in health research approaches, as described in the previous chapter, have been complemented by significant changes to Indigenous health policy.[1]

Our CQI research network has learnt from and contributed to these efforts. Early quality improvement research played an important role in testing the acceptability of CQI approaches and their effect on Indigenous PHC.[2] Important gains have since been made. Quality improvement efforts in PHC have been accelerated and strengthened at multiple levels and contexts.[3] Clinical performance assessment and improvements have been achieved across a range of services[4] and structured health service and systems assessments have been facilitated to support best practice.[5] Quality improvement has increasingly focused on the social, cultural, structural and environmental factors that influence health.[6] As this work has progressed, research teams have adopted a broader agenda to embed Aboriginal and Torres Strait Islander leadership, participation and priorities in health and wellbeing research. Network members have created spaces to safely share their experiences from different viewpoints and learn from each other. These developments are essential for bringing about meaningful change and lasting benefits for communities.

This chapter shares lessons learnt by the research network, which brings together Aboriginal and Torres Strait Islander and non-Indigenous stakeholders to improve healthcare equity. Drawing on publications from network members, we describe some of the structures and mechanisms that are being used to foster culturally safe, strengths-based and transformative PHC and quality improvement research among Aboriginal and Torres Strait Islander communities in Australia. The lessons learnt have informed the principles of CQI implementation and research, and may offer insights for others seeking to improve equity and justice through research.

1   Coalition of Aboriginal and Torres Strait Islander Peak Organisations and Australian Governments 2020.
2   R. Bailie, Si et al. 2007; Si, R. Bailie et al. 2005.
3   R. Bailie, J. Bailie et al. 2017.
4   J. Bailie, Laycock et al. 2016; Gibson-Helm, Rumbold et al. 2016.
5   Cunningham, Ferguson-Hill et al. 2016.
6   Brimblecombe, van den Boogaard et al. 2015; CRE-STRIDE n.d.a.; Standen, Morgan et al. 2020.

Building on strengths to transform research

Research networks provide a forum for experimentation and knowledge creation, information exchange and the spread of good ideas and practice. They can be useful in addressing complex issues or "wicked" problems when solutions go beyond the control and scope of any one agency.[7]

> Research networks ... can be useful in addressing complex issues or "wicked" problems when solutions go beyond the control and scope of any one agency.

Our CQI research network in Aboriginal and Torres Strait Islander PHC has had several iterations (see overview in Chapter 9). Since 2015, the network has used an "innovation platform" approach. Leaders of large-scale change have argued that innovation platforms create an opportunity for people working in different parts of the system to tackle challenging issues together,[8] including entrenched systemic problems.

Centre for Research Excellence in Integrated Quality Improvement

The vision of the Centre for Research Excellence in Integrated Quality Improvement (CRE-IQI) innovation platform, which was funded from 2015 to 2019, was to accelerate and strengthen large-scale primary healthcare quality improvement efforts. To achieve this vision, stakeholders from multiple roles and organisations were brought together to work on shared goals, find solutions to common quality improvement problems, learn from each other, and take collective action. The elements of the CRE-IQI innovation platform are shown in Figure 22.1.

Members included Indigenous and non-indigenous clinicians, researchers, policy and project managers from health services (including community-controlled organisations), regional service support organisations, national support organisations, universities, research institutes and government. As an "open platform", the CRE-IQI encouraged new partnerships and collaborations and provided a vehicle for integrated research and knowledge translation.[9]

"All teach, all learn" approach to research capacity strengthening

One of the goals of the CRE-IQI was to increase the capacity of members to participate in and lead CQI research. It was recognised that this involved capacities for building research skills and confidence, taking ownership and leadership, collaborating, forming research partnerships and working in a culturally safe way, translating research, and building structures and resources.[10]

The CRE-IQI developed a model that drew on capacity strengthening[11] and evidence from capacity building for quality improvement[12] to theorise strategies for strengthening CQI research capacity in Aboriginal and Torres Strait Islander PHC.[13] Consistent with the way of

---

7   J. Bailie, Cunningham et al. 2018.
8   Sustainable Improvement Team and the Horizons Team 2018.
9   J. Bailie, Cunningham et al. 2018.
10   McPhail-Bell, Matthews et al. 2018.
11   Otoo, Agapitova and Joy 2009.
12   Mery, Dobrow et al. 2017.
13   McPhail-Bell, Matthews et al. 2018.

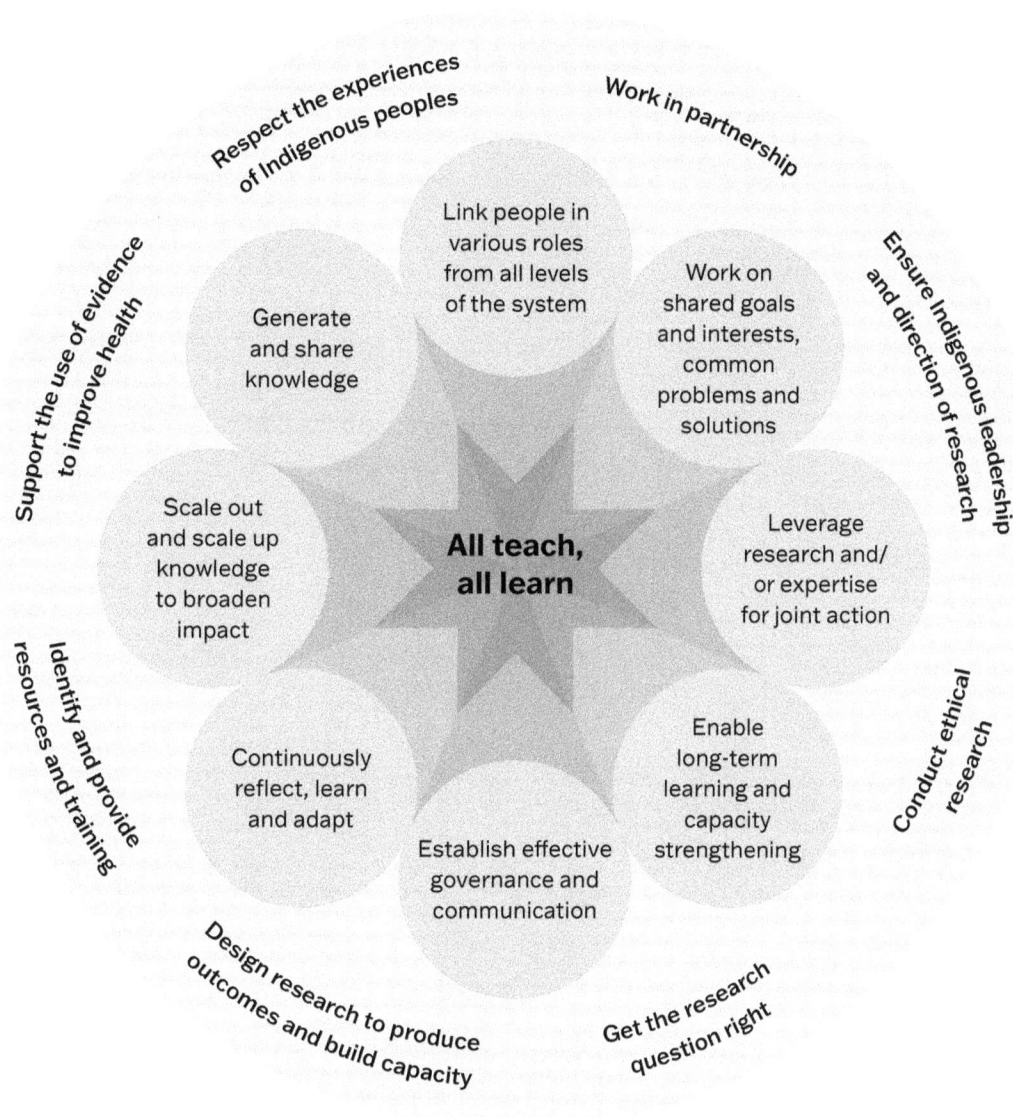

Figure 22.1 Elements of the CRE-IQI innovation platform. Source: A. Laycock, Conte et al. 2020.

working across the research network, an "all teach, all learn" maxim was adopted. "All teach, all learn" embodies the value placed upon mutual learning, where all involved – Aboriginal and Torres Strait Islander and non-Indigenous people, those involved in primary healthcare services, the communities they serve, early career and experienced researchers – are learners and teachers. The strengths-based process used for developing the model identified the need to tackle power imbalances, cultural contexts, relationships, systems requirements and the existing knowledge, skills and experience of all involved to strengthen research capacity.[14]

Four principles were identified for implementing an "all teach, all learn" approach to CQI research capacity strengthening across the network: mutual or two-way learning; Indigenous leadership as core; sharing power and facilitating relationships; resourcing and continuous improvement. The principles are expanded in Box 22.1.

---

14   McPhail-Bell, Matthews et al. 2018.

Box 22.1 Principles of the "all teach, all learn" approach to strengthening capacity for CQI research

Mutual or two-way learning

At the core of the "all teach, all learn" motto is the valuing of Indigenous cultures, knowledge and expertise alongside Western research and knowledge, and recognition that different kinds of capacities are to be developed in different people, processes, organisations and systems. These capacities are influenced by worldview, knowledge, experience and relationships.[15] In the Australian context, mutuality requires valuing Aboriginal and Torres Strait Islander voices, identities and knowledge, and recognising the power held by decision-makers, institutions and structures to improve or undermine Indigenous health.[16]

Indigenous leadership as core

"Indigenous-led research" refers to research that is led and driven by Indigenous researchers, practitioners, policymakers and communities in partnership with community organisations, or through collaborative approaches involving Indigenous community or communities at each stage of the research process.[17] Co-leadership arrangements can bring diverse knowledges in the same way as traditional distributed leadership models. Co-leads are researchers, community members, service providers, and policymakers of varying seniority or position, who support mutual strengthening of research capacity. These co-lead arrangements require culturally safe spaces.

Sharing power and facilitating relationships

A commitment to Indigenous leadership brings considerations and tensions to negotiate collectively for mutually beneficial outcomes. Methodologies that seek to support and value Indigenous knowledge within CQI research, and involve Indigenous people and their interests, are necessary. For non-Indigenous people in leadership roles, this means leading in partnership with Indigenous people and organisations, relinquishing and sharing power over research ownership and associated decisions, processes, outcomes and benefits. Indigenous ownership and respectful relationships from the outset of research enhance the likelihood of research relevance and thus translation and benefit.[18] Allowing sufficient time for building meaningful relationships is essential for quality research and is an activity itself within strengthening research capacity, as it enables respectful engagement with Indigenous knowledge and perspectives.[19]

---

15 Redman-MacLaren, MacLaren et al. 2012; Elston, Saunders et al. 2013.
16 Bond 2009; Evans, Miller et al. 2014; Laycock, Walker et al. 2011; McPhail-Bell, Matthews et al. 2018; Nicholls 2009.
17 Clapham 2011.
18 Tsey, Lawson et al. 2016.
19 Bond, Foley and Askew 2016; Elston, Saunders et al. 2013; McPhail-Bell, Matthews et al. 2018; Tuhiwai Smith 1999.

> **Resourcing and continuous improvement**
>
> Resources (especially staffing) are required to enable the communication, relationships, engagement and training that facilitate the strengthening of capacity for CQI research. Likewise, resourcing and continuous learning are essential to enable co-leadership, which is generally an additional responsibility for busy Indigenous translators, leaders or researchers, or those who combine these roles. Implementation is the responsibility of all within the Centre. A continuous improvement approach is used to test application of the program logic for research capacity-strengthening across the research programs and activities, and to monitor progress against the CQI–research capacity-strengthening priorities.[20]

Guiding principles

When the CRE-IQI was funded in 2015, members agreed that the research network should have an agreed set of operating principles, to guide how Aboriginal and Torres Strait Islander research values[21] would be put into practice in quality improvement research. The principles were adapted, with permission, from a cancer research collaboration in Aboriginal and Torres Strait Islander health, as follows:

- respect the past and present experiences of Indigenous people
- work in partnership
- ensure Indigenous leadership and direction of research – in all stages of the process
- conduct ethical research
- get the research question right
- design research that will be feasible, produce outcomes and build capacity
- identify and provide the right resources and training
- establish systems and practices to support the application of evidence to improve Indigenous primary health care and health outcomes.

Published literature offered little in the way of critical reflection to support the implementation of such principles. The CRE-IQI's management group undertook to evaluate how the principles were implemented and the outcomes over the research network's lifespan.

Evaluating the implementation of the Centre for Research Excellence in Integrated Quality Improvement

Four approaches were used to evaluate the implementation of the CRE-IQI: developmental evaluation; principles-focused evaluation; social network analysis; and framework analysis (Box 22.2).[22] While the resources and expertise required to evaluate this network were considerable, data sources were leveraged for multiple purposes to create efficiency and avoid "evaluation fatigue" amongst participants.

---

20   McPhail-Bell, Matthews et al. 2018.
21   National Health and Medical Research Council 2018a, b.
22   J. Bailie, Cunningham et al. 2022.

Box 22.2 Approaches used to evaluate the implementation of the innovation platform

Developmental evaluation

Developmental evaluation can inform the development and adaptation of innovative and emergent initiatives in complex social environments. The approach uses systems thinking to consider how multiple parts of complex and dynamic systems (such as healthcare systems) are interrelated, focusing on users and use of evaluation findings. In addition to the innovation niche, developmental purpose, systems thinking and utilisation focus, the features of developmental evaluation include a complexity perspective, evaluation rigour, co-creation and timely feedback.[23]

Principles-focused evaluation

Principles-focused evaluation, like developmental evaluation, is an approach rather than a methodology. It examines "(1) whether principles are clear, meaningful and actionable, and if so, (2) whether they are actually being followed and, if so, (3) whether they are leading to the desired results."[24]

Network analysis

Social network analysis is a set of techniques to map, measure and analyse social relationships between people, teams and organisations.[25] Survey methods and software tools are used to collect, visualise, document and analyse interaction data to understand a group's social structure, relationships and interaction patterns.

Framework analysis

Framework analysis is a form of thematic analysis in which an organised structure of concepts or themes is used to analyse data. For example, a framework designed to guide the development or evaluation of quality improvement collaboratives may be used to map and analyse communication, social systems, time span and innovation within the research collaborative, thereby increasing understanding of how the collaborative works and of its strengths and weaknesses.[26]

Applying different methodologies enabled the network to respond promptly to the "emergent" nature of a research system that was complex and dynamic. Together, the four evaluation approaches provided a nuanced understanding of how the collaboration was formed, how it worked, what changes were needed as work progressed, and what it achieved. This would have been difficult to achieve with any single evaluation approach.[27] Specific projects associated with the CRE-IQI were also evaluated using impact and economic evaluation methods[28] and

---

23   Patton 2011, 2016.
24   Patton 2018, 3.
25   Blanchet and James 2012.
26   Nix, McNamara et al. 2018.
27   J. Bailie, Cunningham et al. 2022.
28   Ramanathan, Larkins et al. 2021.

developmental evaluation.[29] The learning that may be drawn from the evaluation of the CRE-IQI innovation platform is an example of how complex research collaborations in health may be evaluated, strengthened and reformed.

Developmental evaluation use and findings

Developmental evaluation was used to inform and support the formation, functioning and outcomes of the CRE-IQI. Innovation platforms have continuous reflection, learning and adaptation as a specific design principle. As developmental evaluation emphasises continuous learning and adaptation, it was well aligned. While rigorous in its use of multiple data sources and varied methods, the developmental evaluation provided scope to move away from a "what is planned needs to be achieved" mindset to one that could continually adapt based on what we were learning and how the collaboration was evolving.

We found the developmental evaluation approach suited to a research collaboration aimed at integrating quality improvement efforts at different levels of the health system in a complex PHC environment. Use of systems thinking (a key principle of developmental evaluation) and attending to relationships and interactions between CRE-IQI members provided insights into how CRE-IQI strategies and processes could be modified to work more effectively. Timely feedback (both opportunistic and at predetermined times) ensured that evaluation data was used to test modifications and make further improvements.[30]

Developmental evaluators need to become embedded within projects to build and maintain evaluator–team relationships, and to know and respond in real time to the evaluation context and innovators' concerns.[31] Having a member of the CRE-IQI staff team in the lead evaluator role met those needs.

Principles-focused evaluation use and findings

A principles-focused evaluation approach enabled critical reflection on how, to what end and whether the guiding principles of the CRE-IQI were being implemented. Interviews with collaboration members and review of documents generated themes that were iteratively discussed with the wider membership, refined and categorised into "strategies" – activities by which implementation of our guiding principles were recognised; "outcomes" – results seen from implementing the principles; and "conditions" – aspects of the context that facilitated and constrained implementation of the principles.[32]

Five strategies were identified as supporting implementation of the principles: honouring the principles, sharing and dispersing leadership across the collaborative, collaborating purposefully, adopting a culture of mutual learning, and being dynamic and adaptable.

> "You have to operationalise [the principles] in some way . . . you've done that . . . reemphasising that these are not static . . . they have to be continually evolving as the work and people and new issues emerge." – researcher, Indigenous, university/ research institute[33]

---

29   Laycock, J. Bailie et al. 2019.
30   J. Bailie, Laycock et al. 2020.
31   Iyamu, Berger et al. 2022.
32   J. Bailie, Laycock et al. 2021.
33   J. Bailie, Laycock et al. 2021, 5.

Outcomes included increased Indigenous leadership and participation, the ability to attract principled and values-driven researchers and stakeholders, and the development of trusting and respectful relationships.

> "I feel like I trust all those [long- standing researchers] that have been around. I trust their values – that you want to be involved with researchers who have similar values." – health service manager, non-Indigenous, Aboriginal community controlled health service[34]

The conditions that facilitated the implementation of the principles were collaborating over time, an increasing number of Indigenous researchers participating in the network and taking an "innovation platform" approach.[35] The strategies, outcomes and conditions are brought together in Figure 22.2.

Having collaboratively developed principles held genuine meaning for members and was important for guiding the network: the principles acted as a compass for navigating complexity and conflict. Implementing the principles within a culture of continuous critical reflection, learning, adaptation and reinterpretation provided focus, direction and a way of working together.[36]

> Having collaboratively developed principles held genuine meaning for members and was important for guiding the research network.

Network analysis use and findings

The CRE-IQI conducted two network analyses over its five-year span. Firstly, cross-sectional surveys of membership were used twice to collect network data. Survey questions captured member feedback on the perceived effect of the CRE-IQI and applied network metrics to examine the functioning of the CRE-IQI over its life cycle.[37] A second network analysis examined collaboration and knowledge generation through the co-authorship of peer-reviewed articles.[38] Findings are detailed in the cited papers. These were the key messages:

- there was a broadening of relationships and a sharing of knowledge not only with existing partners but also new ones; more than a third of sharing occurred outside immediate collaborative partnerships, indicating good network support[39]
- network analysis was useful for evaluating the functioning and collaboration of an innovation platform at individual, organisational and health system levels[40]
- collaboration in publications increased as the network consolidated and expanded
- a need to remedy inequities in female and Indigenous authorship was identified
- diverse authorship and decentralisation of the network appeared to build research impact and advance CQI knowledge and practice
- building long-term relationships facilitated participatory research in CQI.[41]

34   J. Bailie, Laycock et al. 2021, 8.
35   J. Bailie, Laycock et al. 2021.
36   J. Bailie, Laycock et al. 2021.
37   Cunningham, Potts et al. 2022.
38   J. Bailie, Potts et al. 2021.
39   J. Bailie, Cunningham et al. 2022; Cunningham, Potts et al. 2022.
40   Cunningham, Potts et al. 2022.
41   J. Bailie, Potts et al. 2021.

Strategies

Specific activities by which implementation of the principles were recognised

Honouring the principles

Being dynamic and adaptable

Sharing and dispersing leadership

Collaborating purposefully

Adopting a culture of mutual learning

Outcomes

Results observed from implementing the principles

Enabled trusting and respectful relationships

Attracted principled and values-driven people

Increased Indigenous leadership and participation

Conditions

Specific aspects of the context that influenced implementation of the principles

Collaborating over time

Increasing numbers of Indigenous researchers

Taking an innovation platform approach

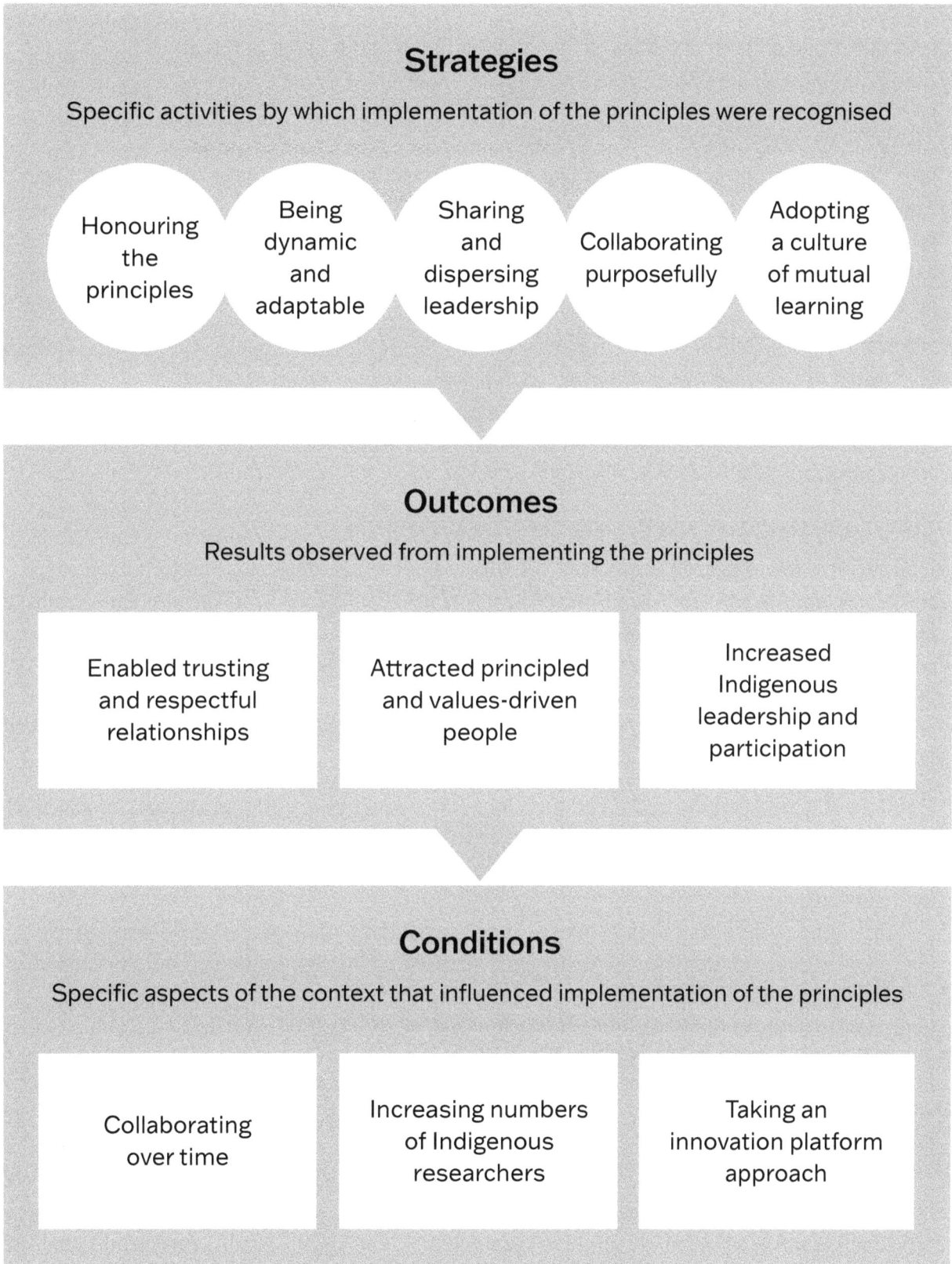

Figure 22.2 Strategies, outcomes and conditions related to how principles were implemented in the research collaboration. Source: J. Bailie, Laycock et al. 2021.

> Building long-term relationships facilitated participatory research in CQI.

Framework analysis use and findings

The evaluation study team used a framework analysis approach to analyse project records, reports and publications, and interviews with stakeholders. Data were mapped retrospectively against the domains of the Agency for Healthcare Research and Quality learning collaboratives taxonomy[42] to understand how and why the CRE-IQI generated innovations.

Findings were detailed by J. Bailie, Peiris and colleagues.[43] These were the key messages:

- The long history of working together enabled trusting relationships, a collective identity and a foundation for new people to join. Time was a crucial element.
- Innovation was stimulated by bringing people together to learn, share ideas and solve problems, with Indigenous participation and leadership at the core of the research agenda-setting.[44]

Impact and economic evaluation of CRE-IQI projects

In addition, a few research projects of the CRE-IQI were evaluated using the "Framework to Assess the Impact from Translational health research" tool. The tool combines quantitative and qualitative measurement techniques to assess effectiveness. It uses a scorecard approach to report research outcomes and impact across five specific domains of benefit, the social return on investment, and case studies.[45]

The use of different evaluation approaches identified generalisable lessons for CQI research networks:

- trusting, respectful research relationships developed over time can support productivity and a collective identity, and provide a foundation for new members
- collectively agreed operating principles help in maintaining direction and navigating complexity
- bringing people together supports learning, sharing of ideas and problem-solving
- diverse participation can be important for advancing innovation, equity and the knowledge and practice of CQI in PHC
- the continuous learning and adaptation that generally characterise CQI can be used to improve the operation of a CQI research network.

Centre for Research Excellence: Strengthening Systems for Indigenous Health Care Equity

The Centre for Research Excellence: Strengthening Systems for Indigenous Health Care Equity (CRE-STRIDE, 2020–25) built on the work and evaluation of the CRE-IQI (2015–19) by strengthening Aboriginal and Torres Strait Islander research leadership, and changing

---

42   Nix, McNamara et al. 2018.
43   J. Bailie, Peiris et al. 2021.
44   J. Bailie, Peiris et al. 2021.
45   Ramanathan, Larkins et al. 2021; Searles, Doran et al. 2016.

Cross-cutting themes   Research approaches   Research programs

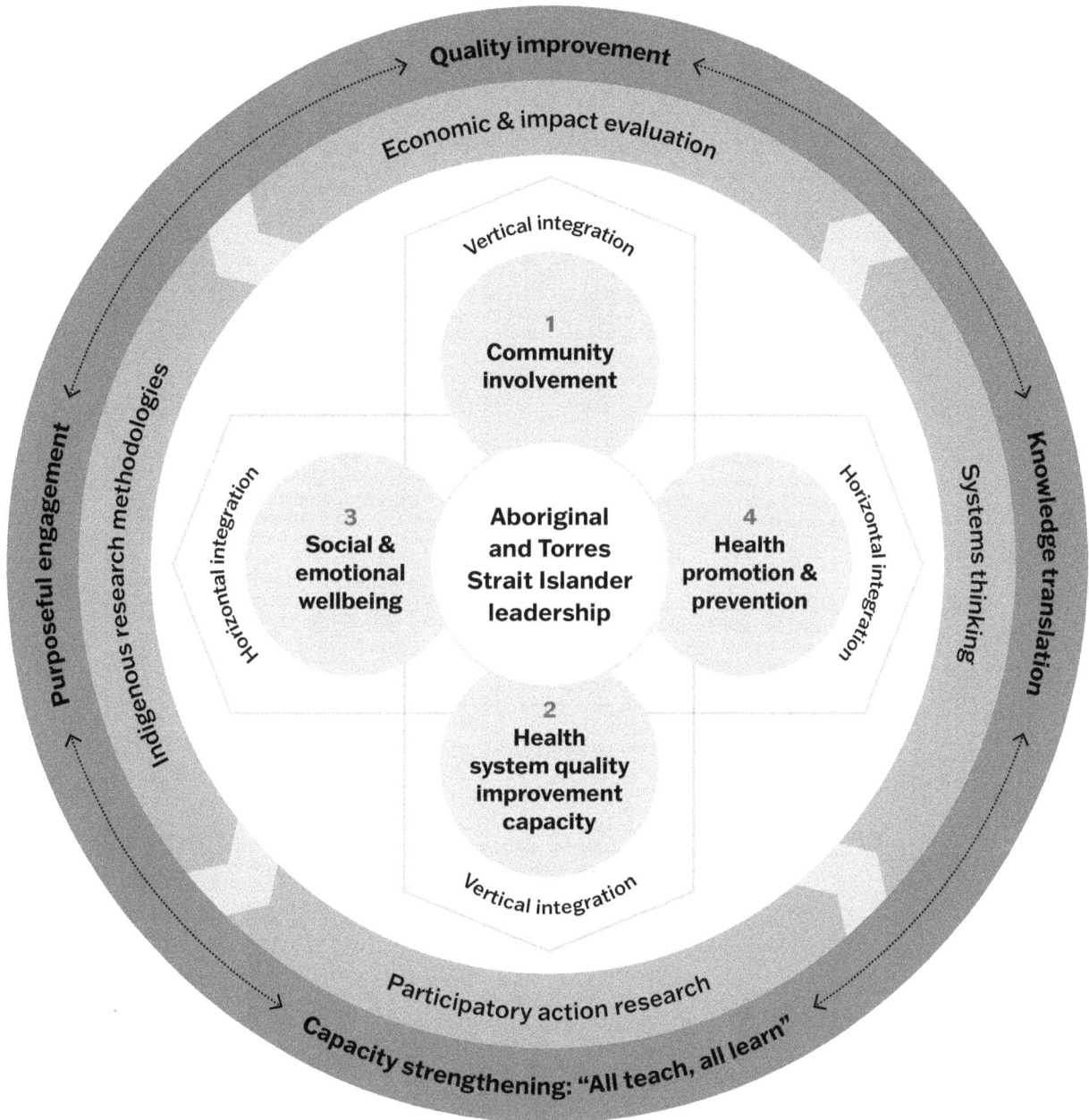

Figure 22.3 CRE-STRIDE Framework. Source: The Centre for Research Excellence: Strengthening Systems for Indigenous Health Care Equity (CRE-STRIDE n.d.a.).

from an advisory group model to one that distributed leadership at all levels, supported by an "all teach, all learn" philosophy between Indigenous and non-Indigenous collaborators. CRE-STRIDE was committed to embedding Indigenous research leadership and methodologies throughout its structures and research programs, which were brought together in the CRE-STRIDE Framework (Figure 22.3).[46]

---

46   The Centre for Research Excellence: Strengthening Systems for Indigenous Health Care Equity (CRE-STRIDE) n.d.a.

The research approaches used in CRE-STRIDE were based on growing evidence of the importance of community-driven, culture-strengthening interventions in Indigenous primary healthcare settings. CRE-STRIDE's way of working put the strengths, needs and aspirations of Aboriginal and Torres Strait Islander people at the centre of the research process, informed by methodologies that reflect Indigenous ways of knowing, being and doing.

CRE-STRIDE vision and guiding principles

CRE-STRIDE's vision was equitable health care for Aboriginal and Torres Strait Islander peoples. Through CQI and collaborative implementation research, the network aimed to strengthen PHC and its interconnections to broader systems that affect health and wellbeing.

Specific strategies for achieving this vision were Aboriginal and Torres Strait Islander research leadership and reciprocal learning; strengthening quality improvement processes within primary healthcare systems and enhancing community engagement; and extending quality improvement processes and collaborations across sectors to promote holistic health outcomes recognising the importance of social and cultural determinants of health and wellbeing.

CRE-STRIDE's guiding principles of practice were modified from the CRE-IQI to reflect active commitments:

- *to respect* – respect the past and present experiences of Aboriginal and Torres Strait Islander peoples
- *to lead* – Indigenous leadership or co-leadership on all projects
- *to learn* – "all teach, all learn" approach to collective capacity strengthening
- *to relate* – collaboration and partnership
- *to share* – sharing research and translation
- *to change* – work alongside community and other stakeholders to generate impactful research.[47]

These principles informed a way of thinking and doing that fosters culturally safe, strengths-based and transformative primary healthcare research with Aboriginal and Torres Strait Islander communities.

An Indigenous research framework for quality improvement research

CRE-STRIDE's Indigenous Research Framework articulated these principles and provided guidance on how the collaboration could operationalise them. The framework brought together key themes from Indigenous research scholarship (as described in the previous chapter) that were important to CRE-STRIDE's goals and work plan. Box 22.3 explains the components of CRE-STRIDE's Indigenous Research Framework.

---

47   The Centre for Research Excellence: Strengthening Systems for Indigenous Health Care Equity (CRE-STRIDE) n.d.b.

Box 22.3 CRE-STRIDE Indigenous Research Framework

Indigenous relationality

Our health and wellbeing encompasses Country, culture, spirituality, community and family. Land is central to our being, we understand and relate to each other by knowing where we come from and, from that, our kinship ties. Indigenous relationality, as described in Indigenous research paradigms, is around us every day. We see it in song, ceremony, throughout our daily lives. It has been intellectualised for academia, but we actually live and feel it. When we think about health and wellbeing, it is not compartmentalised into separate systems (for example, education, legal, health); rather it is a fluid and organic process that connects all elements (both human and non-human).

With this relationality comes responsibility, reciprocity and respect. We are obligated to look after Country and kin. In STRIDE, "thinking relationally" means factoring in these multiple elements into research processes and understanding that Western biomedical gold standards of research evidence alone may not necessarily provide solutions required to address health issues. To strengthen systems for healthcare equity, we must build relationships with community and work with multidisciplinary and intersectoral teams to tailor solutions to context.

Indigenous research leadership

Distributed leadership mirrors traditional forms of Aboriginal and Torres Strait Islander leadership, which is shared amongst people with differing responsibilities. Leaders are recognised based on their knowledge, reputation, personal qualities and ability to look after others (family, Country, systems of law).

Involving Aboriginal and Torres Strait Islander people in STRIDE research will empower and generate leadership at different levels. *Communities* provide leadership through setting research agendas and guiding methodological approaches. *Aboriginal and Torres Strait Islander researchers* provide leadership by sharing knowledge and understanding of Indigenous culture and contexts and facilitating relationships. *Non-Indigenous researchers* provide leadership by being allies, adopting new ways of thinking, critically reflecting on their own positionality and broadening their perspectives on the way knowledge can be generated and viewed. Shared leadership means working alongside each other, requiring respect, responsibility and reciprocity. STRIDE's Indigenous research leadership is not about taking over or duplicating roles; rather it guides a changing narrative so that Indigenous methodologies, community needs, priorities and culture are at the centre of health research, designed to include and deliver benefit to Indigenous peoples.

Indigenous knowledge and sovereignty

Engaging communities in research and quality improvement processes is a foundational process in the work of STRIDE. It is also central to an Indigenous approach of locating research within community: respecting and listening to community; involving and learning from them throughout the research process; and two-way sharing of knowledge for the benefit of community health. It ensures relevance and accuracy of research; that we are working on what the community sees as priorities in a way that they understand and own.

In CRE-STRIDE, we are centring Indigenous knowledge in our research processes. As part of this, we have responsibility to ensure appropriate forms of data collection, use and reporting (Indigenous data sovereignty). This means acknowledging research data belongs to community; disrupting deficit discourses; giving data back in accessible forms (as advised by community); and strengthening the capacity of the community and their health services to act as data custodians. In this way, community is empowered to use their data for their own planning, implementation and monitoring of health and wellbeing issues and for setting research agendas (data self-determination).

"All teach, all learn" capacity strengthening

"Reciprocal learning" reflects the bringing together of different worldviews in a collaborative way, through knowledge sharing, mutual support and openness of hearts and minds to each other's perspectives.

STRIDE's "all teach, all learn" approach consists of mutual learning and valuing of different knowledge systems (Indigenous and non-Indigenous) and different perspectives (researcher, health service provider, community member); co-leadership, power sharing and facilitating relationships underpinned by trust and respect. Designed as a continual process of reflection and review, it requires an ability to consider self in relation to others and to engage in dialogue through constructive learning conversations. As relationality and connectedness are central to our way of life, a particular focus of STRIDE's capacity-strengthening program is how we put inter-sectoral research into action to address social and cultural determinants of health.[48]

> "Reciprocal learning" reflects the bringing together of different worldviews in a collaborative way, through knowledge sharing, mutual support and openness of hearts and minds to each other's perspectives.

A matrix of strategies on how the collaboration can implement STRIDE's principles of practice at an individual, project, collaboration and broader research system level was also developed,

---

48   Indigenous Reference Committee (CRE-STRIDE) 2020.

with the expectation that both the framework and the matrix would evolve over time. These documents formed the basis of regular reflection, evaluation and continuous improvement, with input from the broader collaboration.

Evaluating the Centre for Research Excellence: Strengthening Systems for Indigenous Health Care Equity (CRE-STRIDE)

A developmental evaluation approach was carried forward from CRE-IQI into CRE-STRIDE. The evaluation focused on newer aspects of the research network: increasing the application of Indigenous research methodologies and leadership; strengthening CQI processes within primary healthcare systems with a focus on community linkages; and extending CQI processes across sectors to promote health and wellbeing and to strengthen social and cultural determinants of health. The Ngaa-bi-nya Aboriginal and Torres Strait Islander program evaluation framework[49] guided data collection and analysis in the evaluation. Ngaa-bi-nya takes a strengths-based approach, prompting evaluators to consider the historical, policy and social landscape surrounding Aboriginal and Torres Strait Islander peoples in contemporary settings.

Developmental evaluation findings (not finalised at the time of publication) indicate that the CRE-STRIDE network achieved its goals, despite the early challenges and ongoing effects of the Covid-19 pandemic and weather-related disasters that affected the host organisation and many network members.

- Indigenous leadership became strongly embedded across the network, with Indigenous people represented at all levels.
- The Indigenous Research Framework was accepted and used across many of the STRIDE projects; some members sought guidance for applying the framework in their research. Relationality was highly valued. A focus on Indigenous knowledge and sovereignty strengthened community participation and self-determination in research, broadened members' thinking around data and inclusivity, and expanded the evidence base for Indigenous methodologies in CQI research.
- By integrating Indigenous leadership, knowledges and methodologies throughout the CRE-STRIDE, members were able to enhance community linkages and push the boundaries of CQI to incorporate social, cultural and environmental determinants of health.
- The foundational work of previous iterations of the research network allowed CRE-STRIDE to diversify its research focus and take a more holistic approach to PHC and equity for Indigenous communities. Areas of CQI research included clinical care, social determinants of health, social and emotional wellbeing, environmental and climate change effects.[50]

The next phase of the Indigenous-led CQI research network is STAUNCH – Stronger Together As Unified Nations for Community-led Health. STAUNCH aims to promote sovereign health and wellbeing by centring Indigenous Nation Building to assert local policy and program solutions for improving the quality of comprehensive primary health care. Research activities focus on strengthening First Nations' self-governance, defining new quality and safety standards

---

49   Williams 2018.
50   Benveniste, Laycock et al. 2023.

for care models that include the determinants of health, and guiding policymakers to look at health and wellbeing solutions that holistically consider social, political, economic and environmental issues.

Indigenous data sovereignty

CRE-STRIDE's Indigenous Research Framework (Box 22.3) outlines actions the network took to advance Indigenous data sovereignty, a global movement concerned with the right of Indigenous peoples to govern the creation, collection, ownership and use of data about Indigenous peoples, lands and cultures.[51] In support of these rights, the Global Indigenous Data Alliance has developed the CARE principles for Indigenous data governance, which are framed around collective benefit, authority to control, responsibility and ethics.[52] Case studies, ecosystems and resources for advancing data sovereignty are becoming increasingly available.[53] Indigenous data sovereignty holds messages for CQI research.

The Indigenous data sovereignty movement challenges how governments and institutions have historically captured and used data representing Indigenous peoples to develop policies and programs that do not protect and respect Indigenous interests or worldviews. It also draws attention to the way aggregated and decontextualised data can present people as problematic[54] because they are unable to meaningfully reflect lived experiences, histories and cultural realities. These concerns reflect wider social and global movements calling for a shift from descriptive, problem-focused research about historically disempowered or socially excluded groups, to more action-oriented and solution-focused research that facilitates social inclusion, self-determination and health equity.[55]

The aggregation of data is, at times, necessary for population health approaches such as CQI and epidemic or pandemic management. Aggregated data provide information about the issues communities and populations are dealing with, enable changes in population health to be measured, improvement strategies to be designed and resources to be allocated. When using aggregated population health data to plan policies and improvement interventions, these aspects need to be considered:

- whether the data incorporates and reflects the strengths, values, knowledge systems and practices of the people to whom the policies relate, appropriately as determined by those groups[56]
- how to ensure communities have control over the distribution of resources based on local priorities, existing resources, knowledge, and governance processes[57]
- how data management systems can be used as a resource to serve communities.[58]

---

51   Maiam nayri Wingara Indigenous Data Sovereignty Collective 2019; United Nations 2007, Article 13.
52   Global Indigenous Data Alliance n.d.
53   Kukutai and Taylor 2016; Walter, Kukutai et al. 2021.
54   Walter 2016.
55   Smylie, Lofters et al. 2012.
56   Lovett 2016.
57   Kalinda Griffiths in Phelan 2020.
58   Smylie, Lofters et al. 2012.

Summary

This chapter has described how a CQI and health systems research network in Aboriginal and Torres Strait Islander PHC has actioned key principles and built on learning to transform a CQI research program in Australia. The journey began with a participatory action research project testing the feasibility of CQI in 12 primary healthcare services[59] and evolved into a collaboration involving diverse partners committed to primary healthcare quality improvement. We have shared lessons learnt through two decades of CQI research and evaluation, describing mechanisms and features developed to support innovation and to foster Indigenous-led, strengths-based quality improvement research with Aboriginal and Torres Strait Islander communities.

Equitable, collaborative research relationships have positive relational features that include trust, respect for knowledge and each other, a sense of belonging, and open lines of communication. Positive structural features are also necessary to improve equity in research, including opportunities for capacity building, inclusive decision-making, recognition of contribution (for example, through authorship and distributed leadership), and governance structures that empower participating organisations and communities.[60] These features are important for progressing the network's ongoing research agenda and meeting future research challenges. The capacity to respond and adapt to changing contexts is essential for an equity-focused quality improvement research network and for the effective implementation of CQI.

References

Bailie, J., F. Cunningham, S. Abimbola, A. Laycock, R. Bainbridge, R. Bailie et al. (2022). Methodological pluralism for better evaluations of complex interventions: lessons from evaluating an innovation platform in Australia. *Health Research Policy and Systems* 20(1): 14. DOI: 10.1186/s12961-022-00814-5.

Bailie, J., F. Cunningham, R. Bainbridge, M. Passey, A. Laycock, R. Bailie et al. (2018). Comparing and contrasting "innovation platforms" with other forms of professional networks for strengthening primary healthcare systems for Indigenous Australians. *BMJ Global Health* 3: e000683. DOI: 10.1136/bmjgh-2017-000683.

Bailie, J., A. Laycock, K. Conte, V. Matthews, D. Peiris, R. Bailie et al. (2021). Principles guiding ethical research in a collaboration to strengthen Indigenous primary healthcare in Australia: learning from experience. *BMJ Global Health* 6(1): e003852. DOI: 10.1136/bmjgh-2020-003852.

Bailie, J., A. Laycock, V. Matthews and R. Bailie (2016) System-level action required for wide-scale improvement in quality of primary health care: synthesis of feedback from an interactive process to promote dissemination and use of aggregated quality of care data. *Frontiers in Public Health* 4: 86. DOI: 10.3389/fpubh.2016.00086.

Bailie, J., A. Laycock, D. Peiris, R. Bainbridge, V. Matthews, F. Cunningham et al. (2020). Using developmental evaluation to enhance continuous reflection, learning and adaptation of an innovation platform in Australian Indigenous primary healthcare. *Health Research Policy and Systems* 18(1): 45. DOI: 10.1186/s12961-020-00562-4.

Bailie, J., D. Peiris, F. Cunningham, A. Laycock, R. Bailie, V. Matthews et al. (2021). Utility of the AHRQ learning collaboratives taxonomy for analyzing innovations from an Australian collaborative. *Joint Commission Journal on Quality and Patient Safety* 47: 711–22. DOI: 10.1016/j.jcjq.2021.08.008.

Bailie, J., B. Potts, A. Laycock, S. Abimbola, R. Bailie, F. Cunningham et al. (2021). Collaboration and knowledge generation in an 18-year quality improvement research programme in Australian

---

59   R. Bailie, Si et al. 2007.
60   Faure, Munung et al. 2021; Indigenous Reference Committee (CRE-STRIDE) 2020.

Indigenous primary healthcare: a coauthorship network analysis. *BMJ Open* 11(5): e045101. DOI: 10.1136/bmjopen-2020-045101.

Bailie, R., J. Bailie, S. Larkins and E. Broughton (2017). Editorial: Continuous quality improvement (CQI)—advancing understanding of design, application, impact, and evaluation of CQI approaches. *Frontiers in Public Health* 5: 306. DOI: 10.3389/fpubh.2017.00306.

Bailie, R., D. Si, L. O'Donoghue and M. Dowden (2007). Indigenous health: effective and sustainable health services through continuous quality improvement. *Medical Journal of Australia* 186(10): 525–7. DOI: 10.5694/j.1326-5377.2007.tb01028.x.

Benveniste, T., A. Laycock, R. Bailie, J. Bailie, K. Vine, K. Clancy et al. (2023). Finding our "STRIDE": draft developmental evaluation interim report, vol. 1. Centre for Research Excellence: Strengthening Systems for Indigenous Health Equity. Lismore, NSW: University Centre for Rural Health, University of Sydney.

Blanchet, K. and P. James (2012). How to do (or not to do) . . . a social network analysis in health systems research. *Health Policy and Planning* 27(5): 438–46. DOI: 10.1093/heapol/czr055.

Bond, C. (2009). Starting at strengths . . . an Indigenous early years intervention. *Medical Journal of Australia* 191(3): 175–7. DOI: 10.5694/j.1326-5377.2009.tb02733.x.

Bond, C., W. Foley and D. Askew (2016). "It puts a human face on the researched" – a qualitative evaluation of an Indigenous health research governance model. *Australian and New Zealand Journal of Public Health* 40(S1): S89–S95. DOI: 10.1111/1753-6405.12422.

Brimblecombe, J., C. van den Boogaard, B. Wood, S. Liberato, J. Brown, A. Barnes et al. (2015). Development of the good food planning tool: a food system approach to food security in indigenous Australian remote communities. *Health Place* 34: 54–62. DOI: 10.1016/j.healthplace.2015.03.006.

Centre for Research Excellence: Strengthening Systems for Indigenous Health Care Equity (CRE-STRIDE) (n.d.a.). *Background*. https://cre-stride.org/background/.

Centre for Research Excellence: Strengthening Systems for Indigenous Health Care Equity (CRE-STRIDE) (n.d.b.). *Guiding principles*. https://cre-stride.org/guiding-principles/.

Clapham, K. (2011). Indigenous-led intervention research: the benefits, challenges and opportunities. *International Journal of Critical Indigenous Studies*. 4(2): 40–8. DOI: 10.5204/ijcis.v4i2.63

Coalition of Aboriginal and Torres Strait Islander Peak Organisations and Australian Governments (2020). *National Agreement on Closing the Gap*. Department of the Prime Minister and Cabinet. Canberra: Commonwealth of Australia.

Cunningham, F., S. Ferguson-Hill, V. Matthews and R. Bailie (2016). Leveraging quality improvement through use of the Systems Assessment Tool in Indigenous primary health care services: a mixed methods study. *BMC Health Services Research* 16(1): 583. DOI: 10.1186/s12913-016-1810-y.

Cunningham, F., B. Potts, S. Ramanathan, J. Bailie, R. Bainbridge, A. Searles et al. (2022). Network evaluation of an innovation platform in continuous quality improvement in Australian Indigenous primary healthcare. *Health Research Policy and Systems* 20(1): 119. DOI: 10.1186/s12961-022-00909-z.

Elston, J., V. Saunders, B. Hayes, R. Bainbridge and B. McCoy (2013). Building Indigenous Australian research capacity. *Contemporary Nurse: A Journal for the Australian Nursing Profession* 46(1): 6–12. DOI: 10.5172/conu.2013.46.1.6.

Evans, M., A. Miller, P. Hutchinson and C. Dingwall (2014). Decolonizing research practice: indigenous methodologies, Aboriginal methods, and knowledge/knowing. In P. Leavy, ed. *The Oxford Handbook of Qualitative Research*, 179–91. Oxford: Oxford University Press.

Faure, M., N. Munung, N. Ntusi, B. Pratt and J. de Vries (2021). Considering equity in global health collaborations: a qualitative study on experiences of equity. *PLOS One* 16(10). DOI: 10.1371/journal.pone.0258286.

Gibson-Helm, M., A. Rumbold, H. Teede, S. Ranasinha, R. Bailie and J. Boyle (2016). Improving the provision of pregnancy care for Aboriginal and Torres Strait Islander women: a continuous quality improvement initiative. *BMC Pregnancy and Childbirth* 16: 118. DOI: 10.1186/s12884-016-0892-1.

Global Indigenous Data Alliance (n.d.). CARE Principles for Indigenous Data Governance. https://www.gida-global.org/care.

Indigenous Reference Committee CRE-STRIDE (2020). *Indigenous Research Framework*. Lismore, NSW: Centre for Research Excellence: Strengthening Systems for Indigenous Health Care Equity.

Iyamu, I., M. Berger, S. Fernando, M. Snow and A. Salmon (2022). Developmental evaluation during the COVID-19 pandemic: practice-based learnings from projects in British Columbia, Canada. *Evaluation Journal of Australasia*: 1035719. DOI: 10.1177/1035719X221119841.

Kukutai, T. and J. Taylor, eds (2016). *Indigenous data sovereignty: toward an agenda*. Canberra: ANU Press.

Laycock, A., J. Bailie, V. Matthews and R. Bailie (2019). Using developmental evaluation to support knowledge translation: reflections from a large-scale quality improvement project in Indigenous primary healthcare. *Health Research Policy and Systems* 17(1): 70. DOI: 10.1186/s12961-019-0474-6.

Laycock, A., K. Conte, K. Harkin, J. Bailie, V. Matthews, F. Cunningham et al. (2020). *Improving the quality of primary health care for Aboriginal and Torres Strait Islander Australians 2015–2019: Messages for Action, Impact and Research.* Centre for Research Excellence in Integrated Quality Improvement Lismore NSW: University Centre for Rural Health, University of Sydney.

Laycock, A., D. Walker, N. Harrison and J. Brands (2011). *Researching Indigenous health: a practical guide for researchers.* Melbourne: Lowitja Institute.

Lovett, R. (2016). Aboriginal and Torres Strait Islander community wellbeing: identified needs for statistical capacity. In T. Kukutai and J. Taylor, eds. *Indigenous data sovereignty: toward an agenda*, 213–31. Canberra: ANU Press.

Maiam nayri Wingara Indigenous Data Sovereignty Collective (2019). Indigenous data sovereignty principles. https://mkstudy.com.au/indigenousdatasovereigntyprinciples/.

McPhail-Bell, K., V. Matthews, R. Bainbridge, M. Redman-MacLaren, D. Askew, S. Ramanathan et al. (2018). An "all teach, all learn" approach to research capacity strengthening in Indigenous primary health care continuous quality improvement. *Frontiers in Public Health* 6: 107. DOI: 10.3389/fpubh.2018.00107.

Mery, G., M. Dobrow, G. Baker, J. Im and A. Brown (2017). Evaluating investment in quality improvement capacity building: a systematic review. *BMJ Open* 7(2): e012431–e31. DOI: 10.1136/bmjopen-2016-012431.

National Health and Medical Research Council (2018a). *Ethical conduct in research with Aboriginal and Torres Strait Islander peoples and communities: guidelines for researchers and stakeholders.* Canberra: Commonwealth of Australia.

National Health and Medical Research Council (2018b). *Keeping research on track II: a companion document to* Ethical conduct in research with Aboriginal and Torres Strait Islander peoples and communities: guidelines for researchers and stakeholders. Canberra: Commonwealth of Australia. https://www.nhmrc.gov.au/about-us/resources/keeping-research-track-ii.

Nicholls, R. (2009). Research and Indigenous participation: critical reflexive methods. *International Journal of Social Research Methodology* 12(2): 117–26. DOI: 10.1080/ 13645570902727698.

Nix, M., P. McNamara, J. Genevro, N. Vargas, K. Mistry, A. Fournier et al. (2018). Learning collaboratives: insights and a new taxonomy from AHRQ's two decades of experience. *Health Affairs (Millwood)* 37(2): 205–12. DOI: 10.1377/hlthaff.2017.1144.

Otoo, S., N. Agapitova and B. Joy (2009). *The Capacity Development Results Framework: a strategic and results-oriented approach to learning for capacity development.* Washington, DC: World Bank.

Patton, M. (2018). *Principles-focused evaluation – the guide.* New York, NY: Guilford Press.

Patton, M. (2016). What is essential in developmental evaluation? On integrity, fidelity, adultery, abstinence, impotence, long-term commitment, integrity, and sensitivity in implementing evaluation models. *American Journal of Evaluation* 37(2): 250–65. DOI: 10.1177/1098214015626295.

Patton, M. (2011). *Developmental evaluation: applying complexity concepts to enhance innovation and use.* New York, NY: The Guilford Press.

Phelan, A. (2020). "We need to be seen" – why data is vital in the fight against Covid-19. *University of New South Wales*, 25 March. https://newsroom.unsw.edu.au/news/health/we-need-be-seen-%E2%80%93-why-data-vital-fight-against-covid-19.

Ramanathan, S., S. Larkins, K. Carlisle, N. Turner, R. Bailie, S. Thompson et al. (2021). What was the impact of a participatory research project in Australian Indigenous primary healthcare services? Applying a comprehensive framework for assessing translational health research to Lessons for the Best. *BMJ Open* 11(2): e040749. DOI: 10.1136/bmjopen-2020-040749.

Redman-MacLaren, M., D. MacLaren, H. Harrington, R. Asugeni, R. Timothy-Harrington, E. Kekeubata et al. (2012). Mutual research capacity strengthening: a qualitative study of two-way partnerships in public health research. *International Journal for Equity in Health* 11(1): 79. DOI: 10.1186/1475-9276-11-79.

Searles, A., C. Doran, J. Attia, D. Knight, J. Wiggers, S. Deeming et al. (2016). An approach to measuring and encouraging research translation and research impact. *Health Research Policy and Systems* 14(1). DOI: 10.1186/s12961-016-0131-2.

Si, D., R. Bailie, C. Connors, M. Dowden, A. Stewart, G. Robinson et al. (2005). Assessing health centre systems for guiding improvement in diabetes care. *BMC Health Services Research* 5: 56. DOI: 10.1186/1472-6963-5-56.

Smylie, J., A. Lofters, M. Firestone and P. O'Campo (2012). Population-based data and community empowerment. In Patricia O'Campo and James R. Dunn, eds. *Rethinking social epidemiology: towards a science of change*, 67–92. Dordrecht, the Netherlands: Springer.

Standen, J., G. Morgan, T. Sowerbutts, K. Blazek, J. Gugusheff, O. Puntsag et al. (2020). Prioritising housing maintenance to improve health in Indigenous communities in NSW over 20 years. *International Journal of Environmental Research and Public Health* 17(16). DOI: 10.3390/ijerph17165946.

Sustainable Improvement Team and the Horizons Team (2018). *Leading large scale change: a practical guide*. England: National Health Service.

Tsey, K., K. Lawson, I. Kinchin, R. Bainbridge, J. McCalman, F. Watkin et al. (2016). Evaluating research impact: the development of a research for impact tool. *Frontiers in Public Health* 4: 160. DOI: 10.3389/fpubh.2016.00160.

Tuhiwai Smith, L. (1999). *Decolonizing methodologies: research and indigenous peoples*. London: Zed Books.

United Nations (2007). United Nations Declaration on the Rights of Indigenous Peoples. https://www.ohchr.org/en/indigenous-peoples/un-declaration-rights-indigenous-peoples.

Walter, M. (2016). Data politics and Indigenous representation in Australian statistics. In T. Kukutai and J. Taylor, eds. *Indigenous data sovereignty: toward an agenda*, 79–98. Canberra: ANU Press.

Walter, M., T. Kukutai, S. Russo Carroll and D. Rodriguez-Lonebear, eds (2021). *Indigenous data sovereignty and policy*. London: Routledge.

Williams, M. (2018). Ngaa-bi-nya Aboriginal and Torres Strait Islander program evaluation framework. *Evaluation Journal of Australasia* 18(1): 6–20. DOI: 10.1177/1035719X18760141.

Part IV Summary:
future directions and emerging challenges

Continuous quality improvement (CQI) is generally viewed as an opportunity to reflect on the success of an activity and how it could be improved. As documented here and elsewhere, there have been significant successes in implementing CQI in primary health care (PHC). These successes include measurable improvements in population health outcomes, the adaptation of CQI methodologies to diverse primary healthcare settings, the development of new CQI tools and processes, and recognition of CQI as a core skill for the PHC workforce. New knowledge has emerged for improving the quality of clinical PHC and for tackling the social, cultural and environmental determinants of health through CQI.

When considering the CQI question "How can we do better?", we might first look to core primary healthcare concepts: the place-based context-specific nature of PHC, the right of all individuals, families and communities to health and social justice, the recognition of health as a multi-sectoral social and economic construct, and the empowerment of communities with respect to health services.[1] We can implement CQI in ways that uphold these core concepts: focusing on equity, engaging clients, carers and local communities in CQI processes, and working with agencies in other sectors to improve outcomes.

It is almost half a century since the 1978 Declaration of Alma-Ata identified community-driven, affordable, accessible, safe PHC as key to attaining health for all.[2] Despite remarkable progress in global health, technologies and health care, quality PHC is not universally available, and millions of people die from conditions that should be treatable by health systems.[3] The 2018 Global Conference on PHC[4] reinforced the critical ongoing role of PHC in adapting health systems to respond to our rapidly changing world, addressing the causes and risks for poor health, handling emerging health challenges, and achieving the health-related Sustainable Development Goals.[5] Evidence now confirms climate change as the single biggest health threat facing humanity, and the people whose health is most at risk from the climate crisis are those who contribute least to its causes, and who are least resourced to protect against it: people in low-income and vulnerable communities, displaced people, Indigenous communities, people in places where economies and health infrastructure are weak, and people with

---

1 World Health Organization and the United Nations Children's Fund 2018.
2 World Health Organization 1978.
3 World Health Organization 2018.
4 World Health Organization and the United Nations Children's Fund 2018.
5 United Nations n.d.

underlying health conditions.[6] Health challenges will increase as exposure to threats such as extreme temperatures and weather events, poor air and water quality, food insecurity and disease increase. CQI and quality improvement research have an increasingly important role in strengthening primary healthcare systems and community capacity to adapt to and mitigate these challenges.

There are several significant emerging challenges and opportunities:

- A continuing emphasis on holistic approaches, systems thinking and collaboration for CQI. These competencies will be increasingly important for taking the multi-level, cross-sector approaches needed to meet increasingly complex quality improvement challenges.
- Building skills and relationships to harness the context-specific and diverse knowledges required to achieve high-quality systems, including the lived experiences of primary healthcare clients and Indigenous knowledges about living equitably and sustainably. Definitions of quality need to reflect client and community perspectives, and quality improvement knowledge and practices need to be shared in ways that respect people's rights, sovereignty and dignity.
- Keeping a focus on measuring, reporting and acting on performance against evidence-based best-practice clinical guidelines and best-practice processes.
- Considering the climate crisis when we tackle quality challenges in PHC (for example, through research, by advocating for resources and approaches that protect health, by designing improvement strategies that reduce the environmental footprint of primary healthcare delivery, by modelling sustainable practices).
- Improving the quality of health literacy, health promotion and prevention programs, as a measure to reduce health costs and suffering.
- Prioritising CQI activities and research to reflect the changing needs of service populations. CQI tools and processes will need to respond to emerging health risks and priorities, to meaningfully engage clients and communities, and incorporate the complex social, cultural political and environmental determinants that affect health.
- Effective knowledge translation: putting improvements into practice and sustaining high-quality care; sharing learning in ways that are appropriate to different settings and audiences; and leveraging success to change systems and policies.

This book has aimed to provide an accessible guide to implementing CQI in primary healthcare settings. It has drawn on practical experience and established leadership in this field, the collective learning of many people involved in CQI, and published evidence and resources. It has included stories and findings specific to CQI in Aboriginal and Torres Strait Islander health that are grounded in core PHC, CQI principles and widely accepted CQI approaches. The book shares important learning for implementing quality improvement in primary healthcare settings, but there is much more to learn if we are to truly achieve more equitable people-centred health care.

---

6   World Health Organization 2023.

References

United Nations (n.d.). The 17 Goals. https://sdgs.un.org/goals.

World Health Organization (2023). *Climate change.* https://www.who.int/news-room/fact-sheets/detail/climate-change-and-health.

World Health Organization (2018). *Declaration of Astana.* Global Conference on Primary Health Care: From Alma-Ata towards universal health coverage and the Sustainable Development Goals. Astana, Kazakhstan 25–26 October 2018: World Health Organization and the United Nations Children's Fund (UNICEF).

World Health Organization (1978). *Declaration of Alma-Ata.* International Conference On Primary Health Care, Alma-Ata, USSR: WHO.

World Health Organization and the United Nations Children's Fund (2018). A vision for primary health care in the 21st century: towards universal health coverage and the Sustainable Development Goals. Geneva, Switzerland: WHO and UNICEF.

Index